Voices in Psychosis

Voices in Psychosis

Interdisciplinary Perspectives

Edited by

Angela Woods
Ben Alderson-Day
Charles Fernyhough

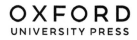

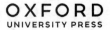

OXFORD
UNIVERSITY PRESS

Great Clarendon Street, Oxford, OX2 6DP,
United Kingdom

Oxford University Press is a department of the University of Oxford.
It furthers the University's objective of excellence in research, scholarship,
and education by publishing worldwide. Oxford is a registered trade mark of
Oxford University Press in the UK and in certain other countries

First Edition published in 2022

Impression: 1

Published in the United States of America by Oxford University Press
198 Madison Avenue, New York, NY 10016, United States of America

British Library Cataloguing in Publication Data

Data available

Library of Congress Control Number: 2022937637

ISBN 978–0–19–289838–8

DOI: 10.1093/oso/9780192898388.001.0001

Printed and bound by
CPI Group (UK) Ltd, Croydon, CR0 4YY

Contents

Cover Acknowledgement   ix
Acknowledgements   xi
List of Illustrations and Tables   xiii
Abbreviations   xv
Contributors   xvii

I. ORIENTATIONS

1. **Voices in Psychosis: Interdisciplinary Listening**   3
   Angela Woods, Ben Alderson-Day, and Charles Fernyhough

2. **Voices in Context: What Do Early Intervention in Psychosis Services Offer?**   17
   Guy Dodgson, Stephanie Common, Peter Moseley, Rebecca Lee, and Ben Alderson-Day

3. **Reflecting on Voices**   32
   Isaac

II. THE EXPERIENCE OF HEARING VOICES

4. **The Quickening**   39
   Gillian Allnutt

5. **The Sound of Fear**   41
   Ben Alderson-Day and Thomas Ward

6. **Affect and Voice-Hearing: Past and Present**   50
   Åsa Jansson

7. **Bodily Sensations During Voice-Hearing Experiences: A Role for Interoception?**   59
   Jamie Moffatt

8. **The Varieties and Complexities of Multimodal Hallucinations in Psychosis**   66
   Peter Moseley and Kaja Mitrenga

9. **Lost Agency and the Sense of Control**   74
   John Foxwell

10. **Pollution and Purity: Understanding Voices as Punishment for Un-Wholly Sins**   82
    Adam J. Powell

III. APPROACHING EXPERIENCE

11. **Voices in Psychosis: A Medieval Perspective**   93
    Hilary Powell

12. **Conspiration in the Archive: Sense-Making and the Research
    Interview Methodology**   101
    Tehseen Noorani

13. **Reading for Departure: Narrative Theory and Phenomenological
    Interviews on Hallucinations**   108
    Marco Bernini

14. **Relating to Leah's Voices**   117
    Angela Woods

IV. LOCATING VOICES IN LANGUAGE

15. **The Phenomenology of Voice-Hearing and Two Concepts of Voice**   127
    Sam Wilkinson and Joel Krueger

16. **Bridging the Gap in Common Ground When Talking about Voices**   134
    Felicity Deamer

17. **Silences in First-Person Accounts of Voice-Hearing:
    A Linguistic Approach**   142
    Elena Semino, Luke Collins, and Zsófia Demjén

V. SPATIAL AND RELATIONAL DIMENSIONS

18. **Household Ghosts and Personified Presences**   153
    Peter Garratt

19. **Voice-Hearing and Lived Space**   161
    Mary Coaten

20. **Vagabond Narratives: To Be Without a Home**   169
    Patricia Waugh

21. **Leah's Voices: Reflections on Auditory Verbal Hallucinations as
    Spiritual and Religious Experience**   176
    Christopher C. H. Cook

22. **'I Just Feel Like There's Just Lots of People in My Head!':
    Reciprocal Roles and Voice-Hearing**   184
    Anna Luce and Nicola Barclay

23. **Learning to Navigate Hallucinations: Comparing Voice Control Ability
    During Psychosis and in Ritual Use of Psychedelics**   194
    David Dupuis

24. 'Then I Open the Door and Walk into Their World':
    Crossing the Threshold and Hearing the Voice   203
    Akiko Hart

VI. VOICE-HEARING AND MENTAL PROCESSES

25. Remembering Voices   213
    Charles Fernyhough

26. Voices and Reality Monitoring: How Do We Know What Is Real?   220
    Colleen Rollins and Jane Garrison

27. Supernatural Presences: Medieval and Modern Narratives of
    Voice-Hearing   229
    Corinne Saunders

28. Maelstrom   239
    David Napthine

Index   249

Cover Acknowledgement

"Missing VI" (July 2020)
Collagraph print on paper.
Original Image size: 440mm x 680mm

Artist Statement:

The scars in the natural landscapes that form mountains, gorges, ravines and valleys that fill with still and moving water are often my starting point. External landscapes that fill the visual field are metaphors for the scars and wounds held in the landscape of the internal world. They changed places back and forth in my mind and hands as I formed the fractured grids and networks that form these printing plates. The energic lines are contours of landscape, fractured by environmental trauma and erosion and at the same time by the shocking impact of loss on the mind and body, neurones, memory, sense of self, sense of selves. Cutting deeply enough, reorienting and disturbing the forms that once were, creates change, new forms and voices of protest and fragmented selves that, forever changed, become part of the new.

Missing VI is the sixth print in a series of 12 collagraph prints exploring the experience of loss, the sense of something missing, the fractures and breaks in contact with others. And, maybe, the shape of new possibilities . . .

Ruth Lafferty
October 2021

Acknowledgements

On behalf of all the contributors to *Voices in Psychosis: Interdisciplinary Perspectives*, we offer our heartfelt thanks to the forty individuals who shared with us their experiences of hearing voices. As participants in the Voices in Psychosis (VIP) study, you gave generously of your time, energy, insight, and expertise, and made it possible for us, and for the readers of this volume, to listen to, and learn from, you.

We would like also to thank all the academic and clinical staff at Durham University, Northumbria University, the Cumbria Northumberland Tyne and Wear (CNTW) NHS Foundation Trust, and the Tees, Esk and Wear Valley (TEWV) NHS Foundation Trust that contributed to the VIP study. Guy Dodgson and Stephanie Common were the clinical leads at CNTW and TEWV, respectively; Ben Alderson-Day and Peter Moseley conducted the phenomenological interviews upon which this book is based; Jahnese Hamilton, Jamie Rea, Sue Bonner, and Bethan Senior played a key role in identifying and supporting people to participate; and Rachel Middleton and Pauline Harrison provided administrative support to the researchers at Durham University. Catherine Exley and Katie Brittain from Newcastle University trained the research team in qualitative methodologies, and Kasia Wilson and Isaac offered valuable input into the research design as voice-hearer consultants to the VIP study.

In its spirit as in its findings, *Voices in Psychosis: Interdisciplinary Perspectives* is a direct product of Hearing the Voice. This interdisciplinary research project, based at Durham University and allied to the Institute for Medical Humanities, was generously funded by the Wellcome Trust from 2012 to 2022. We are particularly grateful to the Trust for its commitment to interdisciplinarity, for recognizing the value of the humanities and social sciences to mental health research, and for enabling this publication to be accessible to readers globally without charge. All the contributors to *Voices in Psychosis* were members or close associates of Hearing the Voice, and participated in regular experimental research meetings convened by the project's Creative Facilitator Mary Robson. We owe Mary a debt of thanks for creating and sustaining the space in which the ideas presented in this volume could be explored and extended collaboratively. Victoria Patton, our Communications, Impact, and Engagement Lead, likewise over many years helped members of the research team, especially those who were new to the field, engage with the experiences and priorities of the voice-hearing community.

While the editors and contributors to *Voices in Psychosis* have learnt much from that community over the course of the project, there are two individuals whose work, ideas, and activism around hearing voices have exerted a particularly strong influence on our collective thinking. Although they could not in the end contribute a chapter, Rai Waddingham and Nev Jones are present throughout this volume and continue to inspire many of its authors. From the project's wider network of collaborators, we thank colleagues from the International Consortium on Hallucinations Research, delegates to the international Personification Across Disciplines conference hosted at Durham in 2018, and Vaughan Bell for his incisive and supportive feedback at key stages in this book's development.

Finally, we would like to thank the individuals who helped make this publication a material reality. John Foxwell worked with us intensively during the Covid-19 pandemic to copy-edit the final manuscript; we benefited tremendously from his editorial precision, rigour, and sophistication. At Oxford University Press, we have been delighted to work with Jade Dixon, Rachel Goldsworthy, and Martin Baum, and thank Martin especially for being an enthusiastic supporter of this innovative interdisciplinary venture from its earliest days. Mary Robson we thank again for producing the line drawings which introduce each of the book's six sections. We encountered Ruth Lafferty's artwork at the conference at which we first presented findings from the VIP study, and are at once humbled and thrilled that her collagraph print *Missing VI* graces the cover of this volume.

Voices in Psychosis is more polyphony than a perfectly harmonious composition; it seeks to proliferate perspectives on hearing voices rather than lay claim to being comprehensive or complete. The volume foregrounds the divergences between different ways of knowing, reading, analysing, and being with the experiences reported by people who hear voices, and in so doing we hope it serves to inspire readers from all disciplines and backgrounds to question their assumptions and deepen their understanding of voice-hearing.

Angela Woods, Ben Alderson-Day, and Charles Fernyhough
June 2022

List of Illustrations and Tables

Figures

2.1   Contexts of voice-hearing used by EIP teams   21

2.2   Illustration of the elements of EIP intervention   24

22.1   Development and enactments of reciprocal roles   186

22.2   Commonly encountered reciprocal roles in psychosis services   188

22.3   Possible reciprocal roles for Nina   189

22.4   Possible reciprocal roles for Grace   191

Images

3.1   Voices   34

3.2   Brain scans 2 normal   35

24.1   Hydra of the State   206

26.1   Brain regions implicated in voice-hearing and reality monitoring   223

Tables

2.1   Comparing the North East with the rest of the UK   20

2.2   Diagnosis by gender for the VIP study   22

16.1   Use of non-literal language in the transcripts   136

Abbreviations

ACC	anterior cingulate cortex
APA	American Psychiatric Association
ARMS	at-risk mental state
AVH	auditory verbal hallucinations
BFT	behavioural family therapy
CAARMS	Comprehensive Assessment of At Risk Mental States
CAT	cognitive analytic therapy
CBT	cognitive behavioural therapy
CBTp	cognitive behavioural therapy for psychosis
CNTW	Cumbria, Northumberland, Tyne and Wear
DID	dissociative identity disorder
DMP	dance movement psychotherapy
DSM-III	Diagnostic and Statistical Manual of Mental Disorders, third edition
DUP	delay in untreated psychosis
DWP	Department of Work and Pensions
EIP	Early Intervention in Psychosis
EMDR	eye-movement desensitization reprogramming
FEP	first-episode psychosis
fMRI	functional magnetic resonance imaging
GP	general practitioner
HTV-PI	Hearing the Voice Phenomenology Interview
IFG	inferior frontal gyrus
KMP	Kestenberg Movement Profile
MMH	multimodal hallucination
mPFC	medial prefrontal cortex
MRI	magnetic resonance imaging
MUSEQ	Multi-Modality Unusual Sensory Experiences Questionnaire
NEVHI	North East Visual Hallucination Interview
NHS	National Health Service
NICE	National Institute for Health and Care Excellence
PANSS	Positive and Negative Syndrome Scale
PCS	paracingulate sulcus
PSYRATS	Psychotic Symptom Rating Scale
PTSD	post-traumatic stress disorder
RR	reciprocal role
RRP	reciprocal role procedure
SMF	Source Monitoring Framework
sMRI	structural magnetic resonance imaging
STG	superior temporal gyrus
TEWV	Tees, Esk and Wear Valley
VIP	Voices in Psychosis
ZPD	zone of proximal development

Contributors

Ben Alderson-Day
Department of Psychology, Durham University, Durham, UK

Gillian Allnutt
Writer, Durham, UK

Nicola Barclay
Cumbria, Northumberland, Tyne and Wear NHS Foundation Trust, UK

Marco Bernini
Department of English Studies, Durham University, Durham, UK

Mary Coaten
South West Yorkshire Partnership NHS Foundation Trust, UK

Luke Collins
Department of Linguistics and English Language, Lancaster University, Lancaster

Stephanie Common
Early Intervention in Psychosis Services, Tees, Esk and Wear Valleys NHS Foundation Trust, UK

Christopher C. H. Cook
Institute of Medical Humanities, Durham University, Durham, UK

Felicity Deamer
Institute of Forensic Linguistics, Aston University, Birmingham, UK

Zsófia Demjén
Centre for Applied Linguistics, University College London, London, UK

Guy Dodgson
Early Intervention in Psychosis Services, Cumbria, Northumberland, Tyne and Wear NHS Foundation Trust, UK

David Dupuis
Research Department, Quai Branly Museum, Paris, France

Charles Fernyhough
Department of Psychology, Durham University, Durham, UK

John Foxwell
Department of English Studies, Durham University, Durham, UK

Peter Garratt
Department of English Studies, Durham University, Durham, UK

Jane Garrison
Department of Psychology, University of Cambridge, Cambridge, UK

Akiko Hart
National Survivor User Network, London, UK

Åsa Jansson
Institute for Medical Humanities, Durham University, Durham, UK

Joel Krueger
Department of Philosophy, University of Exeter, Exeter, UK

Rebecca Lee
Academy of Primary Care, Hull York Medical School, UK

Anna Luce
Crisis, Newcastle, UK

Kaja Mitrenga
Department of Psychology, Durham University, Durham, UK

Jamie Moffatt
Department of Psychology, University of Sussex, Brighton, UK

Peter Moseley
Department of Psychology, Northumbria University, Newcastle upon Tyne, UK

David Napthine
Writer, Durham, UK

Tehseen Noorani
Department of Anthropology, Durham University, Durham, UK

Adam J. Powell
Department of Theology and Religion, Durham University, Durham, UK

Hilary Powell
Department of English Studies, Durham University, Durham, UK

Colleen Rollins
Department of Psychiatry, University of Cambridge, Cambridge, UK

Corinne Saunders
Department of English Studies and Institute for Medical Humanities, Durham University, Durham, UK

Elena Semino
Department of Linguistics and English Language, Lancaster University, Lancaster, UK

Thomas Ward
Institute of Psychiatry, Psychology and Neuroscience, Kings College London, London, UK

Patricia Waugh
Department of English Studies, Durham University, Durham, UK

Sam Wilkinson
Department of Philosophy, University of Exeter, Exeter, UK

Angela Woods
Institute for Medical Humanities and Department of English Studies, Durham University, Durham, UK

PART ONE
ORIENTATIONS

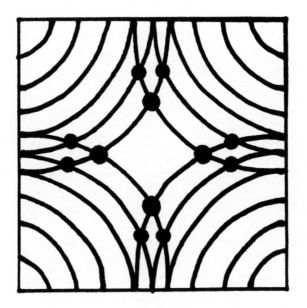

PART ONE

ORIENTATIONS

1

Voices in Psychosis

Interdisciplinary Listening

Angela Woods, Institute for Medical Humanities and Department of English Studies, Durham University

Ben Alderson-Day, Department of Psychology, Durham University

Charles Fernyhough, Department of Psychology, Durham University

This chapter introduces readers to the experience of hearing voices, to the Voices in Psychosis study conducted by Hearing the Voice, and to the aims and trajectories of this edited collection. The twenty-eight chapters in this volume engage a corpus of forty transcripts of interviews conducted with people using Early Intervention in Psychosis services about their experiences of hearing voices. As well as identifying thematic and other trajectories through the volume, this chapter explains its significance to research on voice-hearing, psychosis, and the critical medical humanities. In so doing it extends our argument for the importance of an interdisciplinary approach to the study of human experience.

Over a period of thirteen months in the late 2010s, forty people in the North East of England sat down to speak with a researcher about their experience of hearing voices. For the most part, these conversations took place in domestic settings—across kitchen tables, in bedsits and hostels, front rooms, and lounges—and lasted for between twenty minutes and nearly two hours. The individuals who had chosen to give of their time and insight had all been hearing voices over the previous six months and had all sought help from local Early Intervention in Psychosis (EIP) services. The researchers who arrived with their encrypted voice recorders were gathering data as part of a study seeking a deeper understanding of how voice-hearing experiences in the context of psychosis change over time. The audio recordings of these interviews captured a slice of these embodied multi-perspectival encounters; the transcriptions distilled dialogues in flesh and blood into carefully formatted words on a page. It was this process of transformative recording that makes a certain kind of listening possible.

Angela Woods, Ben Alderson-Day, and Charles Fernyhough, *Voices in Psychosis* In: *Voices in Psychosis*. Edited by: Angela Woods, Ben Alderson-Day, and Charles Fernyhough, Oxford University Press. © Angela Woods, Ben Alderson-Day, and Charles Fernyhough 2022. DOI: 10.1093/oso/9780192898388.003.0001

What is it like to hear voices? This is the question at the heart of Hearing the Voice, a decade-long programme of interdisciplinary research funded by the Wellcome Trust. Based at Durham University, Hearing the Voice has brought researchers in anthropology, cognitive neuroscience, history, linguistics, literary studies, medical humanities, philosophy, psychology, and theology together with clinicians, voice-hearers, and other experts by experience, to generate new knowledge about the experience of hearing voices across scientific, clinical, and cultural contexts. Listening to the experience of people who hear voices constitutes the foundation of our endeavours and is at the centre of this book.

The voices of people who hear voices are growing in number and prominence. Emerging from the narratives shared with family and close friends, with peers in support group and activist contexts, and with mental health professionals, there now exist testimonies about the experience of voice-hearing which are produced for audiences the voice-hearer does not, and may never, know personally. Thanks to the work of the individuals and collectives who make up the international Hearing Voices Movement, it is possible now, in a way it was not thirty years ago, for people to access a wealth of published prose narratives (Knoll, 2017; Romme et al., 2009), TED talks (Longden, 2013), videos, and blogs (Perth Voices Clinic, n.d.). As researchers, theorists, and activists, voice-hearers analyse voice-hearing using a variety of frameworks in leading academic publications, briefings, and reports (Corstens et al., 2014; Jones and Luhrman, 2016; Jones et al., 2016; Kalathil and Jones, 2016; Waddingham, 2015); as artists, voice-hearers communicate powerfully to different audiences through painting, print-making, sculpture, drawing, music, zine-making, and drama (Hearing the Voice, 2019). It does not collapse key distinctions between these distinct formats and modalities to observe that they are all, in an important sense, accounts of experience intended for public consumption.

The transcripts of interviews which are the focus of *Voices in Psychosis* are of a different order. They are the accounts of experience offered on the condition of anonymity, in the knowledge that they would be accessed in full only by the Hearing the Voice research team. They are also records of questions answered spontaneously, testaments to truths it felt possible to share with a particular researcher on a particular day. Experiences of hearing voices are still frequently stigmatized, regarded with suspicion and mistrust, as signs of inherent dangerousness or derangement, as evidence that there is something very seriously wrong. A study about hearing voices which takes care to begin by bracketing prior assumptions about the nature of those experiences, yet still seeks to generate understandings which can help those who are distressed, constitutes a very specific context for conversation.

'I'm happy to help', Violet says towards the end of her interview:[1] 'It makes me feel like, it makes us feel happy because when other people, when like other people hear

---

[1] Note that all voice and voice-hearer names have been changed to preserve anonymity, but are used consistently throughout this volume and in other publications from the Voices in Psychosis study.

what I have to say, it might inspire them.' Mike talks about transforming the suffering he has undergone into something useful for others: 'It's done my head in for so long, so I think fuck it, go and help someone else out.' Emma, when asked if her answers can be used as data in the study, links the value of the forgoing conversation precisely to its taking place within the context of research:

EMMA: Yeah, well I've said more to yous than I've ever said to these [clinicians].
INTERVIEWER: Well we really, really appreciate that, and we do recognise that it's hard.
EMMA: I had an appointment earlier, but this is what I was saying, I was like . . . because I . . . like I find it really hard to talk, and especially to people I don't know.
INTERVIEWER: Mm.
EMMA: But like your case, like it's to do this and then I'll never see you again, if that makes sense?
INTERVIEWER: Yeah.
EMMA: So it's alright to have to like face you, like knowing everything I've just said.
INTERVIEWER: Yeah! (both laugh) That's fine!

'I'm happy to help,' says Ulrik, adding, 'I think more people should be studying mental health.'

Before it is an academic artefact, *Voices in Psychosis* is a work of listening. Our aim as editors was to invite members and close associates of Hearing the Voice to listen, closely, to these forty people's accounts of their experience. We are, as individuals and academics, trained to listen in different ways, to tune in at different frequencies, and thus hear different things. Listening becomes reading, becomes analysis, becomes dialogue—forty conversations about voice-hearing are, in turn, brought into new and long-standing conversations about psychosis, about the ethics of interpretation, about the varieties of human experience and the ways these might be imagined, modelled, mapped, and represented.

The transcripts and recordings of interviews with people about their experience of psychosis and hearing voices fill hard-drives and filing cabinets in universities across the world. The ethical imperative to protect participants from being publicly identified—even in anonymized transcripts—means these qualitative data are only seldom made available to other researchers and only very rarely lodged in data repositories. A successful qualitative research study is one in which the analysis of interview data, usually by a small team of researchers, is reported in, at most, a handful of peer-reviewed academic publications addressing a consequently narrow set of academic and clinical debates. Within this context, *Voices in Psychosis* is exceptional for the diversity of lenses, disciplines, experiences, and methodologies employed by its contributors. At the same time, attending to a single set of sources, a profoundly rich but finite archive of 153,989 words, brings powerful focus to the dialogue between disciplines that are otherwise often talking at cross-purposes (if not about very different things altogether).

The rest of this introductory chapter proceeds as follows. First, we give a brief overview of current research on the experience of hearing voices in the context of psychosis, highlighting some of the outstanding questions which are driving academic and clinical investigations. We then argue for the value of the interdisciplinary approach (Woods et al., 2014) which underpins the work of Hearing the Voice, and we describe in more detail the aims, ethos, and practices of the project as a whole before turning to the Voices in Psychosis (VIP) study. Finally, we introduce the volume itself, identifying various trajectories through its remaining twenty-seven chapters and anticipating some of the conversations to which we offer it as a contribution.

Hearing Voices in Psychosis

Hearing voices is typically seen as a symptom of severe mental illness. Up to 80% of individuals with a diagnosis of schizophrenia hear voices (Aleman and Larøi, 2008), although the prevalence of voice-hearing in people with other psychiatric diagnoses (including post-traumatic stress disorder, bipolar disorder, and borderline personality disorder) has undermined earlier understandings of it as having a special status as a symptom of schizophrenia (Waters and Fernyhough, 2017). While sometimes a source of comfort or companionship, voices in psychotic disorders are more often unsettling, undermining, or abusive, and cause significant suffering and disturbance within people's lives. Despite substantial advances over the last thirty years—by mental health professionals progressing the therapeutic management of distressing voices, by hallucinations researchers in clinical and scientific disciplines, and by voice-hearers and advocates seeking wider societal transformations—experiences of hearing voices in psychosis remain poorly understood and highly stigmatized.

A key feature of current approaches to voice-hearing has been a move away from diagnosis-based analyses to approaches that focus on voice-hearing as an experience that cuts across category boundaries (Bentall, 2003). This has coincided with a growth of interest in complex and frequent voice-hearing experiences that occur in the absence of distress (often termed non-clinical voice-hearing) and that bear important similarities with more everyday experiences such as hearing the voices of fictional or imaginary entities (Foxwell et al., 2020). This experience-based approach has also contributed to a renewed interest in the phenomenology (or subjective experience) of hearing voices, including findings that voices may be largely or entirely lacking in auditory qualities and that they are accompanied by a range of other sensory experiences, including felt presences and bodily sensations (Woods et al., 2015).

A focus of recent research efforts has been on trying to link the varied phenomenology of voice-hearing across different groups to the wide range of cognitive, neural, personal, and sociocultural processes that have been implicated in it (Waters and Fernyhough, 2019). Voice-hearing in psychosis may be best understood as an experience that is partly continuous with everyday inner experience (Toh et al., 2022) and occurs in different forms or subtypes, likely underpinned by distinct mechanisms and aetiological pathways (Smailes et al., 2015). Among the cognitive mechanisms implicated are biases in reality monitoring (see Chapter 26) and source memory (see Chapter 25). Relevant neural features include the integrity of white matter tracts such as the arcuate fasciculus (Whitford et al., 2011)—a key structural pathway connecting parts of the brain thought to be essential in language processing—and atypical patterns of connectivity when the brain is at rest (Alderson-Day et al., 2015). Mechanisms implicated at the personal and sociocultural levels of analysis include the atypical activation of representations of social agents (Wilkinson and Bell, 2016)—thought to contribute to the phenomenon whereby heard voices become personified (Alderson-Day et al., 2021)—the role of trauma and early adversity in the aetiology of voice-hearing (Varese et al., 2012), and the deliberate cultivation of voice-hearing experiences in particular subcultural contexts (Luhrmann, 2017). Researchers have tried to connect these implicated mechanisms to a variety of therapeutic approaches, with a growing assumption that 'one-size-fits-all' therapies will be less effective than those targeted at specific mechanisms and subtypes of voice-hearing.

An Interdisciplinary Approach: Hearing the Voice and the Voices in Psychosis Study

Before being stigmatized as dangerous or classified as a symptom, voice-hearing is a complex, multifaceted phenomenon that takes many different forms and resists reductive explanations. Voices are an important part of human experience—existing in our private, inner lives, but also as part of our shared social and interpersonal worlds—and consequently, the arts, humanities, and social sciences are indispensable to their investigation. Hearing the Voice has grown to be the world's largest interdisciplinary study of voice-hearing, generating new knowledge about what it is like to hear voices, their underlying neural and cognitive mechanisms, the way voices have been interpreted in different cultural and historical contexts, and the relationships among voice-hearing and memory, the senses, creativity, emotion, trauma, language, and social cognition. A key focus for the project has been the frequently distressing voice-hearing experiences reported by people within mental health services, today and in the past. These analyses have been conducted alongside, and in dialogue with, studies of the voices experienced by writers and readers of literary fiction, the spiritually significant voices heard by contemporary Christians, spiritualists, and those taking part in ayahuasca rituals, and the everyday experiences of so-called non-clinical voice-hearers, to name only the most prominent of the project's research areas. Sparking and sustaining a dialogue between these varied investigations was an explicit aim of the fortnightly Voice Club meetings of the research team. One hundred and eighteen Voice Clubs were convened by the project's Creative Facilitator over a period of eight years. They constituted the key space in which to exchange, challenge, and develop ideas, generate interdisciplinary research questions, experiment with new methods, and invite the participation of more than 140 project collaborators. Voice Club educated us in each other's work on voice-hearing by, for example, introducing the cognitive neuroscientists to the most celebrated texts in medieval mysticism, deepening the literary scholars' understanding of contemporary theorization of voice sub-typing, and bringing the full range of disciplinary perspectives to bear on the analysis of new psychotherapeutic approaches to distressing voices. More profoundly, the meetings enabled and encouraged reciprocal influence to develop into novel and interdisciplinary approaches to the study of hearing voices (Bernini and Woods, 2014).

This pattern of interlocking disciplines, in constant dialogue with one another, is reflected in the VIP study. Our aim was to develop a deeper understanding of what it is like to start hearing voices: how voices emerge, their influence and impact on other aspects of experience, their development over time. We wanted to explore if and how voices took on characterful personas, how this fitted with voice-hearers' own understandings, and if the term 'voice' was even an appropriate term for their experience. The scales and measures routinely used in research and in clinical assessments do not capture this complexity, so we devised a phenomenological interview with direct input from people with lived experience of voice-hearing, alongside philosophers, psychologists, linguists, theologians, and literary studies and medical humanities scholars. Taking care not to let our interests and assumptions guide and shape interviewees' descriptions of what can be fleeting and elusive phenomena, the interview starts by inviting a general description before drilling down into more detailed and specific distinctions. The interview was piloted with Isaac, one of this volume's contributors, and further modified in light of his feedback.

Following ethical review and approval of the VIP study, the Hearing the Voice Phenomenological Interview was offered to people hearing voices who were in their first nine months of using EIP services. EIP is the frontline National Health Service (NHS) pathway for people with distressing and unusual experiences, and is introduced in detail in the next chapter. Twenty-three men and seventeen women, aged between 16 and 61, took part in the study. On average, they had been using EIP for four months, and over three-quarters were taking antipsychotic medication to help manage their experiences. All forty were interviewed by one of two psychologists from the team (Ben Alderson-Day and Peter Moseley), and many also took part in different arms of the study that involved having a magnetic resonance imaging (MRI) scan and completing a cognitive assessment.

Some participants in the VIP study had been hearing voices for little over one month, while some had known the company of voices for as long as they could remember. Some talked of imaginary confidantes that became inner critics; others spoke of demonic barks and guardian angels. Each had a unique perspective on what it is to hear a voice. As with the development of the interview protocol, analysis of voice-hearers' accounts involved an interdisciplinary team working together over many months. We discussed excerpts from the interviews in Voice Clubs and presented work in progress in local NHS settings and at Personification Across

Disciplines, an international and interdisciplinary conference organised by Hearing the Voice. The first paper from the VIP study was published in *Schizophrenia Bulletin* in January 2021 (Alderson-Day et al., 2021). Focusing on the personification of voices, it reports on many different aspects of participants' voice-hearing experiences and includes in supplementary materials the full interview protocol and the coding framework used in the analysis. The present volume emerged from the realization that listening carefully to these interviews had led us collectively in more directions that could be captured in a single paper.

Introducing *Voices in Psychosis*

It was to Voice Club that we, as editors, first brought the proposal for *Voices in Psychosis*, and from Voice Club that we identified and invited our contributors. All of the authors featured in this volume are members or close collaborators of Hearing the Voice; the majority have been to dozens of Voice Clubs over many years, including sessions devoted to collective analysis and discussion of the VIP transcripts, as well as pitching and elaboration of the ideas for each of the chapters. This book is about listening to, and learning from, the experiences of voice-hearers, but that listening was, very unusually, a social and embodied practice as much as it was an isolated undertaking in the cells of the ivory tower. Its authors' association with Hearing the Voice is about more than employment or affiliation: it signals a shared experience of conversations held over an extended time frame, of exposure to, and immersion in, different perspectives on hearing voices. There are voices missing from this collection—most notably those of several individuals whose lived experience of hearing voices, academic analysis, and activism opened up new ways of thinking within the project as a whole, but for whom other commitments regrettably took priority. Accepting the loss of their proposed chapters and choosing not to seek alternative contributions was a difficult editorial decision, but one that revealed to us the importance of a shared process to what it is that this volume offers.

Voices in Psychosis is a polyphony, not a perfectly harmonious composition. The number and diversity of disciplines reflected in the book render it a distinctive contribution to the literature on psychosis; the focus of those perspectives on a single data set makes it unique. There has never been, to our knowledge, a publication in which researchers, clinicians, writers, and people with lived experience bring their analytic energies to bear on the same set of primary sources, and it is a further mark of distinction that those original data about voice-hearing richly reward such in-depth inquiry. In order to bring a formal coherence to the volume, we imposed, what were for some contributors quite challenging, editorial restrictions: a length of between 3000 and 3500 words, a maximum of ten references, and a request that technical terminology and explanatory footnotes be kept to an absolute minimum. Within this standardized format, the chapters together foreground the divergences between different ways of knowing, reading, analysing, and being with the experiences reported

in the VIP transcripts. No single disciplinary, practice-based, experiential, or creative perspective has the first or final say—our goal as editors has been to ensure that
the necessary tensions and limitations of *any* inquiry into 'unusual' human experience are acknowledged in a way that also highlights what is distinctive and valuable
about each contribution.

Part One continues with 'Voices in Context: What Do Early Intervention in
Psychosis Services Offer?', a chapter co-authored by the VIP study's clinical leads
Guy Dodgson and Stephanie Common, research leads Ben Alderson-Day and Peter
Moseley, and research assistant Rebecca Lee. This second introduction gives an insight into the specialist mental health services that support people with early experiences of psychosis in the North East of England, including their approaches to the
conceptualization of voice-hearing, diagnosis, medication, and forms of therapy. It
also provides more details about the group of people who participated in the study
and about the interviews conducted with them. In 'Reflecting on Voices', the volume's
third introductory chapter, Isaac, who was an early participant in, and an advisor to,
the VIP study, explores what it is like to read the transcripts of other people's interviews in light of his own voice-hearing experiences.

The remaining chapters of *Voices in Psychosis* are organized thematically. Part
Two, 'The Experience of Hearing Voices', opens with Gillian Allnutt's poem 'The
Quickening', which vividly captures a transformative moment in which the poet's
own childhood self appears to her 'outwith'. Alderson-Day and clinical psychologist Thomas Ward's chapter 'The Sound of Fear' addresses a topic that is surprisingly neglected within research on voice-hearing despite its clinical significance.
Listening to the way participants in the VIP study speak about the fear and existential threat aroused by their voices, their chapter goes on to explore the innovative psychotherapeutic use of computer-generated avatars in helping other
voice-hearers negotiate this terror. In 'Affect and Voice-Hearing: Past and Present',
historian Åsa Jansson argues that the emotional dimensions of voice-hearing have
been underexplored, in part, because early twentieth-century systems of psychiatric classification defined auditory hallucination as belonging to cognitive, rather
than affective, disorders. Attending to the intensity and variety of emotion expressed
by many of its participants, Jansson argues that the VIP study provides grounds
for challenging these psychiatric orthodoxies. Jamie Moffatt, in his chapter 'Bodily
Sensations During Voice-Hearing Experiences: A Role for Interoception?', likewise demonstrates the inadequacy of conventional approaches to voice-hearing as
a strictly auditory phenomenon. Noting that for two-thirds of study participants,
voices were accompanied by a variety of bodily sensations, Moffatt posits that disturbances of interoception—our ability to sense internal bodily states—may play a
more important role in voice-hearing experiences than has previously been recognized. In a similar vein, Peter Moseley and Kaja Mitrenga's chapter 'The Varieties and
Complexities of Multimodal Hallucinations in Psychosis' challenges the tendency
among hallucinations researchers to approach voice-hearing as a unimodal phenomenon. Moseley and Mitrenga's analysis of multimodal hallucinations reported

by VIP participants reveals that temporal synchrony and integration of identity are key to understanding more clearly participants' experiences of seeing, feeling, and being touched by their voices. John Foxwell, in a chapter entitled 'Lost Agency and the Sense of Control', returns us to a longer-standing conundrum posed by the experience of voice-hearing, namely, the way in which voices are distinguished from the individual's own thoughts. Through an analysis that makes use of examples from first-person accounts of literary inspiration, as well as phenomenological psychopathology, he shows how the transcripts disclose fine-grained distinctions between different ways in which voices and thoughts are experienced as being beyond one's control. Concluding Part Two's investigation of the embodied, multisensory, and affective qualities of voice-hearing experiences, Adam J. Powell focuses on the beliefs expressed by two VIP participants that their voices are part of a justified punishment for social transgressions. Powell reads Dan's and Ryan's struggles with feeling guilty, abnormal, and deserving of punishment, through wider cultural dynamics of purity and pollution, and suggests that anthropological analyses of rituals of purification could provide a new way of understanding relational therapies as transforming the 'pollution' of persecutory voices.

What does it mean to seek an understanding of voices through the phenomenological interview? What happens when listening becomes reading? Part Three, 'Approaching Experience', begins by bringing the VIP transcripts into conversation with a very different corpus: the stories found in eighth- to twelfth-century Latin hagiography. 'How', writes Hilary Powell, 'can we ensure that the conversation between past and present moves beyond the small talk of similarities and differences towards a weightier, more mutually enhancing, even transformative conversation?' By focusing on the contexts in which any accounts of 'unusual' experience are produced and shared, Powell's 'Voices in Psychosis: A Medieval Perspective' shows that the modalities of reading practised by medieval monks has much to offer a society that still struggles to listen, openly, to voice-hearers' experiences. Tehseen Noorani's 'Conspiration in the Archive: Sense-Making and the Research Interview Methodology' picks up Powell's interest in the embodied and interpersonal practices that surround, sustain, and are made possible by particular texts, inviting us to attend to what these transcripts reveal about the phenomenological interview itself. Noorani's reading of the encounter as one in which interviewee and interviewer conspire in the production of a narrative that is valued in different ways by both parties challenges the way interviews are commonly regarded across the clinical, psychological, and social sciences. Moving from the collaborative exchange between researcher and participant to the potentially disorienting encounter between reader and transcript, Marco Bernini argues for the value of narratology in the analysis of phenomenological interviews. His chapter 'Reading for Departure: Narrative Theory and Phenomenological Interviews on Hallucinations' attunes us to the complex interplay between hallucinatory experience, its articulation through the interview framework, and the dispositions of the reader, showing that the VIP transcripts have a pedagogic function in helping resist what Bernini describes as the 'intuitive naturalization of unfamiliar experiences'. The fourth and final chapter in this section reflects upon the struggle to understand unusual experiences in ways that resist their naturalization, translation, or theoretical abstraction. A case study and, at the same time, an assemblage of time-stamped fragments, Angela Woods's 'Relating to Leah's Voices' explores how embodied, affective, and multimodal intensities invite very different modes of relation from those of highly personified voices.

'Locating Voices in Language' is a task undertaken by the three chapters that make up Part Four of *Voices in Psychosis*. Philosophers Sam Wilkinson and Joel Krueger begin by addressing the language used to describe voice-hearing experiences, noting that the term 'voice' is used by the VIP participants in a variety of ways. In 'The Phenomenology of Voice-Hearing and Two Concepts of Voice', they unpack the distinction between 'voice' as speech sound and 'voice' as agent, and explore the multiple ways in which the voices no one else can hear are, and are not, like the voices of everyday life. In her chapter 'Bridging the Gap in Common Ground When Talking about Voices', Felicity Deamer also considers the difficulties faced by voice-hearers in conveying, through language, experiences that they feel are highly unusual as well as upsetting. Through her analysis of the different forms of 'non-literal' language used in a subset of the transcripts, Deamer hypothesizes that voice-hearers make use of simile much more than metaphor in locating these unfamiliar experiences within a common conversational ground. Especially within a clinical context, voice-hearing is almost always construed as a problem of presence: voices arrive unbidden, say unwelcome things, and will not leave. In conclusion to this section on language, Elena Semino, Luke Collins, and Zsófia Demjén's 'Silences in First-Person Accounts of Voice-Hearing: A Linguistic Approach' looks first to the high number of instances of negation within the transcripts and then expands upon four distinct kinds and qualities of silence that appear across the interviews.

Peter Garratt's 'Household Ghosts and Personified Presences' is the first of seven chapters to explore the theme of 'Spatial and Relational Dimensions' in Part Five of *Voices in Psychosis*. By 'creating an emotional landscape out of unbidden voices', the ghost stories of Charles Dickens (an author who was fascinated by voice-hearing experiences) resonate with some of the spectral figures described in the VIP study. However, one key distinction between the contemporary and the Victorian literary contexts, Garratt argues, is that these presences could be experienced as hospitable as well as unsettling. In her chapter 'Voice-Hearing and Lived Space', Mary Coaten offers a different perspective on the emotional landscape of voices, one which emphasizes its mytho-poetic dimension. Charting changes in voice-hearers' experiences of space and time—changes which often speak of trauma and dissociation—Coaten reads the VIP transcripts through the lens of her practice as a dance movement psychotherapist attuned to the role of the lived body in psychosis. How might we understand the relationship between the lived body, the spatial qualities of voices, the material realities of domestic life, and home's place within our cultural imaginary? In 'Vagabond Narratives: To Be Without a Home', Patricia Waugh's answer to this question culminates in an analysis of six different types of 'home' materialized in the VIP transcripts.

Christopher C. H. Cook's 'Leah's Voices: Reflections on Auditory Verbal Hallucinations as Spiritual and Religious Experience', the second chapter to concentrate exclusively on Leah's interview, focuses on her voices' spiritual significance. The way Leah relates to her voices—divine and demonic—suggests a religious coping style which Cook argues is largely positive, a form of sense-making in response to trauma. In the next chapter, clinical psychologists Anna Luce and Nicola Barclay introduce concepts from cognitive analytic therapy to show how voice-hearers' early relationships can inform their voice-hearing experiences. '"I Just Feel Like There's Just Lots of People in My Head!": Reciprocal Roles and Voice-Hearing' explores how Nina's and Grace's relations with the different voices they hear could be collaboratively and compassionately explored in a therapeutic setting. Insights from a very different therapeutic setting—the Takiwasi shamanic centre in the Peruvian Amazon—emerge from David Dupuis's chapter 'Learning to Navigate Hallucinations: Comparing Voice Control Ability During Psychosis and in Ritual Use of Psychedelics'. Hearing voices is an important and expected part of 'meeting ayahuasca', and Dupuis's careful comparative analysis shows how the training offered by ritual specialists to help foster individuals' sense of control resonates with the coping strategies reported within the VIP transcripts, which he suggests can, in turn, speak to relational therapies for distressing voices. The final chapter in this section brings both spatial *and* relational dimensions of voice-hearing to the fore. '"Then I Open the Door and Walk into Their World": Crossing the Threshold and Hearing the Voice', Akiko Hart's contribution to *Voices in Psychosis*, is both a deeply personal and an intensely political reflection upon her encounter with the VIP transcripts. While they stimulate analysis and interpretation, participants' descriptions of ghostly shadows and felt presences must also be listened to on their terms; doing so inspires in Hart a new way of relating to her own experiences.

Part Six of *Voices in Psychosis* tackles directly what many of the chapters have so far touched on: the question of what hearing voices can tell us about the ways we understand the human mind. 'Could you tell us a bit about what life was like for you, and how you were feeling, when you first started having these experiences?' is a question asked of all VIP participants. 'Remembering Voices' focuses on their responses to explore the role that memory plays both in the experience of voice-hearing and in talking about those experiences. Voices are seldom straightforward verbatim replays of prior conversations; the VIP transcripts, argues Charles Fernyhough, can deepen our understanding of the variety of complex ways voices 'speak' to and of people's past experiences, especially within the context of trauma. Neuroscientists Colleen Rollins and Jane Garrison's chapter 'Voices and Reality Monitoring: How Do We Know What Is Real?' speaks to another long-standing interest in hallucinations research, namely, the question of how and why voices are experienced as being externally generated. Discussing new research that reveals links between the kinds of voices people hear and particular patterns of folding within the cerebral cortex, Rollins and Garrison suggest that enhancing our knowledge of the cognitive and neural bases of voice-hearing can play an important role in the development of targeted therapies for those who are distressed by their voices.

Might it be the case that enhancing our understanding of how voice-hearing was experienced and perceived in contexts vastly different from our own could also benefit those in distress? In 'Supernatural Presences: Medieval and Modern Narratives of Voice-Hearing', Corinne Saunders offers a detailed comparative phenomenological reading of the VIP transcripts alongside the visionary writings of Julian of Norwich and Margery Kempe. As Saunders's work attests, this kind of attentive literary reading across history and genre 'reveals the complexity of voice-hearing as an experience, its intersections with belief, context, and culture, its profoundly multisensory and embodied aspects, and the deep impulses of those speaking towards not diagnosis but understanding'. *Voices in Psychosis* concludes, fittingly, by refracting this complexity through a new lens, that of myth and epic. In 'Maelstrom', Hearing the Voice writer in residence David Napthine transports us to Corryvreckan, a cave deep beneath the sea in which 'voices' congregate and to which the voices of psychosis might be returned.

There are no linear trajectories through voice-hearing in psychosis—no fixed sequence of experiences, no single or obvious place to start or finish an inquiry, no undisputed hierarchy of explanatory frameworks. The six sections of this volume are a thematic clustering of chapters, intended to concentrate conversations around particular aspects of voice-hearing and the ways in which it can be understood. Other through-lines are possible. Several chapters tune in to the voices heard by individuals living in twenty-first-century North East England by bringing them into conversation with those reported in other times and places: in nineteenth-century asylums (Jansson) and periodicals (Garratt), in Amazonian shamanism (Dupuis), and in the literature and hagiographies of the Middle Ages (Powell and Saunders). Alderson-Day and Ward, Luce and Barclay, Dupuis, and Woods all engage with, and contribute to, the burgeoning interest in relational therapies for people who hear distressing voices; Moffatt, Coaten, and Rollins and Garrison propose new foci in the further development of therapeutic interventions. By virtue of being conceived within the interdisciplinary spaces of Hearing the Voice and being addressed to a diverse and interdisciplinary readership, the chapters in this volume are alive to the frictions, as well as the synergies, generated between different disciplinary approaches to experience, evidence, and scholarly analysis. An invitation to even greater reflexivity with respect to the purposes and practices of reading is made by Noorani, Powell, Woods, and Hart.

Our hope as editors of *Voices in Psychosis* is that this volume will serve to demonstrate the value of multi- and interdisciplinary approaches to the study of human experience. Analysis does not exhaust the work of listening; we can listen long after the utterance itself is no longer heard. We will continue to be with, and be moved by, the voices recorded in the VIP transcripts, and by listening continue to respond to their complex calls.

References

Alderson-Day, B., McCarthy-Jones, S., and Fernyhough, C. (2015). Hearing voices in the resting brain: a review of intrinsic functional connectivity research on auditory verbal hallucinations. *Neuroscience and Biobehavioral Reviews*, 55, 78–87.

Alderson-Day, B., Woods, A., Moseley, P., Common, S., Deamer, F., Dodgson, G., and Fernyhough, C. (2021). Voice-hearing and personification: characterising social qualities of auditory verbal hallucinations in early psychosis. *Schizophrenia Bulletin*, 47, 228–36.

Aleman, A., and Larøi, F. (2008). *Hallucinations: The Science of Idiosyncratic Perception*. Washington, DC: American Psychological Association.

Bentall, R. P. (2003). *Madness Explained*. London: Penguin.

Bernini, M., and Woods, A. (2014). Interdisciplinarity as cognitive integration: auditory verbal hallucinations as a case study. *Wiley Interdisciplinary Reviews: Cognitive Science*, 5(5), 603–12.

Corstens, D., Longden, E., Thomas, N., and Waddingham, R. (2014). Emerging perspectives from the hearing voices movement: implications for research and practice. *Schizophrenia Bulletin*, 40(1), 285–94.

Foxwell, J., Alderson-Day, B., Fernyhough, C., and Woods, A. (2020). 'I've learned I need to treat my characters like people': varieties of agency and interaction in writers' experiences of their characters' voices. *Consciousness and Cognition*, 79, 102901.

Hearing the Voice. (2019). Voices and creativity. https://understandingvoices.com/living-with-voices/voices-and-creativity/ (accessed: 3 March 2021).

Jones, N., and Luhrmann, T. M. (2016). Beyond the sensory: findings from an in-depth analysis of the phenomenology of 'auditory hallucinations' in schizophrenia. *Psychosis*, 8(3), 191–202.

Jones, N., Shattell, M., Kelly, T., Brown, R., Robinson, L., Renfro, R., Harris, B., and Luhrmann, T. M. (2016). 'Did I push myself over the edge?': complications of agency in psychosis onset and development. *Psychosis*, 8(4), 324–35.

Kalathil, J., and Jones, N. (2016). Unsettling disciplines: madness, identity, research, knowledge. *Philosophy, Psychiatry, and Psychology*, 23(3), 183–8.

Knoll, E. (2017). *Emily's Voices*. Knoll Publications.

Longden, E. (2013). Learning from the voices in my head. https://www.ted.com/talks/eleanor_longden_the_voices_in_my_head?language=en (accessed: 15 June 2020).

Luhrmann, T. M. (2017). Diversity within the psychotic continuum. *Schizophrenia Bulletin*, 43(1), 27–31.

Perth Voices Clinic. (n.d). Personal stories from voice hearers. http://perthvoicesclinic.com.au/personal-stories-from-voice-hearers/ (accessed: 15 December 2020).

Romme, M., Escher, S., Dillon, J., Corstens, D., and Morris, M. (2009). *Living with Voices: 50 Stories of Recovery*. Ross-on-Wye: PCCS Books (in association with Birmingham City University).

Smailes, D., Alderson-Day, B., Fernyhough, C., McCarthy-Jones, S., and Dodgson, G. (2015). Tailoring cognitive behavioral therapy to subtypes of voice-hearing. *Frontiers in Psychology*, 6.

Toh, W. L., Moseley, P., and Fernyhough, C. (2022). Hearing voices as a feature of typical and psycho-pathological experience. *Nature Reviews Psychology*, 1, 72–86.

Varese, F., Smeets, F., Drukker, M., Lieverse, R., Lataster, T., Viechtbauer, W., Read, J., van Os, J., and Bentall, R. P. (2012). Childhood adversities increase the risk of psychosis: a meta-analysis of patient-control, prospective- and cross-sectional cohort studies. *Schizophrenia Bulletin*, 38(4), 661–71.

Waddingham, R. (2015). Whose voice are we hearing, really? *European Journal of Psychotherapy and Counselling*, 17(2), 206–15.

Waters, F., and Fernyhough, C. (2017). Hallucinations: a systematic review of points of similarity and difference across diagnostic classes. *Schizophrenia Bulletin*, 43(1), 32–43.

Waters, F., and Fernyhough, C. (2019). Auditory hallucinations: does a continuum of severity entail continuity in mechanism? *Schizophrenia Bulletin*, 45, 717–19.

Whitford, T. J., Mathalon, D. H., Shenton, M. E., Roach, B. J., Bammer, R., Adcock, R. A., Bouix, S., Kubicki, M., De Siebenthal, J., Rausch, A. C., Schneiderman, J. S., and Ford, J. M. (2011). Electrophysiological and diffusion tensor imaging evidence of delayed corollary discharges in patients with schizophrenia. *Psychological Medicine*, 41(5), 959–69.

Wilkinson, S., and Bell, V. (2016). The representation of agents in auditory verbal hallucinations. *Mind and Language*, 31(1), 104–26.

Woods, A., Jones, N., Alderson-Day, B., Callard, F., and Fernyhough, C. (2015). Experiences of hearing voices: analysis of a novel phenomenological survey. *The Lancet Psychiatry*, 2(4), 323–31.

Woods, A., Jones, N., Bernini, M., Callard, F., Alderson-Day, B., Badcock, J. C., Bell, V., Cook, C. C. H., Csordas, T., Humpston, C., Krueger, J., Larøi, F., McCarthy-Jones, S., Moseley, P., Powell, H. Raballo, R., Smailes, D., and Fernyhough, C. (2014). Interdisciplinary approaches to the phenomenology of auditory verbal hallucinations. *Schizophrenia Bulletin*, 40(1), 246–54.

About the Authors

Angela Woods is a Professor of Medical Humanities at Durham University and the Co-Director of Hearing the Voice. Her work in the critical medical humanities focuses on psychosis and narrative.

Ben Alderson-Day is a Research Psychologist at Durham University and Associate Director on Hearing the Voice. He worked as one of the interviewers on the VIP study.

Charles Fernyhough is a Psychologist and Writer. The focus of his recent scientific work has been in applying ideas from mainstream developmental psychology to the study of psychosis, particularly the phenomenon of voice-hearing. He is the Principal Investigator and Director of the interdisciplinary Hearing the Voice project, supported by the Wellcome Trust.

2

Voices in Context

What Do Early Intervention in Psychosis Services Offer?

Guy Dodgson, Early Intervention in Psychosis Services, Cumbria, Northumberland, Tyne and Wear NHS Foundation Trust

Stephanie Common, Early Intervention in Psychosis Services, Tees, Esk and Wear Valleys NHS Foundation Trust

Peter Moseley, Department of Psychology, Northumbria University

Rebecca Lee, Academy of Primary Care, Hull York Medical School

Ben Alderson-Day, Department of Psychology, Durham University

Conducted by Hearing the Voice, in partnership with researchers in the Cumbria, Northumberland, Tyne and Wear (CNTW) and Tees, Esk and Wear Valley (TEWV) NHS Foundation Trusts, the Voices in Psychosis (VIP) study aimed to explore what voices are like when people first start needing help to manage their experiences. In practice, this meant focusing attention on Early Intervention in Psychosis (EIP) services, the frontline pathway by which people receive care when they first develop a sustained period of psychosis. Half of the participants came from EIP services in CNTW—including cities such as Newcastle and Sunderland— while the other half came from TEWV, covering areas such as Durham, Middlesbrough, and Redcar.[1]

In this chapter, we provide an overview of how these services work and the economic and social contexts in which they operate.

The Development of Early Intervention in Psychosis

In the early 1990s, people across the UK with an emerging psychosis faced many problems. As their mental health deteriorated, they often became isolated, with

---

[1] In 2019, Northumberland, Tyne and Wear was joined by Cumbria to become Cumbria, Northumberland, Tyne and Wear NHS Foundation Trust, extending the trust as far west as Whitehaven. As recruitment for the VIP study had finished by this stage, no Cumbrian services were involved in the study.

Guy Dodgson, Stephanie Common, Peter Moseley, Rebecca Lee, and Ben Alderson-Day, *Voices in Context* In: *Voices in Psychosis*. Edited by: Angela Woods, Ben Alderson-Day, and Charles Fernyhough, Oxford University Press. © Guy Dodgson, Stephanie Common, Peter Moseley, Rebecca Lee, and Ben Alderson-Day 2022. DOI: 10.1093/oso/9780192898388.003.0002

families frantically trying to understand what was happening and get help. It typically took eighteen months to get access to mental health services after repeated attempts to secure help. Often access to services was precipitated by a crisis, so the person's first experience of a mental health service was a forced admission to hospital—perhaps in an old Victorian asylum—surrounded by other people who were distressed and who had enduring struggles with their mental health. There was therapeutic pessimism about recovery, with people being told that they had a lifelong illness, that they would be on medication for life, and that they would never work again. Services had little to offer in terms of treatment other than medication and 'monitoring and support'. High levels of stigma around psychotic experiences existed, contributing to fear and avoidance of help-seeking, which in turn led to delays in treatment. The average age of onset of psychosis is around 21 (Kessler et al., 2007), so it was often demoralizing for people early in their adult life.

Early Intervention in Psychosis services were an attempt to address these problems. Initially developed in Melbourne, Australia by Patrick McGorry, they were first deployed in Birmingham in the UK in the mid-1990s. The Labour government invested heavily in the National Health Service (NHS) and in mental health services, prioritizing the development of EIP services (Kings Fund, 2005). EIP services had an age range of 14–35 (to ensure that they also covered the peak onset for women, which is later than for men), and therefore crossed the traditional transition from child to adult health services at 18. They were tasked to reduce the duration of untreated psychosis (DUP), working on the basis that there was a critical period at the start of psychosis during which interventions could change the long-term course of illness. EIP services worked with people for three years in order to cover this critical period and also to ensure consistency of care. The services were designed to be 'youth-friendly', actively promoting hope of recovery and working closely with the family to ensure everyone was working together to help the young person.

At its inception, EIP had face validity, but little empirical evidence to support its basis. The growth of EIP services across the 2000s changed this, with robust evidence demonstrating both improved outcomes and cost saving. Improved recovery outcomes in comparison to standard care have been found in engagement, symptom reduction, vocational and social functioning, and reduced incidence of suicide (Chen et al., 2011; Correll et al., 2018). McCrone et al. (2009) identified that the introduction of an EIP service achieved a cost saving per patient of £5000 in year one, increasing to £14,000 by year three, through the reduction of admission and readmission rates to inpatient services.

Despite the demonstrated cost saving for the wider health economy, EIP remains a more costly option in the immediate term. Therefore, in the 2010s, with the reduction in public spending and impact of austerity, EIP services were in a perilous state and many services closed. Their possible demise overall was halted in 2016, when the government introduced an Access and Waiting Time Standard for EIP services. This standard promised additional investment for EIP services, stretched EIP services to extend the age range to 14–65, and offered services to people presenting with a potential psychotic prodrome (i.e. people 'at risk' of developing a full psychosis). Crucially, a more responsive service was offered: a target was set for everyone with an emerging psychosis to be seen within two weeks of referral to secondary mental health care, and to be able to access evidenced treatment recommended by the National Institute for Health and Care Excellence (NICE) guidance Quality Standards (QS102 and QS180).

EIP: The Local Context

The clinical catchment area for the VIP study, termed here as the 'North East', included the eastern half of England from the city of York up to the Scottish border, incorporating the regions of North Yorkshire, Teesside, County Durham, Tyne and Wear, and Northumberland. EIP services were developed in the North East between 2002 and 2004. Most services are specialist teams, with some adaptions for more rural patches ('spoke' workers are based in rural areas and are linked to the 'hub' where the full team is based and where there is a more concentrated population). The North East is a mixed urban and rural patch, with a combined population of approximately 2.6 million, rising to over 3 million with the inclusion of North Yorkshire. Many jobs were in coal mining, heavy industry, or shipbuilding, but these have reduced over the last fifty years, leaving an area with higher unemployment, lower average wages, and higher deprivation, compared to the national average of the UK (see Table 2.1). The depressed job market has limited the attractiveness of the area, so the North East has a relatively stable population, with low levels of racial and ethnic diversity. This fact is reflected in the statistics for EIP use: at least 92% of TEWV service users identified as being white British or from another white background.

How Do Voice-Hearers Come into Contact with EIP Services?

Voice-hearing and unusual beliefs are the most common presenting issues for which someone would be referred to an EIP service, most frequently by the person's general practitioner (GP). GP services form part of what is termed the primary care area of the NHS. Ideally people experiencing distressing symptoms that are potentially psychotic would receive rapid referral from primary care to an EIP team based in mental health secondary care services. To make sure referrals happen quickly, EIP services maintain an open referral policy by which anyone can refer directly to EIP teams (individuals, concerned relatives, or other agencies such as criminal justice or drug and alcohol services). Though treatment delays are much reduced, compared to the 1990s, there are still circumstances by which access to EIP services can be delayed both in primary care (e.g. symptoms not recognised) and in secondary care

Table 2.1 Comparing the North East with the rest of the UK

	North East		UK	
Population	2,657,909		66,435,550	
Unemployment	5.7%		3.8%	
Gross domestic product (GDP) per head	£23,569		£31,976	
Deprivation	34%		20%	
Ethnicity	Asian	2.9%	Asian	7.5%
	Black	0.5%	Black	3.3%
	Mixed race	0.9%	Mixed race	0.6%
	White British	93.6%	White British	80.5%
	White other	1.7%	White other	4.4%
	Other	0.4%	Other	1.0%
Life expectancy	Males	Females	Males	Females
	77.9	81.7	79.3	82.9

Data reflect 2020 reports for 2019, apart from GDP (2018 estimate) and life expectancy (2017–2019 estimate). North East deprivation figure is an average of each local authority's Index of Multiple Deprivation Score.

Source: Office for National Statistics licensed under the Open Government Licence v.3.0. Northern Ireland End User Licence (103.4 kB doc).

(e.g. an acute admission psychiatric ward only referring to EIP services at the point of discharge). The Access and Waiting Time Standard introduced in 2016 borrowed a model from NHS cancer care to reduce these potential delays. Currently, in the North East, approximately 60–80% of people reach EIP services within two weeks of seeking help from health care services.

How Do EIP Services Conceptualize Voice-Hearing?

EIP teams are multidisciplinary. The largest cadre of staff are termed 'care coordinators', who are either mental health community nurses or mental health social workers, or occupational therapists. In addition, there are psychologists and psychological therapists, psychiatrists, support workers, and increasingly staff with expertise in employment. All people who are referred to EIP services receive an assessment, generally carried out by a care coordinator, which focuses on an exploration of the person's experiences. Some services use a psychometric assessment to inform this process—such as the Positive and Negative Syndrome Scale (PANSS) (Kay et al., 1987), or CAARMS, a tool for the Comprehensive Assessment of At Risk

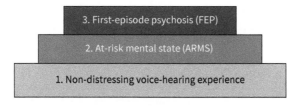

Figure 2.1 Contexts of voice-hearing used by EIP teams.

Mental States (Yung et al., 2005)—and consideration of these assessments by the multidisciplinary team will lead to a decision about whether this person is offered a service from the EIP team. The conceptualization of voice-hearing at assessment by EIP clinical services is shown in Figure 2.1.

Regarding group 1, it is known that there is a significant number of people in the general population who hear voices but are not distressed or troubled by these experiences. Although they may come into contact with health services, the fact that they hear voices would not warrant intervention in some cases but may indicate a need for support further down the line. Often, their presentation causes concern in wider health settings, prompting a referral to EIP services, but they then do not receive intervention (and may be referred to another service).

Group 2 refers to those in an 'at-risk mental state' (ARMS), which is perhaps more clearly termed as a presentation of a potential psychotic prodrome. Since the 1990s, researchers have attempted to identify the pathognomonic features of a psychotic prodrome in order to intervene to prevent the onset of first-episode psychosis (FEP). Variants of these criteria have been identified in North America (Addington et al., 2011), continental Europe (Bijl et al., 1998), and Australia (McGorry et al., 2009). In the UK, we use the Australia criteria, and the local criteria is a modified version of this (see Box 2.1).

In terms of voice-hearing, examples of an ARMS would include either hearing a voice infrequently, but with perceptual clarity, or having a diffuse voice-hearing

---

Box 2.1 ARMS criteria used in TEWV and Northumberland, Tyne and Wear NHS Foundation Trusts

Someone who is:

- aged 14–35 **AND**
- help-seeking **AND**
- has chronically poor, or a recent decline in, functioning **AND**
- has intense, but infrequent, psychotic symptoms **OR**
- has frequent, but low-intensity, psychotic symptoms **OR**
- has recently recovered from a brief psychotic episode.

Table 2.2 Diagnosis by gender for the VIP study

Diagnosis	Males (N = 23)		Females (N = 17)	
	n	%	n	%
Psychosis (unspecified)	7	17.5	3	7.5
Depression with psychotic features	2	5	2	5
Schizophrenia	2	5	0	0
Post-traumatic stress disorder	0	0	2	5
Emotionally unstable personality disorder	0	0	2	5
Substance-induced psychosis	1	2.5	0	0
Delirium	0	0	1	2.5
None	11	27.5	7	17.5

experience that happens with high frequency. It has been demonstrated that intervention with a form of cognitive behavioural therapy (CBT) for psychosis can be effective, for some people, in preventing the transition to a first episode of psychosis (Van der Gaag et al., 2019), and on this basis, the identification of an ARMS is recommended by NICE.

For the VIP study, only two out of forty voice-hearing participants were with the service via an ARMS pathway, reflecting the fact that most participants in the study were having both frequent and well-defined psychotic experiences. Such experiences constitute group 3 of Figure 2.1: those experiencing FEP. This group is the original focus of EIP work, and their voice-hearing experiences characteristically pass a threshold in terms of frequency, intensity, and negative life impact (as would be identified by a clinical psychometric such as the PANSS (Kay et al., 1987)). However, it is not required that people show evidence of these experiences having an enduring nature, or any of the associated 'negative symptoms' necessary for psychiatric diagnosis of a psychotic disorder (such as social withdrawal or anhedonia). A key tenet of the EIP approach is intervention in the absence of diagnostic certainty, on the basis that immediate intervention at this time may prevent the onset of a diagnostic disorder. For the VIP study, eighteen out of forty voice-hearing participants were with services on this basis, with the most common diagnosis being one of an unspecified psychosis (see Table 2.2). It should also be emphasized that their admission would not have been based purely on the presence of voices—instead, admission would depend on voices occurring in a context of distress and a decline in functioning.

Voice-Hearing and Diagnosis

It would be remiss here not to make reference to the issue of diagnosis and psychotic experience. The therapeutic pessimism that existed in relation to distressing psychotic experience for much of the nineteenth and twentieth centuries was underpinned by a diagnostic classification of this experience which often inferred a biological aetiology and a poor prognosis. Strong challenges to this always existed in service user-led and critical psychiatry movements, but in the 1990s and 2000s, this challenge was joined by influential critique from clinical psychology. Concerns were raised about the validity and reliability of psychotic disorder classification and the extent to which this acted as a barrier to the development of effective treatment (e.g. Bentall, 1990). The evolution of EIP has been influenced by these ideas and context, and many staff are attracted to work in EIP services on the basis of their role in the 'social movement' of change to mental health treatment provision. However, a degree of variance and debate exists on the issue of 'diagnostic uncertainty' within EIP services, contributed, in some degree, by the multidisciplinary nature of EIP. For some, EIP's role is to target those individuals who are on a trajectory to an inevitable psychotic disorder diagnosis and intervene in an attempt to ameliorate the impact of the disorder. In such a context, a 'full remission' of symptoms may be retrospectively interpreted in terms of a false positive presentation and incorrect acceptance by the EIP service. The alternative perspective would view EIP's role as providing intervention for distressing experiences, irrespective of the potential diagnostic profile.

This can lead to inter- and intra-team variance in EIP services. For voice-hearing, some teams may offer intervention to individuals who have had long-standing voice-hearing experiences since childhood, whereas others may not. Some teams may exclude voice-hearers for whom this experience co-occurs with a presentation consistent with an Emotionally Unstable Personality Disorder diagnosis (a highly contentious diagnostic category associated with long-term problems with mood and behaviour). An added factor is that EIP services exist within a wider context of mental health care and social security support which is diagnosis-based, so this tension is often one that is difficult for service users and staff to navigate.

What Does the Service Offer for Voice-Hearers?

'Care Coordination' Work

On acceptance into EIP services (see Figure 2.2), a service user is allocated a care coordinator who provides the initial orientation and engagement with the service. A key focus of the EIP model is smaller caseloads for care coordinators, compared to traditional community mental health teams, so that they have the capacity to meet with service users more frequently and flexibly.

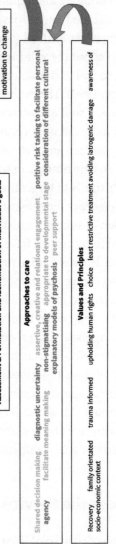

Figure 2.2 Illustration of the elements of EIP intervention.

Socio-economic disadvantage is significantly represented in EIP service users, and the transitions of late adolescence and early adulthood can be fault lines for difficulties in housing and financial circumstances. Co-occurring substance dependency can also contribute to social and financial adversity and instability. For a proportion of service users, their own experience of being parented or being a parent has brought them into contact with local authority children's support services. The impact of austerity policies introduced from 2010 in the North East has been a significant retraction of voluntary services and local statutory services (e.g. Sure Start programmes), leading to an even greater need in this area. This means that for many, the initial priority and focus of work with the care coordinator are targeted at primary needs in order to establish a stable foundation from which they can then be in a position to access interventions.

EIP service users are often characterized as 'hard to engage'. Societal concerns about dangerousness associated with experiences like voice-hearing lead people to be fearful of opening up about these experiences, and thus a focus of the initial care coordination role is 'assertive engagement'. Here, assessment of the individual's needs—while also respecting their choices with regard to involvement in mental health services and any potential short- or long-term risks that would arise from non-engagement—presents a challenge that requires a degree of creativity. A key element of such early engagement has traditionally been the normalization of voice-hearing experiences in the context of immediate stressful circumstances and the conveyance of a hopeful message about prognosis. In recent years, this has been augmented in the light of the recognition of the correlation between voice-hearing and early life adversity and trauma, with an opportunity for meaning-making in terms of how 'What has happened to me?' might lead to 'What I am experiencing?'. The care coordinator's early work focuses on supporting the identification of goals in relation to personally meaningful recovery, rather than on a unitary aim of symptom reduction.

Medication and Physical Health

The NICE guidelines for psychosis (National Institute for Health and Care Excellence, 2014) do not privilege medication above psychosocial interventions. In reality, however, most voice-hearers on the FEP pathway do receive antipsychotic medication as their first treatment (NICE recommends that antipsychotic medication is not used for people in an ARMS) and this was reflected in our study, with thirty-two out of forty participants currently receiving antipsychotics. The types of antipsychotic medication most commonly prescribed are known as 'atypical' antipsychotics. These medications first became available in the 1990s and were heralded as a major breakthrough by having a significantly lower side effect profile than the traditional antipsychotic medications (e.g. chlorpromazine). However, it has since come to light that atypicals carry a different, but also serious, side effect profile of increased risk to cardio-metabolic health (Üçok and Gaebel, 2008). This factor, coupled with poorer physical health profiles for people who experience psychosis, means that close monitoring of health markers and support with lifestyle decisions, such as diet and smoking, are now key services provided by EIP teams. Moreover, prescribing decisions now take into account a careful risk–benefit ratio analysis to balance symptom relief with maintaining physical health.

Psychosocial Interventions

Until recently, the availability of psychosocial interventions beyond medication has been limited, even in relatively well-resourced services like EIP. A key focus of the Access and Waiting Time Standard was to address this. Owing to different levels of investment and existing service provision, however, some variance in the availability of interventions remains.

Cognitive Behavioural Therapy for Psychosis
The development and availability of talking therapies for psychosis in routine health care came relatively late, compared to other conditions such as anxiety and depression. This is often attributed in large part to the conceptualization of hearing voices and other psychotic experiences as 'ununderstable' and therefore unamenable to talking therapy. This persisted late into the twentieth century in NHS care, where psychotic experiences such as voice-hearing were identified as exclusion criteria for trials of talking treatments for affective disorders or trauma. The role of clinical psychology in the delivery of behavioural approaches was to manage the impact of long-term conditions, and engagement with people regarding their voice-hearing experiences was discouraged. Clinical trials of therapeutic approaches designed specifically to target voice-hearing commenced in the UK in the 1990s. Clinical trials have indicated a degree of effectiveness that has led NICE to recommend cognitive behavioural therapy for psychosis (CBTp) as a treatment (Turner et al., 2020), even though efficacy is not found to be on par with CBT treatments for anxiety and depression. CBTp employs a 'traditional' CBT model, in which the cognitive appraisal of experiences leads to distressing emotional responses and sometimes unhelpful behavioural responses, which in turn maintain distress. In the case of voice-hearing, the conceit is that it is not the voices themselves that cause distress, but the interpretation of this experience that is the primary concern. Distress is maintained by counterproductive strategies used in response, and these can be targeted via classical cognitive behavioural methods. In the study, eleven participants had been given access to CBTp at the time of participation.

Other Individual Therapies
During the course of involvement with EIP services, some voice-hearers may also receive an alternative or additional type of talking therapy, which is determined

by individual goals and local availability. Examples include CBT for anxiety or depression, cognitive analytic therapy (CAT), or trauma-focused therapies such as eye-movement desensitization reprogramming (EMDR). In the study, only one participant out of forty had received CAT, while one other had received EMDR.

Family Intervention for Psychosis

Alongside CBTp, NICE (National Institute for Health and Care Excellence, 2014) recommends access to family-based interventions for people with psychosis. It does not specify a particular therapeutic model of family intervention, but the elements it describes are contained in behavioural family therapy (BFT). The model has three components: *psychoeducation*, *communication skills*, and *problem-solving*. The focus of the original BFT model was on educating families in how to understand and manage a life-long, largely biological illness which would be primarily treated with medication. Its current iteration has shifted to focus on the family developing a shared understanding. Family intervention for psychosis has the strongest evidence base of all recommended interventions, but it traditionally has had a low delivery rate (The Schizophrenia Commission, 2012). This may be understood in terms of a combination of factors such as: (1) families' reluctance to take part in something that they perceive may blame them for their loved ones' difficulties; or (2) care coordination staff can feel relatively unskilled in delivery by virtue of its brief training requirements. In the North East, a model is used according to which specialist systemic family therapists support and supervise generic care coordination staff and provide systemic family therapy when indicated. In areas where this model has been implemented, we have seen an increase in delivery rates. In keeping with its limited availability overall, relatively few participants in the study had received any form of family intervention—only two out of forty participants had taken part in family therapy at the time of the study.

The Course and Ending of EIP

Service users with FEP can remain under the care of EIP for up to three years, although in some cases, people leave earlier if they feel they have achieved their recovery goals or if they disengage from the service. A key tenet of the service model is that people should have availability up to three years. In times of increased pressure on teams, maintaining this for all service users can be challenging. In comparison, the ARMS pathway is shorter, with service users remaining under care for six months, during which time the focus is on psychological therapy (with less focus on assertive engagement). Over half of all EIP service users are discharged back to their GP, while some of the remainder are transferred to other secondary care services. Evidence from research trials has shown the effectiveness of EIP, but there are increased attempts to routinely collect outcome data, both on symptom reduction and from service users about their quality of life and whether they feel they have recovered. Although many people make good recoveries, a small number have long-term difficulties with distressing symptoms and often spend long periods of time in psychiatric hospitals. EIP is seen as a very successful development in psychiatric services, but there remain areas in which outcomes for service users could be improved.

Taking Part in Research: The VIP Study

A key aim of the VIP study was to talk to people about their voices as early as possible. However, as we would expect, many people using EIP face a range of challenges that they must tackle before they are in a position to take part in research. For that reason, on average, our research team ended up seeing people for the first time around 3–4 months after their first contact with EIP, and usually after they had been through an intense period of care coordinator liaison, medication prescription (and re-prescription), and, in some cases, psychological therapy.

We initially approached people who were within the first six months of using EIP services, although this was later extended to nine months as some people needed longer before feeling able to take part. Participants had to be aged 18–65 and to have been hearing voices at least once a week for a month in order to take part in the study. People who had been unwell for a long time before becoming known to services—having a suspected duration of untreated psychosis of over five years—were not included in the study, to retain a focus on voices in psychosis in their relatively early stages. In addition, diagnoses relating to a neurological disorder or damage—such as stroke—were an exclusion criterion on the basis that hallucinatory experiences are frequently quite different in such cases. Potential participants were first identified by their care team and asked if they would give consent to be contacted by the Durham University research team. With the help of the clinical research network (a body that supports research in the NHS), arrangements were then made for fully briefing participants, obtaining consent, and running the first interview.

The majority of the interviews were conducted in participants' homes, although they could also choose to take part at Durham University or at an NHS site. Interviews took place all year round, through all kinds of weather, in the company of dogs and cats, and often after repeated rearrangements. Some people engaged fully and noted that this was one of only a few opportunities they had been given to really talk in depth about their voices. Others participated with differing degrees of apprehension; talking about voices can be hard, and it can be difficult—if not sometimes impossible—for other people to understand. It was therefore crucial for interviewers to choose the right questions, asking them in an open and flexible way, and allowing the space and time for people to describe their experiences in a way that worked for them.

The semi-structured, but intentionally open-ended, interview that we used was developed through interdisciplinary debate and discussion within the Hearing the

Voice team over a number of years. It drew on our prior studies of emotional experience in depression and on the experience of hearing voices (Woods et al., 2015), and on extensive consultation with experts by experience and with world-leading anthropologists of psychosis. The interview was structured around eight core questions, and begin with an open invitation to describe the experience in the participants' own terms.

The Hearing the Voice Phenomenology Interview

1. Could you try to describe to me some of the voice (or voice-like) experiences you've been having?
2. Could you tell us a bit about what life was like for you, and how you were feeling, when you first started having these experiences?
3. How does it feel when you have the experience?
4. Do your experiences contain messages of any kind?
5. Does it feel as though the experiences have their own character or personality?
6. Have your experiences changed at all since they first started?
7. Why do you think these experiences are happening?
8. Is there anything else we haven't talked about yet, but is an important part of your experience?

Each core question was followed by optional prompts used by the interviewer to explore particular aspects of the experience. For instance, question 1 included prompts relating to the number of voices, their position in space, and the potential presence of voices in any other sensory modalities (such as vision). Following the interview, a standardized rating scale of hallucinations was deployed: the Psychotic Symptom Rating Scale (PSYRATS) (Haddock et al., 1999). This allowed phenomenological exploration to be conducted alongside validated scoring used elsewhere in research. As part of the wider study, participants were also asked to complete questionnaires on various topics (such as the qualities of their inner speech), cognitive tasks examining the potential mechanisms underlying unusual perceptual experiences, and a magnetic resonance imaging (MRI) scanning session. The results of these aspects of the study are reported elsewhere (e.g. Moseley et al., 2020). In this volume, we focus only on the interviews collected, the stories of the voice-hearers involved, and our responses to them as an interdisciplinary team.

References

Addington, J., Cornblatt, B. A., Cadenhead, K. S., Cannon, T. D., McGlashan, T. H., Perkins, D. O., Seidman, L. J., Tsuang, M. T., Walker, E. F., Woods, S. W., and Heinssen, R. (2011). At clinical high risk for psychosis: outcome for nonconverters. *American Journal of Psychiatry*, 168(8), 800–5.

Bentall, R. P. (1990). The illusion of reality: a review and integration of psychological research on hallucinations. *Psychological Bulletin*, 107(1), 82–95.

Bijl, R. V., Ravelli, A., and Van Zessen, G. (1998). Prevalence of psychiatric disorder in the general population: results of The Netherlands Mental Health Survey and Incidence Study (NEMESIS). *Social Psychiatry and Psychiatric Epidemiology*, 33(12), 587–95.

Chen, E. Y. H., Tang, J. Y. M., Hui, C. L. M., Chiu, C. P. Y., Lam, M. M. L., Law, C. W., Yew, C. W. S., Wong, G. H. Y., Chung, D. W. S., Tso, S., Chan, K. P. M., Chee Yip, K., Fong Hung, S., and Honer, W. G. (2011). Three-year outcome of phase-specific early intervention for first-episode psychosis: a cohort study in Hong Kong. *Early Intervention in Psychiatry*, 5(4), 315–23.

Correll, C. U., Galling, B., Pawar, A., Krivko, A., Bonnetto, C., Ruggeri, M., Craig, T. J., Nordentoft, M., Srihari, V. H., Guloksuz, S., Hui, C. L. M., Chen, E. Y. H., Valencia, M., Juarez, F., Robinson, D. G., Schooler, N. R., Brunette, M. F., Mueser, K. T., Rosenheck, R. A., Marcy, P., Addington, J., Estroff, S. E., Robinson, J., Penn, D., Severe, J. B., and Kane, J. M. (2018). Comparison of early intervention services vs treatment as usual for early phase psychosis: a systematic review, meta-analysis and meta-regression. *JAMA Psychiatry*, 75(6), 555–65.

Haddock, G., McCarron, J., Tarrier, N., & Faragher, E. B. (1999). Scales to measure dimensions of hallucinations and delusions: the psychotic symptom rating scales (PSYRATS). *Psychological Medicine*, 29(4), 879–889.

Kay, S. R. F., Fiszbein, A., and Opler, L. A. (1987). The Positive and Negative Syndrome Scale (PANNS) for schizophrenia. *Schizophrenia Bulletin*, 13(2), 261–76.

Kessler, R. C., Amminger, G. P., Aguilar-Gaxiola, S., Alonso, J., Lee, S., and Ustün, T. B. (2007). Age of onset of mental disorders: a review of recent literature. *Current Opinion in Psychiatry*, 20(4), 359–64.

Kings Fund. (2005). An independent audit of the NHS under Labour (1997–2005). https://www.kingsfund.org.uk/publications/independent-audit-nhs-under-labour-1997-2005 (accessed: 15 July 2021).

McCrone, P., Knapp, M., and Dhanasiri, S. (2009). Economic impact of services for first-episode psychosis: a decision model approach. *Early Intervention in Psychiatry*, 3(4), 266–73.

McGorry, P. D., Nelson, B., Amminger, G. P., Bechdolf, A., Francey, S. M., Berger, G., Riecher-Rössler, A., Klosterkötter, J., Ruhrmann, S., Schultze-Lutter, F., Nordentoft, M., Hickie, I., McGuire, P., Berk, M., Chen, E. Y. H., Keshavan, M. S., and Yung, A. R. (2009). Intervention in individuals at ultra high risk for psychosis: a review and future directions. *Journal of Clinical Psychiatry*, 70(9), 1206–12.

Moseley, P., Alderson-Day, B., Common, S., Dodgson, G., Lee, R., Mitrenga, K. J., Moffat, J. A., and Fernyhough, C. (2022). Continuities and discontinuities in the cognitive mechanisms associated with clinical and non-clinical auditory verbal hallucinations. *Clinical Psychological Science,* https://doi.org/10.1177/21677026211059802

National Institute for Health and Care Excellence. (2014) Psychosis and schizophrenia: treatment and management. (Clinical guideline 178.) 2014. http://guidance.nice.org.uk/CG178].

The Schizophrenia Commission (2012). *The Abandoned Illness: A Report from the Schizophrenia Commission*. London: Rethink Mental Illness.

Turner, D. T., Burger, S., Smit, F., Valmaggia, L. R., & van der Gaag, M. (2020). What constitutes sufficient evidence for case formulation–driven CBT for psychosis? Cumulative meta-analysis of the effect on hallucinations and delusions. *Schizophrenia Bulletin*, 46(5), 1072–1085.

Üçok, A. L. P. and Gaebel, W. (2008). Side effects of atypical antipsychotics: a brief overview. *World Psychiatry*, 7(1), 58–62.

Van der Gaag, M., van den Berg, D., and Ising, H. (2019). CBT in the prevention of psychosis and other severe mental disorders in patients with an at risk mental state: a review and proposed next steps. *Schizophrenia Research*, 203, 88–93.

Woods, A., Jones, N., Alderson-Day, B., Callard, F., and Fernyhough, C. (2015). Experiences of hearing voices: analysis of a novel phenomenological survey. *The Lancet Psychiatry*, 2(4), 323–31.

Yung, A. R., Pan Yuen, H., McGorry, P. D., Phillips, L. J., Kelly, D., Dell'Olio, M., Francey, S. M., Cosgrave, E. M., Killackey, E., Stanford, C., Godfrey, K., and Buckby, J. (2005). Mapping the onset of psychosis: the comprehensive assessment of at-risk mental states. *Australian and New Zealand Journal of Psychiatry*, 39(11–12), 964–71.

About the Authors

Guy Dodgson is a Consultant Clinical Psychologist and the Clinical Lead for EIP services in CNTW NHS Foundation Trust. He was the Principal Investigator for the VIP study within CNTW and the overall Chief Investigator for the study.

Stephanie Common is a Consultant Clinical Psychologist and the Clinical Lead for EIP services in TEWV NHS Foundation Trust. She was the Principal Investigator for the VIP study within TEWV.

Peter Moseley is a Senior Research Fellow in Psychology at Northumbria University. He is interested in linking phenomenology, cognition, and brain processes associated with voice-hearing.

Rebecca Lee is a PhD Researcher at Hull York Medical School who specializes in mental health and homelessness. She was a Research Assistant on the VIP study from 2019 to 2020.

Ben Alderson-Day is a Research Psychologist at Durham University and an Associate Directoron Hearing the Voice. He worked as one of the interviewers on the VIP study.

3

Reflecting on Voices

Isaac

I am a male, who is, while typing this, twenty-five years of age. I have heard voices for five years now. I took part in the Voices in Psychosis (VIP) study initially as a voice-hearer and 'pilot' participant. I told the research team about my voice-hearing experiences, which were put on record. I had my brain scanned also and took part in various tests such as having my IQ tested. I have also been a consultant over the past few months as someone who has read many of the VIP interviews and has offered feedback.

I have learnt a great deal after reading over twenty interviews from people who experience hearing voices, of one kind or another. There are many similarities to those that I am experiencing . . . and some important differences. Reading about other voices is something that I believe will help me move forwards in self-reflection, and be a way to combat the trauma that they have become in my life, so much so that they are impeding the development of personal relationships and radically impeding my career goals.

How Voices Begin

> I've had a few different things throughout like friendships and that, a couple of friendships, loss of a close mate's mam. . . . So around that period, so I don't know whether that was all, it was a collaboration of everything. . . . Stress or whatever you know. (Alex)

Many of the voices in the VIP study at first began in sufferers during times of extreme stress. This is exactly how mine first began, while I was trying to complete university coursework. Whatever the shock to the system, it seems that, in all cases, the sufferer was not able to control events and felt helpless. It reminds me of Harry, whose voice 'comes out of nowhere' during stress.

Isaac, *Reflecting on Voices* In: *Voices in Psychosis*. Edited by: Angela Woods, Ben Alderson-Day, and Charles Fernyhough, Oxford University Press.
© Issac 2022. DOI: 10.1093/oso/9780192898388.003.0003

Some accounts also mention how the sufferer wasn't sleeping much during such stressful times, when they first began hearing voices:

Ehm, a lot, a lot, I mean I have a lot of anxiety, because I'm restless and eh, I don't sleep and me mind goes wandering. . . . And like I get to a point where I'm trying to, there's that much anxiety, I have to go and try and find out if sommat is going on. . . . It's just I can't go to sleep, my head's all over . . . And eh I just don't switch off, even if I go and lie in my bed, I, I, I can't, [just] toss and turn till I get back up. (Fred)

What these accounts go on to describe mirrors my first experience, in which I couldn't quite comprehend what was happening. I remember being significantly stressed out and very sleep-deprived, while trying to meet university coursework deadlines. In these case studies, sleep deprivation and insomnia were mentioned several times. If you are worried and anxious, then you won't sleep, it seems. My case is similar to Alex's, who mentions that he 'wasn't getting much sleep . . . maybes only two to three hours' sleep' a night when he first started hearing voices.

Some of the people in the interviews had been bullied by their contemporaries and peers while at school. This was not addressed by those with a duty of care, resulting in it continuing over time. It seems that the trauma of being picked upon in a school environment, and there being no support coming, is a major factor in developing hearing voices. Many had fallen out with close friends. I also had such experiences at school before the onset of my voices at university.

What It Feels Like

Jane from the VIP interviews mentions how she has a little girl's voice which comes into her head and talks through her like some kind of demonic possession. This also happens to me, except that it is in the form of a man who torments me when I am highly stressed. Jane says that she gets muscle spasms when the voice is 'talking through' her. I do not, however, get muscle spasms when the voices talk through me.

Another voice-hearer Sean also started hearing voices coming from outside of his head, thinking they were coming from outside of him, so he went out to investigate. When I started hearing voices, it sounded like a woman was talking about me from another room. This was while at university, after suffering my first psychotic break from reality. My first experience of hearing voices entailed hearing the voices of a group of lads who appeared to be talking from downstairs about me. I went to investigate in the common room and there was nobody there. This is very similar to Sean, who lived in a flat and heard the voices of what appeared to be people upstairs talking about him, when this was not the case (see Image 3.1).

And then when I walked outside, before I go, the voices had started, I heard the word 'dickhead' and I thought . . . I went like outside and I thought, why that's a bit strange, unless like I say somebody upstairs just said it randomly. (Sean)

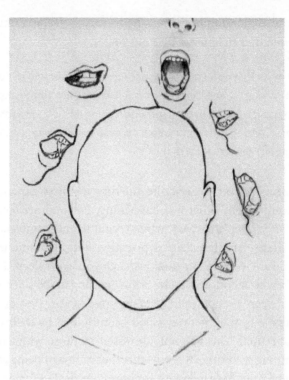

Image 3.1 Voices.
Credit: E Lightfoot, 2021.

I also experience, like some, tactile hallucinations. One person in the interviews mentions a feeling of being hit on the head, which is similar to what I experience, although there is never any bruising or evidence of physical harm. Hearing my voices is very much like having a radio or phone planted inside the head, without any crackling or noises due to bad reception. During the early first stages of hearing, these voices sounded like they were coming from another room. I literally had to check whether they were coming from that room, and upon investigation they were not.

> But there's been a few times where I've thought I could hear it here and had to go outside and check . . . and then my mum's been like, there's no one there Gail. . . . It's quite different, difficult to differentiate between what is real and what isn't and . . . what are my thoughts and . . . then . . . I don't know how much I have control over these kind of things which come into my head. (Gail)

In my experience, when you hear voices, you become less aware of reality due to the perpetual distraction inside your head. It might also be necessary for a voice-hearer to ask another person, whose voice has been in their head, if that person was actually part of that experience, rather than their voice having been hallucination which was conjured up by the voice-hearer's brain. Voice-hearers may do this because telling

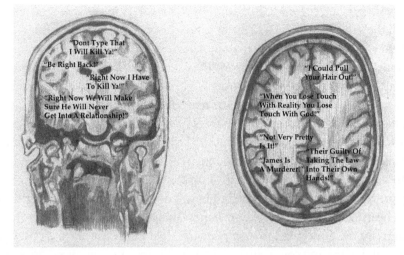

Image 3.2 Brain scans 2 normal.
Credit: E Lightfoot, 2021.

the difference between the two might be hard. This kind of checking was, for me, best tested out between myself and a professional, such as a counsellor or family member, since it is common for me to hear such people in my head. The answer so far from real people has always been 'no', 'we did not have the same experience in our head', and so on (see Image 3.2).

I would commonly hear the voices of whoever I had interacted with after I had interacted with them. This is why such experiences seem to be like telepathic communication. Many of the hallucinations are based on fears, so maybe I hear such people in my head because of paranoia. I have no paranoia about my family being inside my head, so I do not hear their voices inside my head like I once did anymore.

Personal Challenges

While it is useful to identify the similarities between the VIP accounts and my voice-hearing experiences, identifying the differences has been just as key. They have caused me to wonder at the uniqueness of the individual, which creates a challenge for all those parties and professionals who have to help and support sufferers.

I have never taken drugs.
I experience my voices constantly with no let-up.
I feel pain when believing that I am being hit over the head, although this is not the feeling which comes with the voice.

When I watch TV, the actors will take on a new life inside my head. I know that for many, the voices come in times of stress, which appears to trigger the onset of hearing voices, when there was previously a silence. Writing as someone who hears voices all the time, I would like to know more about people whose voices do not always speak; I would like to know what they are doing, thinking, and feeling and what is generally happening in such a person's life when the voices are not around.

Sharing stories between voice-hearers is intriguing and a bit disturbing. I would encourage people who experience voices to share such experiences with counsellors for support, but not with strangers. It might be something to do when in support groups with other people who hear voices. Voice-hearers may learn to manage or even treat their voices this way. I think that it is important for people to understand how stress, bullying, and sleep deprivation can bring on voice-hearing, in order to help prevent it. I would have liked to have known such coping strategies before I started hearing voices. I see now how important things like relaxation are.

My aims for the future are to keep practising what I have learnt from my cognitive behavioural therapy and counselling. Also I am to continue my counselling sessions and to stick with my medication. I continue to live a healthy lifestyle. I would like more people to be talking about what can cause voice-hearing in 10–20 years' time. I had one assembly at school when I was younger concerning how bullying can cause serious mental health conditions to people, but I would also like awareness to be made at university where some young adults develop these kinds of conditions. This is because university years can be stressful times and young adults are more likely to deprive themselves of sleep to get assignments done, which can lead to these breaks from reality.

I hope that people are better able to treat and cure such conditions in the future, although there are people who fully recover.

PART TWO
THE EXPERIENCE OF HEARING VOICES

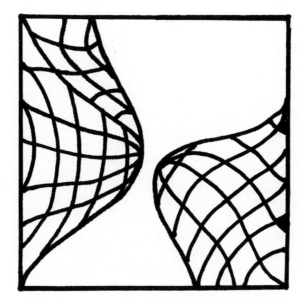

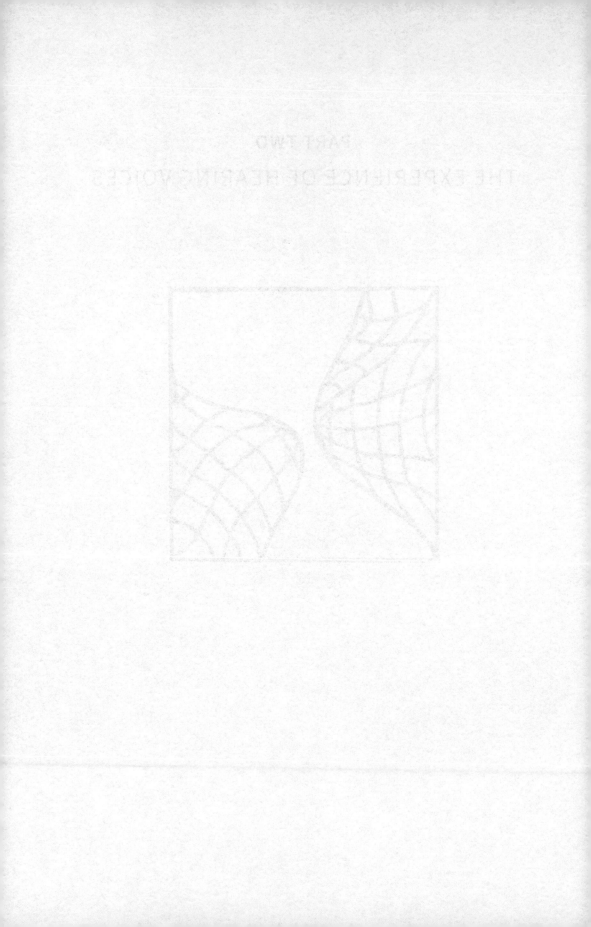

4

The Quickening

Gillian Allnutt, Poet in Residence with Hearing the Voice

She came to me during the last week of April, 1988.
I was alone in Alison's council flat

in Islington, the corner of Newington Green
and Green Lanes.

She didn't say anything then and hasn't spoken since—
despite the appearance

in time of those old pretenders,
words and what they think they are

in their imperial new clothes.
For she who mourned the emperor, her father, in his shabby original clothes

in truth
was older than the moon, outwith

the onset and the setting of imagination.
All alone

she came
and sometimes

she was three and sometimes seven
and then

she was both.
She was, as I said, outwith.

I kept looking over my shoulder
for her—

Gillian Allnutt, *The Quickening* In: *Voices in Psychosis*. Edited by: Angela Woods, Ben Alderson-Day, and Charles Fernyhough, Oxford University Press.
© Gillian Allnutt 2022. DOI: 10.1093/oso/9780192898388.003.0004

I knew she was and I knew she wasn't there
any more than her father

with his *sure as eggs is eggs*
and his beggar's bag.

But when I felt about me for her fear—
knowing her

then, as if for
the first time, as my fleet familiar—

I knew that if I listened for her
she'd be there.

A Note on the Poem 'The Quickening'

In 1988, I was approaching forty, maybe halfway through my life. And it was then that she—the child in the poem, the child in myself—came to me and I named her Small Gillian. I thought she was both myself at three years old and myself at seven; she was outwith time and, in a way, ageless. Since then, she has taught me so much about how hard it is to trust and how hard it is to listen and about what love must be.

I'd like to thank Jade, Leah, Orla, and Zara whose courage and honesty gave me permission to write a poem about one of the strangest, and ultimately most helpful, experiences of my life.

About the Author

Gillian Allnutt has published nine collections of poetry, including *How the Bicycle Shone: New & Selected Poems* (Bloodaxe, 2007) and *wake* (Bloodaxe, 2018). She was awarded The Queen's Gold Medal for Poetry in 2016. Since 2016, she has worked as a poet with Hearing the Voice and, during the academic years 2018/19 and 2019/20, held a Royal Literary Fund Fellowship at York University.

5

The Sound of Fear

Ben Alderson-Day, Department of Psychology, Durham University

Thomas Ward, Institute of Psychiatry, Psychology and Neuroscience, Kings College London

A stranger threatens to torture your children unless you do exactly what he says. A demon penetrates your mind, distorting how you perceive the world in front of your eyes. A dark presence waits at the boundary of your awareness, watching. These experiences, freighted with fear, are common tropes of the horror genre, and yet are daily experiences for some voice-hearers. Popular notions of voice-hearing—in stories, media, and the wider cultural imagination—emphasize the wild, paranoid, and uncontrollable features of the experience. Cognitive psychological models, in which hallucinations are primarily framed as a kind of perceptual error, emphasize points of misattribution and salience. Clinically, the focus may be placed on the meaning-making and appraisals that shape responses to a voice. One thing that is sometimes missed is the role of fear as a primary and potentially enduring emotion in the context of hearing distressing voices. The aim of this chapter is to reconsider the role of fear in the voice-hearing experience, its presence in the interviews of the Voices in Psychosis (VIP) study, therapeutic approaches to fear when working with voices, and how fear pervades not only the experience of a voice, but one's whole sense of being in the world.

Fear in the VIP Study

In the psychological literature, fear is typically distinguished from anxiety and other states of distress by being focused on a specific object of threat. Psychological therapy might involve targeted work with the object using techniques like graded exposure, in which people gradually habituate to the presence of what they fear and find ways to manage it. In the case of voice-hearing, the 'voice' could be considered as an object (i.e. an entity or agent that brings threat), or the event of voice-hearing itself could be considered as a threatening situation. But keeping this object in focus, as something tractable and concrete, poses a different kind of challenge.

Reports of fear and terror are evident throughout the accounts of voice-hearers in the VIP study. Sixty per cent of participants reported fear in connection with their voices, which in the study included voices that 'prompt specific feelings of fear or

Ben Alderson-Day and Thomas Ward, *The Sound of Fear* In: *Voices in Psychosis*. Edited by: Angela Woods, Ben Alderson-Day, and Charles Fernyhough, Oxford University Press. © Ben Alderson-Day and Thomas Ward 2022. DOI: 10.1093/oso/9780192898388.003.0005 dread', as well as voices 'elicited or exacerbated by fearful states'. Fear has been noted as a feature of voice-hearing in prior phenomenological work, but perhaps not to the same degree. Nayani and David (1996), for example, observed that only 16% of their participants reported fear in association with, or prompting the onset of, their voices. For the VIP participants, fear can be elicited in different ways. Most notably, the voices themselves can take 'demonic' and frightening forms (for instance, one participant, Bill, heard a 'barking' voice), and the voices may make explicit and violent threats to the voice-hearer or others. Swearing, physical threats, and coercion towards suicide or self-harm are rife in the VIP interviews and in accounts of distressing voice-hearing more broadly. The accounts suggest an emotional response that goes beyond the fear one might feel towards an actual object or situation; instead, the fear is of something more diffuse, intangible, and existentially unsettling. Here, we will briefly outline and explore three key ways in which fear can be amplified in the context of voice-hearing: realization, loss of reality, and potentiality.

Realization

On average, the interviewees in the VIP study had been using clinical services for only 3–4 months. Sometimes the involvement of services closely followed the onset of voices, but in other cases, people reported hearing voices for a number of years before deciding to seek help. Fear was not always the prevalent emotion at the time of the interview (at least, when compared to feelings of anxiety or depression), but it may have been a key part of the experience when the voices first started, driving subsequent meaning-making and other responses. This could be because the experience itself was fear-inducing (e.g. hearing threats and commands to harm oneself), or because, not long after, the individual realized that others could not hear the voices too—and that they were alone in facing this unfamiliar and threatening terrain.

Particularly if the voices they heard were realistic and congruent with their environment, people often could not pinpoint a moment of realization, but rather spoke of a creeping sense of a new and unnerving reality:

It's frightening. Totally frightening the way I feel . . . Because once I knew who like, like . . . once I knew that that was in me head and the policeman had told us, all I got then was just [the voice] repeating it. . . . the lad upstairs repeating that 'dickhead' word all the time. (Sean)

In the beginning it was, it was absolutely, it was really terrifying, because I didn't understand what was happening to us. (Leah)

It was scary at first, because I was asking me older brother and he was like, no, I can't hear them, so I'm like . . . well there's one said I can't hear them. And I asked me little sister, I ask me little sister all the time, can you hear that? She's like, no. (Toby)

Loss of reality

For others, once it had been established that they were hearing voices, the ongoing uncertainty of what was real and what was not became deeply unsettling. In some instances, it seemed less that there was a clear sense of an *alternative* reality (e.g. a strongly held belief about the nature of the threat or persecution), and more like a fog of doubt about what could be trusted in the outside world. Moreover, where things started to improve, the stark contrast between experiences of reality and un-reality could itself be unnerving. There could be fear in recollecting what it was like to be 'lost' in voices, which could be amplified by a terror of return:

> I think because I am that much better now that it's, it's more scary than when I was re-ally unwell, because when I was so unwell, everything was going wrong and I didn't care, whereas now I do want to get better and be able to come home and live a normal life. (Gail)

> It's something that, it scares you every time, when you realise that there's nobody there, it's a scary thought to be left with. And you're always left anxious, you know, and con-fused. (Bill)

For ten voice-hearers in the study (25%), fear co-occurred with *boundary voices*—voices that are experienced as coming from locations that were 'just beyond per-ception' or 'just out of earshot', such as through walls, doors, and windows or round corners. Here the imminent threat is often located at the uncertain limits of one's own sense of immediate space. In this respect, the position of voices (and their status as fear objects) relies less on the objective space that voice-hearers inhabit, and more the perceived space that they occupy and can be sure of (what some phenomen-ologists have termed 'lived' space (Merleau-Ponty, 1962)). For these people, fear thrived at the borders of what could be perceived with certainty.

Potentiality

This sense of potential threat pervaded accounts in which fear was *the* prominent emotion during the interview. For example, Fran frequently experienced a bellowing voice that she would liken to a character from a horror movie. In sound, meaning, and impact, the voice evoked sheer terror. During her interview, questions had to be frequently paused or specifically redirected away from a specific voice. Even talking about the voice elicited strong feelings of distress and current threat, with the fear at times becoming overwhelming.

> It's when I'm feeling really anxious, I'll have like this dark, deep, bellowing voice, what I never, I've never heard like outside of the head. Like human interaction, I've never heard that voice before. . . . it's a voice what is very scary, it wakes me up . . . like I don't know

it's . . . it's hard talking about it already. . . . like you know when you have a nightmare, and there's, you just, like I don't even know if I can explain it, if you watch a horror movie . . . and that person, that horror movie kind of thing, it's that kind of thing, what you would think, oh . . . Just someone, someone deep and dark and the things what he comes out with, it's . . . quite scary, it's . . . not [a] nice experience. (Fran)

The voice that Fran experienced would frequently say extremely derogatory things to her, but, importantly, it would also act in a terrorizing way. Later in the interview, she described the voice as a black shadow that could creep up on her from behind and then scream in her ear while she was sitting at work, or even wake her from sleep. Voices disrupting or preventing sleep in this way were reported by other participants as well, often where the potential for the voice to speak or 'act' in other ways filled the voice-hearer with dread of what was about to happen.

Sometimes I get that scared, well I used to get that scared when I was in my bed that I couldn't move and I'd lay there for like six hours without being able to move. . . . Because every time, as soon as I moved, I could hear the voice or I could hear the banging start again. (Carl)

Like I try and explain psychosis to people, it's like your mind has all the information of all your vulnerabilities and all the things that will make you uncomfortable, scared, then uses them to vocate [sic] and make a kind of almost like a horror film around you with the things you can see in here. So it will, they'll kind of say, you know you don't want to be here or . . . insinuating to kill myself and all sorts of stuff (Olivia)

In this context, the intentionality of the voice, its perceived omnipotence (including possible supernatural powers to harm), and the unreality of the ongoing situation appears to make some voice-hearers prey to their very worst fears. Fear in this context involves the capacity of the mind to terrorize itself not only with what is known, but often more importantly, with what is not known about this powerful 'other'. The deepest fears that many of us hold are not limited to the realms of physical harm, no matter how explicit the threat of violence may be. For many, the fear is fundamentally social; it is the fear that our most shameful secrets and most unacceptable thoughts will be accessed and broadcast to others, leading to humiliation, rejection, and social annihilation.

The voice itself may be frightening and unusual, but the loss of the mooring of reality and the potential for the voice to act in any way, at any time, create fear in the form of an existential threat which can be extremely hard to escape. In the next section, we will consider therapeutic approaches to helping people escape this terror.

Working with Fear

Psychological approaches to working with voices typically adopt a cognitive understanding of the experience (Chadwick and Birchwood, 1994). Morrison (2001) connected voice-hearing to clinical approaches to anxiety, placing voices within the broad array of phenomena that intrude into consciousness. Consequently, the maintaining role of threat-focused attention and voice-hearers' use of safety-seeking behaviours (such as avoidance and hypervigilance) became foci for therapeutic intervention. Within traditional cognitive approaches, one is typically working one step removed from emotion, focusing on the associated meaning-making, attentional focus, or behavioural response. Such approaches thus risk operating at a purely intellectual, rather than emotional, level—an observation sometimes referred to as the 'head–heart lag'. There is therefore increasing recognition of the importance of bringing emotion 'into play' within cognitive approaches to psychosis.

Yet addressing fear in voice-hearing raises certain difficulties. In contrast to contexts in which the feared object is directly accessible (e.g. fear of heights, spiders, or social situations), the challenge in managing voices is how to bring this intensely private, affect-laden experience into therapy. Several techniques offer ways to connect with the experience and emotion of hearing a voice, including the 'empty chair' (in which people are invited to address the voice as if it were sitting with them in the room), imagery re-scripting (where repetitive and intrusive mental imagery is explored and reshaped in a guided and supported way), and various forms of roleplay. For example, in the Talking with Voices approach (Corstens et al., 2012), a facilitator engages in direct dialogue with the voice(s), working relationally on social–emotional dilemmas that may manifest in the voice experience. Another example is AVATAR therapy, a relational approach that involves 'face-to-face' dialogue with a computerized representation of the persecutory voice (the avatar) which the hearer creates (Leff et al., 2013). The therapist—switching between speaking as themselves and voicing the avatar—facilitates a dialogue in which the aim is for the voice-hearer to develop an increased sense of power and control (Craig et al., 2018).

Fear plays a crucial role within the AVATAR therapy approach. Consistently high ratings for sense of 'presence'—the extent to which the avatar dialogue was like hearing and speaking to the actual voice—highlight the potential for working with emotional meanings *in vivo*.[1] Prior to the first dialogue, an initial session involves sensitive assessment of the person's voice(s) which is used to establish verbatim content and voice characterization. The person then creates their avatar using specially designed software to match both auditory voice characteristics and the image they associate with their voice. This assessment and avatar creation can be a powerful experience ('you're the first person to hear what I hear') and there can be a sense of taking control inherent in 'creating my avatar'.

The therapy that follows involves two broad phases. Phase 1 focuses on exposure to the avatar speaking verbatim voice content while the person is supported to take

---

[1] The use of presence in digital and virtual reality-based methods is typically used to indicate whether an experience feels truly present in a veridical sense (i.e. 'it sounds *just like* the voice I hear'). This is to be distinguished from experiences of 'felt' or 'sensed' presences that are sometimes described by voice-hearers in which their voices 'have' a presence beyond what can be heard. Felt presence phenomena are known to occur in a range of contexts, including bereavement, sleep deprivation, survival situations, and neurological change.

power and control within the dialogue. The words spoken by the persecutory voice frequently have the power to terrify, shame, and silence the person (often associated with a stress response, which reinforces this relational experience of fear and powerlessness). The act of working directly on verbatim content begins a process of breaking this shame/silence cycle, with the voice-hearer turning to face experiences that may have been feared and avoided for many years. Phase 2 moves into more extended use of dialogue and a focus on relational and autobiographical themes that are reflected in the voice experience.

AVATAR therapy shares common ground with other approaches to working with fear by allowing direct exposure to a realistic representation of the voice, i.e. the object of fear. This embodied representation of the voice may help crystallize an amorphous shape-shifting sense of threat into something tangible. Initial sessions can provoke strong feelings of fear and associated concerns of harm to self, voice retaliation, and loss of control. High levels of anxiety and physiological arousal typically reduce over the course of the sessions, suggesting possible processes of desensitization or habituation to the feared stimulus. Enacting changes in relating to the voice (moving from submissive to assertive responding), including a focus on non-verbal aspects such as voice tone, posture, and eye contact, may also facilitate ways of learning to inhibit immediate reactions—an important part of targeting the conditioned fear response (Craske et al., 2014).

An explicit narrative of change, involving taking back power and control over terrifying experiences, facilitates engagement in these potentially challenging early sessions. Within a recent large-scale trial of AVATAR therapy (Craig et al., 2018), shifts were observed early for some people, raising the possibility that this exposure work may be sufficient for important change in some cases. Examples from the trial include Claire, who faced a terrifying, vividly realized demonic presence hell-bent on punishment (verbatim content: 'You're a stupid useless cunt'; 'I'm taking you to a dark dark place'), or Anne, who after decades of imposed silence in a voice-relationship of coercion and control (verbatim content: 'You will be raped'; 'You should shut your mouth . . . don't say anything'), took courage from facing an abuser.

However, and as noted above, voice-hearing is often not reducible into a simple object of fear, but rather experienced in relation to a powerful and threatening social 'other'. Fear can become amplified by voices with their own intentionality. Phase 2 AVATAR work involves more elaborated dialogue enacting the characterized nature of the feared voice. The concept of potentiality is relevant to dialogues which attempt to illuminate the limits of the voice's capacity to harm, undermining the threat 'from within' the agency of the perceived voice ('I only wield the power to confuse, to make you hate yourself, to stop you living your life'). Dialogues, which contextualize the voice-relationship within the person's life history, can add a clarity and understanding which may, at least for some, mitigate the confusion and fear associated with the original 'loss of reality'. As in the Talking with Voices approach (Corstens et al., 2012), there is an opportunity for resolution of relational and emotional conflict. For example, during dialogues targeting self-forgiveness and compassion

(Ward et al., 2020), Claire started to let go of guilt and shame, voicing a view of herself as a 'good person' (a loving mother and daughter) not deserving of demonic punishment. In this phase of therapy, the interpersonal modus operandi of the voice is brought to the fore ('I say the things you believe about yourself deep down'). For Anne, the voice came to be understood as her deceased father—a dominant and abusive presence. First exposure to the avatar was notable for triggering responses which echoed a younger terrified self (a marked 'shrinking' in both tone of voice and posture). Over time, Anne related to the avatar (and voice) from a new position of power and control, and the threat and terror started to diminish ('I am not a little girl anymore. . . . I'm a grown woman . . . I have the right to say how I feel . . . you cannot harm me' (Ward et al., 2020)).

Working dialogically with the avatar allows the voice, as experienced, to come into a therapy with an immediacy and emotional potency: the fear is *in* the room in a way that goes beyond traditional approaches. Learning to be with this potentially terrifying presence and riding out the initial fear reaction in a safe and supported way can be a crucial step towards changing the relation to a voice. At least for some people, the AVATAR approach seems to offer crucial access to emotion and emotional meaning-making ('hot' cognition), and the potential for meaningful and lasting change.

Fear, Agency, and the Ineffable

In the context of voice-hearing, fear is often in the background, positioned as an understandable emotional response to the meaning-making around the voice. This chapter has attempted to bring fear back into the conversation around voice-hearing. As we have noted, the voice is not a simple object of fear. Rather, voice-hearing is a deeply personal experience which is at once social and isolative, in the sense that it is not shared with others outside of the voice-hearer relationship. The object of fear cannot be externalized or pointed to, and yet it is always with you.

Fear can become heightened when voices are highly characterized and present with a strong sense of intentionality and potential to harm. Such voices may, at times, resemble experiences of domestic violence and abusive, controlling relationships, with potentially similar relational rhythms of fear, dread, and destabilization, and the steady erosion of autonomy and sense of self. Conversely, non-personified voices have the potential to terrorize in other ways: for instance, as an amorphous shape-shifting presence located at the borderlands of one's sense of 'lived' space, delivering an ineffable sense of threat, both imminent and immanent. For some, the essence of the voice experience can unmoor the hearer from a previously unquestioned confidence in the reality they typically perceive. The unspoken fear relates to a loss of connection with the world the person previously inhabited, the world shared with others; this leaves the person feeling not only afraid, but also completely alone.

Why, then, might fear not always be thought of as central in how we think about voices? One reason may be timing. The VIP interviews highlight how fear may be particularly relevant around the onset of voice-hearing, where it can drive patterns of responding and relating which crystallize over the following weeks and months. The immediacy of the fear response may decrease over time as other emotions (including anxiety, depression, shame, guilt, and anger) come increasingly to the fore and become targets for therapy. However, as shown in the AVATAR approach, the potential for strong, fearful reactions to voices can remain even after decades. Fear, in direct or refracted forms, may underpin ways of understanding and responding to the voices, and potentially block opportunities for engagement or change. In this context, fear is not simply a momentary reaction, but also one that is deeply embedded in the overall experience of voice-hearing. Experimental evidence highlights how fear disrupts subjective feelings of intentional control (Christensen et al., 2019); in terror, we often lose our sense of agency or may feel it has been taken from us. With voice-hearing, the first blow is the loss of volition inherent in the voice-hearing experience, which can induce terror. The manner in which this can itself undermine agency delivers a perfect storm, within which voices and fear fuel each other amidst an ever-diminishing sense of personal agency, power, and control. The unspoken question becomes: without one's moorings, without certainty or confidence, where is the foothold to start taking power and control over these experiences?

Within a clinical context, there are intersecting reasons for the backgrounding of fear. Cognitive therapy for psychosis emphasizes gradual, sensitive engagement as a necessary precursor to targeted work, and concerns can be expressed about the potential for unhelpful 'destabilization' of the voice-hearer. It should be acknowledged that clinicians are also human beings and exposure to the true nature of voice-hearing, even at one step removed, can provoke fear and avoidance. The clinician may at times (with or without awareness) steer sessions away from the lived reality of the experience, including the violence and derogation of verbatim content, and into domains where emotion may be more readily 'contained'. Similar concerns have been voiced in the context of discussions of past trauma and abuse.

There is also the practical challenge of bringing the voice into therapy. We have presented AVATAR therapy as a novel approach—involving embodiment of the feared voice, and direct dialogic work—in which the person takes back control over previously feared and disempowering experiences. In clinical research, it is important to bear in mind that cognitive, emotional, attentional, and behavioural processes operate as dynamic complexes within the flux of daily life, and not as neatly delineated processes. Significant advances in treatments using virtual reality present exciting opportunities for developing therapeutic contexts, which can mirror the way in which emotional and cognitive processes 'bleed' into each other within real-world situations.

Fear is a crucial, but historically under-acknowledged, aspect of what it means to hear a voice. Fear in this context is not a simple emotion. Rather, voices can represent profound physical, social, and existential threats, delivered in myriad forms, both explicit (that which is said) and implied (that which is left unsaid). Fear can evolve over time, driving meaning-making and response. It can be amplified by a creeping realization of isolation, a loss of confidence in reality, and a sense of dread regarding potential harm. Our discussion of AVATAR therapy has highlighted the potential of clinical approaches in which fear, in all of its visceral and varied forms, is brought directly into the therapeutic context. Such techniques have the promise of enabling people to face their fears and find new agency and meaning in the world.

References

Chadwick, P., and Birchwood, M. (1994). The omnipotence of voices: a cognitive approach to auditory hallucinations. *British Journal of Psychiatry*, 164(2), 190–201.

Christensen, J. F., Di Costa, S., Beck, B., and Haggard, P. (2019). I just lost it! Fear and anger reduce the sense of agency: a study using intentional binding. *Experimental Brain Research*, 237(5), 1205–12.

Corstens, D., Longden, E., and May, R. (2012). Talking with voices: exploring what is expressed by the voices people hear. *Psychosis*, 4(2), 95–104.

Craig, T. K., Rus-Calafell, M., Ward, T., Leff, J. P., Huckvale, M., Howarth, E., Emsley, R., and Garety, P. A. (2018). AVATAR therapy for auditory verbal hallucinations in people with psychosis: a single-blind, randomised controlled trial. *The Lancet Psychiatry*, 5(1), 31–40.

Craske, M. G., Treanor, M., Conway, C. C., Zbozinek, T., and Vervliet, B. (2014). Maximizing exposure therapy: an inhibitory learning approach. *Behaviour Research and Therapy*, 58, 10–23.

Leff, J., Williams, G., Huckvale, M., Arbuthnot, M., and Leff, A. P. (2013). Avatar therapy for persecutory auditory hallucinations: what is it and how does it work? *Psychosis*, 6(2), 166–76.

Merleau-Ponty, M. (1962). *Phenomenology of Perception*. Translated from French by C. Smith. London: Routledge.

Morrison, A. P. (2001). The interpretation of intrusions in psychosis: an integrative cognitive approach to hallucinations and delusions. *Behavioural and Cognitive Psychotherapy*, 29(3), 257–76.

Nayani, T., and David, A. (1996). The auditory hallucination: a phenomenological survey. *Psychological Medicine*, 26(1), 177–89.

Ward, T., Rus-Calafell, M., Ramadhan, Z., Soumelidou, O., Fornells-Ambrojo, M., Garety, P., and Craig, T. K. (2020). AVATAR therapy for distressing voices: a comprehensive account of therapeutic targets. *Schizophrenia Bulletin*, 46(5), 1038–44.

About the Authors

Ben Alderson-Day is a Research Psychologist at Durham University and a Co-Investigator on Hearing the Voice. He worked as one of the interviewers on the VIP study.

Thomas Ward is a Clinical Psychologist and Researcher with Kings College London and the South London and Maudsley NHS Foundation Trust. He has worked as a Lead Therapist on trials of AVATAR therapy for voices and of SlowMo therapy for paranoia.

6

Affect and Voice-Hearing

Past and Present

Åsa Jansson, Institute for Medical Humanities, Durham University

While affect and voice-hearing were seen as closely linked in the early decades of psychiatry, this relationship is marginalized in contemporary diagnostic literature, largely as a result of the gradual separation in the twentieth century of affective (mood) and cognitive (schizo-) disorders. However, recent studies emphasize the significance of affective states in voice-hearing. A close relationship between affect and the experience of hearing voices is equally suggested by the Voices in Psychosis (VIP) interviews. In this chapter, I ask how the phenomenological, data-driven, and person-centred approach of the VIP study can contribute to a dynamic understanding of the relationship between affect and voice-hearing that is both clinically relevant and cognizant of historical shifts in the perception and experience of hearing voices. The VIP data suggest that the role of affect in the experience of hearing voices is complex and multifaceted, challenging the dominant psychiatric narrative that emphasizes voice-hearing as a symptom of schizophrenia while downplaying its relationship to affective states and mood disorders. I suggest that the VIP data encourage further phenomenological research into affect and voice-hearing, and that such an approach can contribute to the de-stigmatization of voice-hearing as well as of the schizophrenia spectrum disorders.

> It's when I'm feeling really anxious, I'll have like this dark, deep . . . voice, what I never, I've never heard like outside of the head. (Fran)

Fran started to hear voices when she was thirteen, at a time of intense emotional upheaval—she faced bullying at school, and at home she was living through her parents' separation. When she speaks about her voices, she is unequivocal that they emerged from a place of anxiety and emotional distress. Describing her experience, Fran explains that 'I've always had depression and I've also had anxiety . . . And I always thought with my anxiety it was just someone there'—that someone appearing as a dark, deep voice. Having lived with her voices for a number of years, Fran notes that they often escalate when she's 'feeling down or upset'.

In twenty-first-century psychiatry, voice-hearing is widely regarded as a sign of psychosis. Conceptualized as 'auditory verbal hallucinations' (AVHs), it is primarily

Åsa Jansson, *Affect and Voice-Hearing* In: *Voices in Psychosis*. Edited by: Angela Woods, Ben Alderson-Day, and Charles Fernyhough, Oxford University Press. © Åsa Jansson 2022. DOI: 10.1093/oso/9780192898388.003.0006 (but not exclusively) perceived as a key symptom of the schizophrenia spectrum disorders. In this context, affective states, such as depression and anxiety, are often considered secondary from a diagnostic point of view. In the early decades of psychiatry, however, it was widely accepted that there was a strong (and often causal) relationship between affect and voice-hearing. Diagnostic descriptions of severe and debilitating low mood and anxiety usually included both auditory and visual hallucinations. These were often mood-congruent but could also manifest in ways that would today be described as bizarre. The link between affect and voice-hearing was, however, gradually weakened from the turn of the twentieth century onward, a process that was driven by the classification of mental disorders introduced by the German psychiatrist Emil Kraepelin in 1899 and which culminated with the publication of the third edition of the American Psychiatric Association (APA)'s *Diagnostic and Statistical Manual of Mental Disorders* (*DSM-III*) in 1980. In the sixth edition of his influential textbook, Kraepelin divided mental disorders into dementia praecox and manic–depressive insanity, with 'psychotic' symptoms such as paranoid and bizarre delusions and voice-hearing primarily assigned to the former, which subsequently became schizophrenia. In the decades that followed, more severe psychotic symptoms, such as persistent auditory verbal hallucinations, were gradually marginalized as diagnostic criteria for mood disorders. Consequently, the relationship between affect and voice-hearing today receives far less attention in clinical research and theoretical works than it did during the first decades of psychiatry.

In contrast to this, a strong link between affect and voice-hearing, such as expressed by Fran, is cited by several participants in the Voices in Psychosis (VIP) study. This chapter asks what we can learn about the relationship between affect and voice-hearing from the VIP study's phenomenological, person-centred approach to voices. While a relationship between emotional states and voice-hearing is evident from the VIP data, it is not the focus of the study, and analysis to date has not investigated affect as a cause or an effect of voices, leaving the nature of the relationship underexplored. I argue, however, that phenomenological studies such as VIP offer a valuable space for interrogating the link between affect and voice-hearing. In this way, I hope to contribute to a decentralization of the current dominant narrative in psychiatry that downplays the role of affect in psychosis, by adding a critical historical perspective to attempts to restore and renew the role of emotional states such as depression and anxiety in the emergence of voices.

Affect and Voice-Hearing: A Very Brief History

Since its inception, psychiatry has been a discipline fraught with disagreement over how to classify and diagnose mental disorders. Throughout the nineteenth century, when psychiatry was gradually being established as a branch of medicine and a modern academic discipline, multiple systems of classification and conflicting illness categories were in use across Europe and North America. Nevertheless, it was widely believed that affect played a key role in the development and progression of insanity, and that emotional disorders such as melancholia and mania (two of the most commonly diagnosed disorders across asylum populations in Britain and Western Europe) often manifested with delusions and hallucinations, particularly in the later stages of illness. Many people who arrived in the asylum suffering from low mood and anxiety expressed what doctors considered to be 'false' beliefs. These were commonly associated with guilt and shame (primarily of a religious nature), but could also be of a more bizarre character such as believing oneself to be royalty. Equally, people suffering from affective disorders were seen as prone to both visual and auditory hallucinations such as hearing commands from God, seeing angels or the devil appear, or hearing the voices of dead relatives. Paranoid hallucinations were also frequently noted such as hearing the voices of 'detectives' or of neighbours conspiring and gossiping.

At the time, doctors did not always distinguish between delusions and hallucinations in diagnostic literature, sometimes using the former as an umbrella term for both false beliefs and visual or auditory experiences. Equally, when describing patients' experiences, it was often not specified whether voices were explicitly heard or if patients felt themselves to be communicated to in other ways. For instance, Thomas Clouston, superintendent at the Royal Edinburgh Asylum, listed among the most common delusional experiences in patients diagnosed with melancholia 'being conspired against', 'being acted on by spirits', 'being followed by the police', and 'being called names by persons' (Clouston, 1883, pp. 87–9). Patient case notes from the asylum during Clouston's time there suggest that voice-hearing appeared to be common among patients with melancholia and mania; one man, for example, claimed that he 'constantly hears voices talking to him, and that he sees ladies floating in the air who come to speak to him' (Royal Edinburgh Asylum, 1872–1873), whereas another heard the voices of people conspiring against him, and several patients reported hearing or seeing God, angels, and the devil. Similar cases appear in the records of other asylums across Britain. Most commonly, patients with affective disorders would hear voices with a religious undertone, but they equally reported hearing voices with no divine associations such as those of detectives, neighbours, famous people, or voices apparently lacking in personification. This was mirrored in published literature where both mania and melancholia were described as frequently manifesting with auditory experiences, sometimes described as delusions and sometimes as 'hallucinations of hearing'.

Towards the end of the century, medical writers were increasingly arguing for the categorical separation of delusions and hallucinations as diagnostically different phenomena, and simultaneously started to pay more attention to patients' 'voices' as a distinct symptom separate from other hallucinations. In the early 1890s, one psychiatrist suggested that hallucinations in affective disorders, particularly melancholia, were qualitatively different from similar experiences in non-affective, 'constitutional' disorders such as paranoia (Krafft-Ebing, 1890, p. 431). This view was more firmly articulated by Emil Kraepelin, who, at the turn of the century, divided mental disorders into dementia praecox, which later became schizophrenia, and manic–depressive insanity, a precursor to bipolar disorder. In doing so, he distinguished between the kinds of hallucinations experienced in the different forms of mental disease. While he noted that voices were frequently a symptom of severe depressive illness, these were generally different from the hallucinations of hearing manifesting in dementia praecox, which had a more bizarre quality (Kraepelin, 1899). In the early twentieth century, Karl Jaspers further cemented this distinction when arguing that delusions and hallucinations in psychotic disorders such as schizophrenia were 'un-understandable'—that is, not explicable with reference to the patient's mood and life history. These were symptoms of 'madness proper' and, as such, should be distinguished from pathological experiences in mood disorders (Jaspers, 1923, pp. 110–11).

In this way, voices were gradually downplayed as a symptom of affective disorders, a process that culminated with the publication of *DSM-III* in 1980. In the third, much revised edition of the APA's widely used manual, voice-hearing was heavily marginalized in mood disorders, while presented as a defining symptom of schizophrenia. While psychiatry never entirely did away with a close link between affect and voice-hearing, it does not fit the dominant narratives of the *DSM* or the World Health Organization's *International Classification of Diseases*. The overwhelming focus on voices as a symptom of schizophrenia has contributed to the perception of this disorder as madness proper. This has important implications for people so diagnosed, as well as for voice-hearers more broadly, as it works in a circular way to further entrench the stigma of schizophrenia and the stigma of voice-hearing, as well as a diagnostic approach in which the presence of voice-hearing is likely to result in a diagnosis of schizophrenia.

Nevertheless, the link between affect and voice-hearing has received more attention in recent years. For instance, a 2006 study on psychosis and affect suggested tangible links between depressed mood and the severity of auditory verbal hallucinations, as well as some types of delusions in schizophrenia (Smith, 2006). Similarly, building on this research, Łukasz Gawęda, Paweł Holas, and Andrzej Kokoszka noted in a more recent study that depression impacted on both AVHs and delusions in schizophrenia, but that the severity of these were also mediated by metacognitive beliefs, which are imbued with affective reasoning about one's own thought processes (Gawęda et al., 2013). Finally, Matthew Ratcliffe and Sam Wilkinson have mapped on an experiential level how anxiety can trigger verbal hallucinations, which they note occur in schizophrenia as well as in depressive conditions, post-traumatic stress disorder, borderline personality disorder, and non-clinical populations (Ratcliffe and Wilkinson, 2016).

The Phenomenology of Affect and Voice-Hearing

It is evident from the research cited above that hearing voices is—or can be—a highly emotional experience. But how should this be investigated? The relationship, or relationships, between voice-hearing and affect that emerge in the VIP study suggest that a phenomenological approach has much to offer as a tool with which to better understand how emotion features in the experience of hearing voices. Phenomenology is concerned with the investigation of subjective experience and requires the suspension of preconceived beliefs or judgements about the object studied. When applied to clinical research, a phenomenological approach therefore asks that we direct our attention towards the patient's experience from their own perspective, instead of towards aetiological or diagnostic considerations.

Participants in the VIP study were interviewed using the Hearing the Voice Phenomenology Interview (HTV-PI), which is based on an earlier study carried out by Hearing the Voice researchers investigating the phenomenology of voice-hearing. The first study used an online thirteen-item questionnaire comprising a combination of open- and closed-ended questions, which were designed 'to be unbiased, non-leading, and non-hierarchising prompts that aimed to elicit phenomenologically rich data' (Woods et al., 2015, p. 324). The questions were developed in consultation with a local voice-hearing group and other experts by experience. Responses were coded using inductive thematic analysis, in which analytical themes are drawn from the data itself, rather than being imposed a priori by researchers. Inductive thematic analysis, in other words, prompts researchers to approach the data with an open mind and develop codes based on the nature and content of the information provided by interviewees. However, it is crucial to remember that themes do not simply 'emerge' from the data unaided and unmediated. Researchers are not without bias and preconceptions, meaning that the coding of data in inductive thematic analysis is both open and data-driven, and at the same time also directed by the (conscious or unconscious) bias of researchers.

Affect was not central to the design of the online study, but the presence of emotional states in relation to voices emerged as a key theme. The study reports the number of participants who expressed a link between their voices and a range of emotions, such as depression, anxiety, fear, sadness, and shame, as well as positive and 'neutral' emotions. While the coding of the data does not indicate whether affect is experienced as a cause or an effect of hearing voices (or both), the study demonstrates a strong relationship between emotional states and hearing voices for the majority of participants. 'Anxiety' is most frequently cited (65%), followed by 'fear' (60%), and 'depression' (52.5%). A strong relationship between negative affect and voices was equally suggested by the earlier study carried out by Hearing the Voice, where fear emerged as the most common emotion (41%), followed by anxiety (31%) and depression (29%) (Woods et al., 2015, p. 326).

What can this tell us? Both studies used both open- and closed-ended questions, allowing for interview subjects' own words and perspectives to guide the research. Affect emerged as a core feature of voice-hearing, but with variations in types of emotional states. Moreover, the question of whether voices are more likely to be preceded or precipitated by affect is only partially addressed, but its importance is indicated by the VIP interview transcripts. It follows, then, that existing phenomenological research indicates that a strong relationship between affect is far from unusual, but that this relationship is often complex and ambivalent.

Several participants in the VIP study cite negative affect as playing a key causal or triggering role in the appearance of voices, but voices are equally experienced as generating difficult emotions. For instance, Jade says of her voices that they tend to appear when she feels 'a bit nervous or a bit anxious', whereas 'as long as I'm not anxious about anything, and nothing's upsetting me, I don't really hear them'. For others, however, hearing voices appears to trigger or escalate negative affect that was not present, or present but not previously dominant. Alex, for example, explains that he has developed anxiety and panic attacks in anticipation of his voices appearing in certain contexts. Liam notes that he had not felt distressed or experienced emotional trauma immediately prior to his first voice-hearing experience, but rather that it occurred after a visual experience where he perceived that the sky was going to swallow everything up. He suggests that 'everything was alright' until that moment, but that the experience of hearing voices makes him feel 'scared and worried' (further descriptions of participants' voice-hearing experiences can be found in Box 6.1).

Box 6.1 Emotions associated with the experience of hearing voices, as described by VIP participants (names have been changed to preserve anonymity)

I have . . . suffered from depression . . . and . . . I think that's what triggered it, because me doctors says, sometimes with depression, it can turn into psychosis.

[It can] happen from having depression, so I was thinking like well it's just part of depression, that's why I'm getting this, and the stress of living through what I've had up there. (Sean)

I just feel . . . angry and sad. I feel like, like kicking off and just smashing everything. But then sometimes when I hear the voices and I get, when I get like that, I know that I don't want to smash me house up, because I've got OCD as well. . . . So then I just start cleaning, so that's made us, me OCD get worse. (Iris)

Sometimes when I'm, I feel upset, ehm . . . sometimes eh there's one, there's one voice that likes to, he likes to eh nag me and he likes to make me feel worse.

[N]ormally I get upset about myself but sometimes I'm upset about something else, he'll start pointing out negative things about me and ehm . . . he'll make me feel bad and . . . it's gotten really bad before, that I felt really, really bad, I've hurt myself before and . . . (Nina)

I guess sometimes it's like induced by stress or certain situations, where it just seems like your brain goes into overload or . . . sometimes it comes out of nowhere.

But ever since this happened I was trying to think if I've always heard these voices in me head since me anxiety and stuff started in middle school . . . nay (?) high school, sorry. (Harry)

I was at work, and I felt a little bit angry, there was something that my manager said that I didn't agree with, and then all of a sudden they were just there, and it was very intense, very loud.

[I associate the voices with] low moods, really scared, afraid, I get really upset.

[I[t happened quite a lot more when I was at work, because I was under stress and I was under pressure. Ehm . . . sometimes when there's . . . arguments and conflict, they get worse then. (Grace)

A similarly complex and multifaceted cause and effect relationship between affect and voice-hearing is vividly portrayed by Emily Knoll in *Emily's Voices*, an autobiographical book detailing the author's experience of hearing voices. Knoll (2017, p. 16) describes growing up in a household where arguments and strong emotions were taboo, forcing her to learn 'to hold in my emotions' and feeling 'as if I was not allowed to show my sadness'. Knoll developed anxiety and obsessive–compulsive behaviours before the voices started to appear, and the latter are described as both originating in emotional distress and causing further negative affect, including shame and fear associated with the stigma of voice-hearing perceived as mental illness, and with the diagnosis of schizoaffective disorder that she was given.

When Knoll starts working as a researcher on a project investigating voice-hearing, however, her own lived experience becomes a valuable asset. As the VIP data suggest, an approach that both utilizes existing expertise provided by voice-hearers and aims at a non-biased interpretation and analysis of the experience of voice-hearing can produce novel data about how hearing voices is experienced and understood, which is not pre-limited by existing medical views on what voice-hearing is (or is not). Following from this, the VIP data crucially suggest that there is often (but not always) a strong relationship between affect and voice-hearing, but that this relationship is anything but simple and one-directional. Emotional trauma or distress, or pre-existing emotional states such as depression, can be experienced as the source and/or the trigger of a voice-hearing episode, but voices can equally be felt to appear with little or no prior negative affect. Equally, the experience of hearing voices can itself be a traumatic event, giving rise to new, or escalating existing, emotional distress.

This suggests that the dominant diagnostic approach in which voice-hearing is primarily understood as a symptom of schizophrenia risks overlooking the central role of affect in voice-hearing. This inevitably restricts the language available for both patients and clinicians in expressing and making sense of the often complex and sometimes conflicting relationship between affect and voice-hearing. Moreover, the lack of focus within existing diagnostic definitions on understanding how affect and voice-hearing are experienced in conjunction marginalizes the role of subjective meaning and self-reflection. However, as the VIP data suggest, meaning-making and reflective thinking are central to how people who hear voices make sense of their lived experience, and the emotional states associated with that experience are often a key part of the reflective process.

It follows that a phenomenological approach to understanding voice-hearing can shed much needed light on the relationship between affect and voice-hearing. The VIP data provide a compelling argument for further research into the role of emotion in the experience of hearing voices, suggesting that such research can be of significant clinical value, not least in terms of indicating ways of providing support (when needed) that fully addresses both emotional distress and the hearing of voices in a way that is most helpful to each individual. This is likely to include strategies that treat affect and voice-hearing as a single, dynamic, and complex experience, rather than as two separate phenomena. In this way, further phenomenological research into affect and voice-hearing has the potential to help expand and transform current psychiatric conceptualization of this relationship, which may be limiting how experience can be expressed, understood, and supported in mental health services.

Finally, the stigma associated with the schizophrenia spectrum disorders is closely tied to the diagnostic separation of affective and cognitive disorders in which voice-hearing is marginalized as a symptom of the former, and emotional states perceived as secondary in the latter. This current separation reinforces a circular process of stigmatization, in which schizophrenia is perceived as 'madness proper', voices are primarily read as a symptom of schizo- disorders, and both voice-hearing and schizophrenia are stigmatized or perceived as stigmatizing. Mapping the often close and complex relationship between affect and voice-hearing on an experiential level can help challenge existing medical labels associated with voice-hearing, and in this way can also contribute to the destigmatization of voice-hearing with or without diagnosis, as well as of the schizophrenia spectrum disorders.

References

Clouston, T. S. (1883). *Clinical Lectures on Mental Diseases*. London: J. & A. Churchill.

Gawęda, L., Holas, P., and Kokoszka, A. (2013). Do depression and anxiety mediate the relationship between meta-cognitive beliefs and psychological dimensions of auditory hallucinations and delusions in schizophrenia? *Psychiatry Research*, 210(3), 1316–19.

Jaspers, K. (1923). *Allgemeine Psychopathologie, für Studierende, Ärzte und Psychologen*, 3 Aufl. Berlin & Heidelberg: Springer-Verlag.

Knoll, E. (2017). *Emily's Voices*. Knoll Publications. Oxford.

Kraepelin, E. (1899). *Psychiatrie: ein Lehrbuch für Studirende und Aerzte*, 6 Aufl. Leipzig: J. A. Barth.

Krafft-Ebing, R. (1890). *Lehrbuch der Psychiatrie auf Klinischer Grundlage für Praktische Ärzte und Studirende*, 4 Aufl. Stuttgart: Ferdinand Enke.

Ratcliffe, M., and Wilkinson, S. (2016). How anxiety induces verbal hallucinations. *Consciousness and Cognition*, 39, 48–58.

Royal Edinburgh Asylum (1872–1873). *Male Casebooks, 1872–1873*. Lothian Health Services Archives, Edinburgh University Library, Ref: LHB 7/51/23.

Smith, B., Fowler, D. G., Freeman, D., Bebbington, P., Bashforth, H., Garety, P., Dunn, G., and Kuipers, E. (2006). Emotion and psychosis: links between depression, self-esteem, negative schematic beliefs and delusions and hallucinations. *Schizophrenia Research*, 86(1–3), 181–8.

Woods, A., Jones, N., Alderson-Day, B., Callard, F., and Fernyhough, C. (2015). Experiences of hearing voices: analysis of a novel phenomenological survey. *The Lancet Psychiatry*, 2(4), 323–31.

About the Author

Åsa Jansson is a historian of psychiatry and psychology. Her research interests include the history of hallucinations and delusions, the history of emotion regulation, and the diagnostic separation of affective and cognitive disorders. Her monograph *From Melancholia to Depression: Disordered Mood in Nineteenth-Century Psychiatry* (Palgrave, 2021) maps how melancholia was reconceptualized in the nineteenth century as a biomedical illness and the first modern mood disorder. She works in alternative provision education.

7

Bodily Sensations During Voice-Hearing Experiences

A Role for Interoception?

Jamie Moffatt, Department of Psychology, University of Sussex

One of the clearest lessons to learn from participants in the Voices in Psychosis (VIP) study is that voice-hearing experiences are much more than simply auditory phenomena. When asked in the interview whether their body felt any different during voice-hearing experiences, two-thirds of participants reported that their voices were accompanied by unusual bodily sensations. For example, Dawn frequently hears a stern female voice that causes a shudder: 'I just . . . I feel like I shudder . . . That's a sense I can . . . she makes me shudder', or a feeling of tightness: 'Mm, maybe I feel like my body's like . . . you know when you get anxious and your body kind of goes tight'. At other times, she describes feeling separated from her body: 'I like feel really detached, like, like a ghost, like I'm not in the room but I am there, like . . . I'm just watching everyone else do what they're doing.' The bodily effects described by participants range from relatively minor experiences, such as an elevated heart rate, to more disruptive states, such as feeling a complete loss of control over one's own body. As in Dawn's case, some people report experiencing several different types of bodily sensations.

The frequent occurrence of bodily sensations in experiences of voice-hearing implies that interoception is playing a significant part in such experiences. The term interoception refers to the ability to sense internal bodily states and sensations. Interoceptive ability is thought to be important in many psychological processes, such as emotions and representations of the self (Seth, 2013), and is increasingly being understood as central to several physical and mental health issues (Quadt et al., 2018). However, at the time of writing, there is little published research exploring how interoception relates to voice-hearing, or to psychosis more broadly.

In this chapter, I will describe how interoceptive ability is measured in psychological studies. I will then highlight two types of bodily sensations which were frequently reported by VIP participants and which related to emotion and feelings of dissociation from the body, before explaining what is already known about their relationship with voice-hearing. I will conclude by considering how research on interoception may provide fresh insights to the experience of voices in psychosis.

Jamie Moffatt, *Bodily Sensations During Voice-Hearing Experiences* In: *Voices in Psychosis*. Edited by: Angela Woods, Ben Alderson-Day, and Charles Fernyhough, Oxford University Press. © Jamie Moffatt 2022. DOI: 10.1093/oso/9780192898388.003.0007

Interoception

Interoception is the ability to sense and interpret information which arises internally from the body. This is in contrast to the traditional exteroceptive sensations of hearing, vision, touch, smell, and taste, which reveal information about the external world, or proprioception, which is the ability to sense the location and movement of one's own body in space. Examples of interoceptive sensations include feeling the heart pounding, feelings of hunger or thirst, and feelings of breathlessness.

Individual differences in interoceptive ability are typically assessed with heartbeat detection tasks, the two most common of which are the heartbeat tracking task and the heartbeat discrimination task. In the tracking task, participants count their heartbeats over a certain period and their total count is compared to the actual number of heartbeats. In the discrimination task, participants listen to several sequences of auditory tones presented either in time or out of time with their own heartbeat and must decide whether each sequence was in or out of time with their heartbeat. Performance on either task is taken to be an indicator of interoceptive accuracy or of an individual's objective competence in detecting their bodily state. Another aspect of interoceptive ability is an individual's personal belief in their ability to detect bodily states. This aspect is known as interoceptive sensibility, and is measured by using self-report measures such as questionnaires or by assessing confidence when completing the heartbeat detection tasks. A final aspect of interoceptive ability can be defined as the extent to which interoceptive accuracy and interoceptive sensibility align, and is referred to as interoceptive awareness (Garfinkel et al., 2015). Somebody with minimal interoceptive awareness may be very poor at the heartbeat detection tasks but believe that they are very good at detecting their own heartbeat, or vice versa.

Interoceptive accuracy, sensibility, and awareness relate to an individual's ability to consciously access their bodily states and sensations. However, individual differences in interoception can also be found below the level of conscious awareness. All major biological systems convey information to the brain about the state of the body. In the case of the cardiovascular system, this could be information about the strength and timing of each heartbeat. The brain then stores and uses this information to maintain the biological stability needed to survive, through automatic reflexes or motivational drives such as hunger, or by generating explicit sensations of bodily states. Therefore, individual differences in interoceptive ability may also be present in the ability of the biological system to convey information to the brain or in the quality of the neural representation of interoceptive information. It is important to note that all biological systems convey interoceptive information to the brain, but the majority of research on interoception has focused on the ability to detect heartbeats. This is mainly for practical reasons, as heartbeats are regularly occurring signals that can be easily tracked with non-invasive sensors such as electrocardiograms or pulse oximeters. However, it also reflects an assumption that different interoceptive modalities share the same underlying processes. This assumes that someone good at detecting heartbeats will also be more sensitive to changes in temperature, for instance, when this may not be the case.

Increasingly, interoceptive ability is understood to have a profound influence on mental well-being (Quadt et al., 2018), but currently there are only a few published studies which have measured interoceptive ability in psychosis. Across these studies, people with a diagnosis of schizophrenia demonstrated worse interoceptive accuracy on a heartbeat detection task than people with no diagnosis (e.g. Ardizzi et al., 2016). This suggests that interoception is generally reduced in people with psychosis. 'Positive' symptoms of schizophrenia, such as hallucinations and delusions, were more frequent and severe in people who were more accurate at detecting their heartbeats (Ardizzi et al., 2016). In contrast, no association was found between interoceptive accuracy and 'negative' symptoms. This suggests that interoception has specific associations with different experiences within psychosis. For example, interoception was particularly elevated in people who experienced symptoms of grandiosity, defined as heightened self-focus and exaggerated opinions of the self (Ardizzi et al., 2016). Similarly, the bodily effects reported by voice-hearers in the VIP study suggest that interoception may also play a crucial role in the voice-hearing experience.

Emotional Processing

Idioms such as 'butterflies in the stomach' and 'a shiver running down the spine' remind us that bodily sensations and the ability to sense them are an integral aspect of any emotional experience. Intuitively, it may seem as if bodily changes that are frequently associated with emotions are caused by those emotions. For example, when watching a horror film, our heart may beat faster because we are afraid. However, since at least the time of William James, philosophers, psychologists, and neuroscientists have argued that it is the other way around. Instead, the experience of emotion appears to be based upon our ability to sense bodily changes—we may feel fear when watching a horror film because our heart is beating more quickly. This is an important distinction because it places the perception of bodily states and sensations at the centre of emotional processing. This has been reflected in psychological research. People with better interoceptive accuracy tend to have more intense experiences of emotion (Pollatos et al., 2007), and interoception also appears to be important for implementing emotion regulation strategies (Füstös et al., 2013). Reports of emotion-related bodily experiences in the VIP study suggest that interoception may also be important for understanding the role of emotion in voice-hearing experiences.

Several participants in the VIP study describe emotion-related bodily effects that occur during voice-hearing experiences. As Page, for example, explained: 'I also feel really like hot and flushed because I'm, my heart's beating quickly and stuff'. Others describe bodily sensations such as shaking, feeling sweaty, and feeling tight or tense. These strong emotional reactions are perhaps unsurprising, as every single participant in the VIP study had experienced distress in relation to their voices. However, the descriptions of bodily effects are a sharp reminder that it is important to consider the role of the body when attempting to understand emotional experiences related to voices. Furthermore, if these sensations are the result of an emotional situation that has triggered the voice, rather than as a response to the voice itself, interoception may also be important for understanding how voices occur.

The experience of emotions is thought to be highly related to interoceptive ability. As noted, people who perform well on heartbeat detection measures tend to be more sensitive to emotional stimuli than those who perform poorly, rating their emotions as more intense (e.g. Pollatos et al., 2007). Emotional sensitivity is elevated in psychosis, and heightened emotional sensitivity in daily life predicts the occurrence of psychosis symptoms, such as voices (Myin-Germeys and van Os, 2007). Heightened emotional sensitivity in psychosis may therefore be the product of enhanced interoceptive ability. Whether this is the case is currently unclear—although people with schizophrenia tend to have reduced interoceptive accuracy, heightened interoceptive accuracy appears to be associated with more frequent and severe positive symptoms (Ardizi et al., 2016). More recent work suggests that it is interoceptive awareness—the correspondence between interoceptive accuracy and interoceptive sensibility—that is related to emotional sensitivity. Garfinkel et al. (2016) demonstrated that interoceptive awareness, rather than accuracy or sensibility alone, was related to a measure of emotional sensitivity in autistic and non-autistic individuals. In other words, the extent to which somebody is consciously aware of their bodily sensations predicted their sensitivity to emotions. It may be this aspect of interoceptive ability which is related to the elevated emotional sensitivity in psychosis.

Most participants in the VIP study report strong, negative emotional responses to their voices which are often accompanied by bodily sensations. However, despite other similarities in voice phenomenology, there is a subsection of the population who do not find their voices to be distressing and do not seek or require clinical care. Although the content of a voice-hearing experience is a considerable factor in determining whether a voice is distressing, cognitive models of psychosis emphasize the importance of interpretations and appraisals of voice-hearing experiences. Appraisals may be highly dependent on one's ability to regulate emotions. Generally, people with good interoceptive ability are more aware of their emotions and are more successful in identifying and implementing effective emotional regulation strategies. One such emotional regulation strategy is reappraisal, which involves attempting to reinterpret negative emotional memories in a less negative way. People with better interoceptive accuracy are more successful in their reappraisals (Füstös et al., 2013). This suggests that interoceptive ability may be an important factor in the extent to which people are able to reappraise their negative voice-hearing experiences, and therefore may be crucial in determining the distress caused by voices.

Dissociative Experiences

Another type of unusual bodily sensation that many participants report in the VIP study is the experience of disconnection from their own body or from the world around them. Anthony describes this feeling eloquently:

> I feel like I've taken a seat . . . in the back of my mind. . . . And I just feel like I'm watching, you know kinda myself do things. So I'm watching through my eyes, but I feel . . . sat back, I don't feel like I'm fully in control. Ehm, and there's quite a lot of kinda time distortion and things there as well, ehm, sometimes you know an hour could have passed, a couple of hours could have passed, or it could feel like an hour's taken kinda three hours.

These experiences are descriptively similar to dissociative experiences. Dissociation occurs on a continuum of severity, from relatively benign experiences, such as becoming absorbed in a good book, to more disruptive and distressing experiences often reported in the VIP study, such as a lack of ownership over the body or feeling alienated from reality. Subjective senses of the reality of the world and of selfhood are thought to be highly reliant on interoceptive ability (Seth, 2013).

One technique that researchers have for studying what may cause an experience of dissociation is by experimentally recreating the experience. The most well-known of these techniques is the rubber-hand illusion. In the rubber-hand illusion, the participant places their hand out of sight, next to a visible fake rubber hand. Then, using a brush, the researcher will simultaneously stroke the fake hand and the real hand in the same areas. After several seconds of this, many people report a strange sensation of ownership over the fake hand and a sense of disownership over their actual hand. Susceptibility to this effect appears to be related to interoceptive ability. People with heightened interoceptive accuracy tend to be less susceptible to the illusion (Tsakiris et al., 2011). This suggests that dissociative experiences may be related to interoceptive ability. However, the rubber-hand illusion is a short, temporary, and relatively benign experience of body disownership. Interoception does also appear to be related to experiences of dissociation that are more severe and occur in the course of people's daily lives. Dissociation is the core component of dissociative disorders, such as depersonalization–derealization disorder. Research has demonstrated that people with a diagnosis of dissociative disorder tend to show reduced interoceptive ability, compared to non-clinical participants (Schäflein et al., 2018). Interoception may therefore be involved in the aetiology of more severe and distressing dissociative experiences, such as those that appear to accompany some experiences of voice-hearing.

Other Bodily Sensations

A third type of bodily sensation—reported by nearly one-quarter of participants in the VIP study—can be thought of as a sensation of touch, or as a tactile hallucination. For example, when asked about bodily sensations that accompany her voices, Kate reports that 'I've had somebody throw . . . water at me legs before, when I've had a pair of shorts on, but there's no water there, and it's just that . . . water sensation'. It is a topic of debate within the interoception literature as to whether perceptions of touch can be classified as interoception. Traditional definitions emphasize that interoception concerns the perception of internal bodily states and sensations, whereas touch provides information about the external world. However, more recent definitions of interoception argue for the inclusion of certain types of touch, such as pain, itching, and tickling sensations. This is based on findings that these are processed by similar areas of the brain as other interoceptive sensations. Although the relevance of interoception for understanding tactile perceptions is currently unclear, the reports of tactile sensations during voice-hearing provide further evidence that bodily sensations may be crucial to understanding voice-hearing experiences.

Finally, some people report no bodily sensations alongside their voices, or as Violet puts it: 'I'm not too sure! . . . Because I don't, I don't really focus on my body!' It is clear from the VIP interviews that voices are a varied experience and, as such, interoception may have no influence on some voice-hearing experiences. I have focused here on the influence of interoception on emotional processing and dissociation because these are directly relevant to bodily sensations that were reported in the VIP study. However, interoception is also an integral part of other psychological processes, such as cognition, decision-making, and memory (Quadt et al., 2018). Future research should also consider the influence of the body on these processes in relation to voice-hearing. Furthermore, much of the influence of interoception may occur below the level of conscious awareness. Individual differences in interoceptive ability may be found at the biological or neural level and, as such, may not translate to explicit bodily sensations. Therefore, the lack of bodily effects alongside voice-hearing may not mean that interoception has no influence on the experience.

In conclusion, the study of interoception—defined as the ability to sense internal bodily states and sensations—may play an important role in understanding voice-hearing experiences. Voice-hearers in the VIP study reported emotion-related bodily changes, as well as feelings of separation from the body or reality which may be classed as dissociative experiences. Interoception is an integral aspect of emotional processing and is particularly related to emotional sensitivity and the use of emotion regulation strategies. Research also suggests that it is required for maintaining intact senses of reality and selfhood. The key role that interoception plays in these psychological processes, as well as the frequent reports of bodily sensations during voice-hearing, suggest a substantial influence of interoception on voice-hearing which should be the subject of further interdisciplinary investigation.

References

Ardizzi, M., Ambrosecchia, M., Buratta, L., Ferri, F., Peciccia, M., Donnari, S., Mazzeschi, C., and Gallese, V. (2016). Interoception and positive symptoms in schizophrenia. *Frontiers in Human Neuroscience*, 10. https://www.frontiersin.org/articles/10.3389/fnhum.2016.00379/full (accessed: 12 April 2022).

Füstös, J., Gramann, K., Herbert, B. M., and Pollatos, O. (2013). On the embodiment of emotion regulation: interoceptive awareness facilitates reappraisal. *Social Cognitive and Affective Neuroscience*, 8(8), 911–17.

Garfinkel, S. N., Seth, A. K., Barrett, A. B., Suzuki, K., and Critchley, H. D. (2015). Knowing your own heart: distinguishing interoceptive accuracy from interoceptive awareness. *Biological Psychology*, 104, 65–74.

Garfinkel, S. N., Tiley, C., O'Keeffe, S., Harrison, N. A., Seth, A. K., and Critchley, H. D. (2016). Discrepancies between dimensions of interoception in autism: implications for emotion and anxiety. *Biological Psychology*, 114, 117–26.

Myin-Germeys, I., and van Os, J. (2007). Stress-reactivity in psychosis: evidence for an affective pathway to psychosis. *Clinical Psychology Review*, 27(4), 409–24.

Pollatos, O., Herbert, B. M., Matthias, E., and Schandry, R. (2007). Heart rate response after emotional picture presentation is modulated by interoceptive awareness. *International Journal of Psychophysiology*, 63(1), 117–24.

Quadt, L., Critchley, H. D., and Garfinkel, S. N. (2018). The neurobiology of interoception in health and disease: neuroscience of interoception. *Annals of the New York Academy of Sciences*, 1428(1), 112–28.

Schäflein, E., Sattel, H. C., Pollatos, O., and Sack, M. (2018). Disconnected—impaired interoceptive accuracy and its association with self-perception and cardiac vagal tone in patients with dissociative disorder. *Frontiers in Psychology*, 9. https://www.frontiersin.org/articles/10.3389/fpsyg.2018.00897/full (accessed: 12 April 2022).

Seth, A. K. (2013). Interoceptive inference, emotion, and the embodied self. *Trends in Cognitive Sciences*, 17(11), 565–73.

Tsakiris, M., Tajadura-Jiménez, A., and Costantini, M. (2011). Just a heartbeat away from one's body: interoceptive sensitivity predicts malleability of body-representations. *Proceedings of the Royal Society*, 278, 2470–6.

About the Author

Jamie Moffatt is a Doctoral Researcher based at the University of Sussex, investigating the use of methods to experimentally induce anomalous experiences such as hallucinations and feelings of dissociation. Jamie previously worked at Hearing the Voice as a Research Assistant investigating the cognitive and neural mechanisms underlying voice-hearing experiences.

8

The Varieties and Complexities of Multimodal Hallucinations in Psychosis

Peter Moseley, Department of Psychology, Northumbria University[*]

Kaja Mitrenga, Department of Psychology, Durham University[*]

While research on auditory verbal hallucinations in psychosis is well established, comparatively little attention has been paid to hallucinations in other modalities or to hallucinations in more than one sensory modality. Several names have been proposed to describe hallucinations occurring in multiple sensory modalities, including polymodal, polysensory, polysensual, intersensorial, or fantastic hallucinations (Lim et al., 2016). This variety hints at the complexity of the phenomena and a lack of specificity when asking about or describing these experiences in hallucinations research. For example, it is not always clear if these definitions refer to hallucinations occurring in multiple sensory modalities separately and sequentially (i.e. at different points in time) or simultaneously (i.e. hallucinations occurring at the same time). Those hallucinations that register in multiple modalities simultaneously are also sometimes described as *fused* or *string* hallucinations, and are often characterized by hearing voices and seeing relevant, congruent visual images. Recent studies have attempted to better define multimodal hallucinations (MMHs) by taking into account the different dimensions of these experiences (Dudley et al., 2018; Montagnese et al., 2021). Here, we use the term multimodal hallucinations in its broadest sense to refer to any descriptions of hallucinations occurring in more than one sensory modality, either perceived simultaneously or sequentially, and including those hallucinations which are or are not linked to the same identity or agent. In this chapter, we aim to describe complexities and understudied aspects of MMH, and discuss ways in which hallucinations in different modalities do and do not seem to co-occur.

Out of all sensory modalities, auditory verbal hallucinations (or *voices*) are the most prevalent modality of hallucinations, followed by visual, tactile, and olfactory experiences (Lim et al., 2016). Voices are experienced by nearly 80% of people with a diagnosis of schizophrenia, and are additionally sometimes reported in the general population without a psychiatric diagnosis (Lim et al., 2016). Research shows that for visual hallucinations (or *visions*), the prevalence is reported to be between

---

[*] The authors contributed equally to this work.

Peter Moseley and Kaja Mitrenga, *The Varieties and Complexities of Multimodal Hallucinations in Psychosis* In: *Voices in Psychosis*. Edited by: Angela Woods, Ben Alderson-Day, and Charles Fernyhough, Oxford University Press. © Peter Moseley and Kaja Mitrenga 2022. DOI: 10.1093/oso/9780192898388.003.0008

4% and 65%, with a mean prevalence of around 27% among people with a diagnosis of schizophrenia—suggesting that auditory hallucinations might be almost twice as common as visual (Waters et al., 2014). However, the reported prevalence of hallucinations across modalities in psychosis has also been called into question. For example, research using experience sampling—where participants record their experiences at different time-points during a day—has shown that visual hallucinations can be experienced *more* frequently than auditory hallucinations (Delespaul et al., 2002). Interestingly, when it comes to hallucinations experienced in more than one modality, 53% of people with a diagnosis of schizophrenia reported MMHs, and 23% reported only unimodal hallucinations (Lim et al., 2016). Considering the co-occurrence of different modalities, it seems that visual and auditory modalities are the most likely to co-occur together, while the prevalence of co-occurrence in other modalities, e.g. in visual–tactile or visual–olfactory hallucinations, is much lower (McCarthy-Jones et al., 2017). This suggests that auditory hallucinations are more likely to be unimodal experiences, while experiences of visual hallucinations are more likely to be a part of a multimodal experience. The evident inconsistencies in the reported prevalence of these experiences might be due to, for example, different methodological approaches used or research bias towards studying hallucinations in the auditory modality. Varied prevalence reports can be a result of looking at the lifetime prevalence or point prevalence (e.g. monthly) of these experiences. Lifetime prevalence of hallucinations in different modalities is relatively high—for example, point prevalence is often below 5% for visual, tactile, and olfactory modalities (McCarthy-Jones et al., 2017). This highlights the need for consistency in studying MMHs in future research to avoid disparity in prevalence reports.

Furthermore, higher prevalence of reported auditory hallucinations over other modalities may be because research has largely focused on studying hallucinatory experiences in the auditory modality. Underestimating and understudying these experiences may have serious implications for people who frequently deal with these experiences. Hallucinations research should make the best effort to thoroughly understand the dimensions of hallucinatory experience across all sensory modalities. Unfortunately, lack of interest in modality specificity (or focus on just one modality of hallucination at a time) is reflected, as well as reinforced, in methods of studying hallucinations, such as in currently used symptom rating scales—the widely used Psychotic Symptom Rating Scale (PSYRATS) measures the incidence of auditory verbal hallucinations only, and the North East Visual Hallucination Interview (NEVHI) only records the occurrence of visual hallucinations. A more recent scale designed to be used in both clinical and non-clinical populations, the Multi-Modality Unusual Sensory Experiences Questionnaire (MUSEQ), looks at the hallucinatory experiences across different sensory modalities, including auditory, visual, gustatory, and olfactory hallucinations, and sensed presences, although it does not consider co-occurrences of different modalities. Considering the discrepancies in the prevalence of different modalities of hallucinations reported, a standardized tool for use in clinical and non-clinical practice would be a positive step for reporting realistic prevalence of different sensory modalities of hallucinations.

Variation in Multimodal Hallucinations

If, in psychosis, hallucinations in more than one modality are not the exception, but the norm, further research into the forms, phenomenology, and underlying cognitive neuroscientific mechanisms of MMHs is urgently needed. Dudley et al. (2018) address the issue of phenomenology, proposing that MMHs can be serial or simultaneous, related or unrelated (i.e. hallucinations reported as coming from the same person/entity), and congruent or incongruent (i.e. hallucinations that are feasible in reality). Focusing on the visual modality, they recruited 22 people with psychosis, all of whom reported visual hallucinations, investigating how often these co-occurred with experiences in other modalities, and the relation between these different modalities. The data suggested that almost all participants reporting visual hallucinations also reported auditory hallucinations, that most individuals experience both simultaneous and serial MMHs, and that the different modalities are often attributed to the same agent. It seems, then, that in people with visual hallucinations, the extent to which hallucinations in other modalities can be treated as a completely 'separate' experience is questionable.

Here, we outline and expand upon two attributes in which MMH can differ, which we term *temporal synchrony* and *integration of identity*, and explore their prevalence in the Voices in Psychosis (VIP) interviews ($N = 40$). We will provide some examples from the VIP interviews and pose questions for future research.

Temporal synchrony refers to whether hallucinations in different modalities occur at the same point in time (i.e. simultaneously), or at separate points in time (i.e. serially). For example, in a serial MMH experience, an individual might hear a voice at one point in time and separately report seeing shadows or faces at different points in time. In a simultaneous experience, the voice and face may be perceived at the same point in time. However, even within simultaneous MMHs, there may be important variation in, for example, whether the hallucinations act at the same time (e.g. when hearing a voice, the individual may also report seeing shadows moving randomly; in contrast, the shadows could move in a way perceived to be connected to the voice speaking), and in the case of fused hallucinations, whether movements of the mouth are fully synchronous with a heard voice.

Integration of identity refers to the extent to which experiences in different modalities are attributed to the same agent. For example, an individual might hear a voice they attribute to a specific family member or friend, yet report visual experiences of different individuals or objects (i.e. incongruent hallucinations). Alternatively, someone could hear the voice of the family member, as well as seeing a figure that they believe is that family member (i.e. congruent hallucinations). Note that in the case of visions, the visually perceived agent may not correspond to a full percept of

Table 8.1 Proportion of hallucinations in different modalities and the number of modalities reported in the VIP sample

Modality	Percentage
Auditory	100
Visual	75
Tactile	23
Olfactory	38
Gustatory	0

Number of modalities	Percentage
1	15
2	45
3	30
4	10

an individual, instead simply being a disembodied face or shadow. This attribute refers instead to the belief expressed by the individual regarding the identity attributed to hallucinations in different modalities.

What Don't We Know about Multimodal Hallucinations?

The VIP interviews provide a rich insight into the variability of the phenomenology of MMHs. The examples given here (see Boxes 8.1, 8.2, 8.3 and 8.4) as well as previous research on MMHs, show that these experiences can vary in synchronicity, as well as in the extent to which different modalities are attributed to the same agent. There are, however, a number of issues that have not been addressed in the current literature, which should be addressed going forward.

As already noted, there has been little detailed work on the prevalence or phenomenology of different kinds of MMHs, suggesting that MMHs may be the rule, rather than the exception, in people with psychosis. Montagnese et al. (2021) make an important contribution by outlining the framework for classification of multimodal experiences based on their different characteristics. Research on hallucinations

Box 8.1   Orla

Orla reports synchronous auditory, visual, and tactile hallucinations that she attributes to a single named older woman whom she has heard, seen, and felt since the age of six. Now a 19-year-old woman, Orla offers vivid descriptions of hearing and seeing the older woman—she can see her mouth change shape as she speaks and see her move in the room, and she sometimes feels the woman grab her by the throat. She also reports that she often hears the woman's voice even when she cannot see her (but nonetheless feels that she is present), and sometimes will feel her sit silently at the end of the bed at night. She was not distressed by these experiences until she was a teenager, when the woman began to focus on aspects of Orla's physical appearance and self-esteem, and to encourage her to attempt suicide. Orla's experience, then, is of strongly fused hallucinations across three modalities, which occur synchronously and are attributed to the same identity. Nevertheless, Orla also describes these experiences occurring non-synchronously; further, she describes sometimes hearing mumbling male voices that she cannot see or identify.

Box 8.2   Page

Page is a 25-year-old woman who reports hearing a distinct male voice inside her head. The voice is often angry or aggressive, and has occurred since she was approximately twelve years old, although she now believes it belongs to an ex-partner. At other points in time, Page hears whispering voices that feel like they are located outside of her head and close to her ear, or sometimes from 'just round the corner'. Page also describes how 'sometimes along with the whispering, I will . . . see like little shadows out of the corner of me eye, or like someone will be like waving at us like that, and I'll look and there'll be nothing there . . . they tend to go together'. These experiences are described as typically being synchronous, but there is no hint that Page ascribes her visual hallucinations to the same identity as the voice she hears (her ex-partner), despite their co-occurrence in time.

Box 8.3   Zara

Zara, a 45-year old woman, reports hearing a number of different voices, including voices belonging to her deceased grandmother, a fetus from a pregnancy she was forced to terminate as a teenager, and non-identifiable voices that keep 'banging on in her head' which encourage her to self-harm or attempt suicide. She also reports visual hallucinations, such as seeing a man whom she refers to as Roger, and seeing her deceased brother-in-law. However, these individuals never speak and sometimes appear simply as a shadow. These multimodal hallucinations are described as distinctly separate experiences: they occur at different points in time (i.e. non-synchronously) and are not attributed to the same identity.

Box 8.4 Leah

Leah describes hearing a number of different commanding voices, some belonging to people she has known in her life. She also hears a voice she refers to as the archangel Michael, who acts as her protector. She reports visual hallucinations, including 'shadows and spirits', and once or twice has seen large black wings that she feels to be part of Michael. Although she does not typically describe seeing Michael at the same time as hearing him, sometimes the voice instructs her to look at images which she interprets as being a part of his identity.

---

should take these into account to improve our understanding regarding how often MMHs are synchronous or non-synchronous, how often they are attributed to the same identity, and how synchronicity might be linked to identity integration, if at all. Furthermore, we do not know the relative frequencies of various modalities within individuals (e.g. if an individual reports auditory and visual hallucinations, this will count as an MMH—but it is possible that individual auditory hallucinations occur on a daily basis, whereas visual hallucinations occur only very rarely). Nor do we know the relative complexity of experiences in different modalities with MMH; for example, Page (see Box 8.2) describes highly personified and complex experiences of voice hearing, but her visual experiences are much more fleeting and 'simple', often consisting of shadows seen out of the corner of her eye. In contrast, Orla (see Box 8.1) describes complex visual hallucinations of the same older woman whose voice she hears.

Second, with the issue of integration of identity across modalities, it is difficult to untangle when MMHs are reported as such because they are genuinely multimodal, and when they are instead the result of post hoc reasoning or beliefs about their content. One possibility is that in some MMHs, the auditory and the visual (for example) come packaged together—if generated by the same underlying cognitive or neural process (e.g. being linked to social agency, or 'person-selective' brain regions such as the posterior superior temporal sulcus (Tsantani et al., 2019)), hallucinations might therefore be identified as the same agent (for more discussion, see Fernyhough, 2019). However, if an individual hears a male voice and regularly sees a male figure that others cannot, it would seem a reasonable logical step to assume they are the same person, despite being generated by at least partially distinct cognitive mechanisms (e.g. relating to auditory and visual perception, respectively). These possibilities may be identical, or extremely similar, at the level of phenomenology, and it will therefore require a combination of careful and detailed phenomenological work, and nuanced cognitive neuroscientific paradigms, to begin to understand these possibilities.

Complicating this is the relative lack of understanding of the cognitive neuroscientific mechanisms that may underlie MMHs. Current hallucinations research tends to focus on modality-specific tasks that are thought to assess relevant constructs such as source monitoring, self-recognition, or top–down processing (often embedded in a predictive processing framework). Since most research focuses on auditory hallucinations, these tasks typically require participants to complete auditory tasks (e.g. auditory signal detection, voice recognition, memory for spoken words, etc.). More recent research has also applied similar paradigms to other sensory modalities (e.g. Aynsworth et al., 2017), to investigate whether similar mechanisms could underlie visual or olfactory hallucinations. While these studies give promising results and could speak to a modality-general process underlying these experiences, they do not address the issue of integration (in time or in identity) across modalities. Some previous research has indicated that people with a diagnosis of schizophrenia show deficits in audio-visual integration, such as in the McGurk effect (de Gelder et al., 2003), although to our knowledge, these paradigms have not been used with individuals with MMHs (compared to individuals without MMHs); of particular interest would be comparisons between individuals with synchronous and those with non-synchronous MMHs, for example.

Finally, at a clinical level, it will be key to understand if and how MMHs may lead to heightened distress in people with psychosis. As a preliminary observation, in the VIP sample, people with both visual and auditory hallucinations scored no higher on the 'emotional' subscale of the PSYRATS, which assesses distress associated with hallucinations, than did people with only auditory hallucinations.[1] In contrast, people who reported MMHs in which multiple modalities were attributed to the same identity scored significantly higher than did people without such MMHs.[2] These groups did not differ in other aspects of the symptom rating scale (the 'cognitive' and 'physical' subscales, and delusion ratings). Although comprising a small sample size, this hints that MMHs with integrated identities may be particularly distressing for individuals with psychosis, suggesting that this should be a key area for future research.

Overall, it seems that MMHs may be much more frequent than commonly acknowledged. The simultaneously detailed, yet open-ended, nature of the VIP interviews may have encouraged participants to describe experiences that typically would not have been asked about. Untangling the complexities of MMHs, as outlined in this chapter, will not only enable a fuller understanding of psychosis, but also enable interventions to be developed and targeted where most appropriate.

References

Aynsworth, C., Nemat, N., Collerton, D., Smailes, D., and Dudley, R. (2017). Reality monitoring performance and the role of visual imagery in visual hallucinations. *Behaviour Research and Therapy*, 97, 115–22.

---

[1] Visual and auditory hallucination group ($n = 30$), PSYRATS – $M = 9.93$, $SD = 4.05$. Auditory hallucinations group ($n = 10$), PSYRATS – $M = 10.00$, $SD = 4.52$, $t(38) = 0.04$, $p = 0.97$, $d = 0.02$.
[2] MMHs attributed to the same modality ($n = 11$), PSYRATS – $M = 12.6$, $SD = 2.42$. Other MMHs ($n = 29$), PSYRATS – $M = 8.93$, $SD = 4.19$, $t(38) = 2.75$, $p = 0.009$, $d = 0.97$.

Delespaul, P., deVries, M., and van Os, J. (2002). Determinants of occurrence and recovery from hallucinations in daily life. *Social Psychiatry and Psychiatric Epidemiology*, 37(3), 97–104.

Dudley, R., Aynsworth, C., Cheetham, R., McCarthy-Jones, S., and Collerton, D. (2018). Prevalence
and characteristics of multi-modal hallucinations in people with psychosis who experience visual
hallucinations. *Psychiatry Research*, 269, 25–30.

Fernyhough, C. (2019). Modality-general and modality-specific processes in hallucinations.
Psychological Medicine, 49(16), 2639–45.

Lim, A., Hoek, H. W., Deen, M. L., Blom, J. D., Bruggeman, R., Cahn, W., de Haan, L., Kahn, R. S., Meijer,
C. J., Myin-Germeys, I., van Os, J., Wiersma, D., and GROUP Investigators. (2016). Prevalence and
classification of hallucinations in multiple sensory modalities in schizophrenia spectrum disorders.
Schizophrenia Research, 176(2–3), 493–9.

McCarthy-Jones, S., Smailes, D., Corvin, A., Gill, M., Morris, D. W., Dinan, T. G., Murphy, K. C.,
O'Neill, F. A., Waddington, J. L., Australian Schizophrenia Research Bank, Donohoe, G., and Dudley,
R. (2017). Occurrence and co-occurrence of hallucinations by modality in schizophrenia-spectrum
disorders. *Psychiatry Research*, 252, 154–60.

Montagnese, M., Leptourgos, P., Fernyhough, C., Waters, F., Larøi, F., Jardri, R., McCarthy-Jones, S.,
Thomas, N., Dudley, R., Taylor, J.-P., Collerton, D., and Urwyler, P. (2021). A review of multimodal
hallucinations: categorization, assessment, theoretical perspectives, and clinical recommendations.
Schizophrenia Bulletin, 41(1), 237–48.

Tsantani, M., Kriegeskorte, N., McGettigan, C., and Garrido, L. (2019). Faces and voices in the
brain: a modality-general person-identity representation in superior temporal sulcus. *NeuroImage*,
201, 116004.

Waters, F., Collerton, D., Ffytche, D. H., Jardri, R., Pins, D., Dudley, R., Blom, J. D., Mosimann, U. P.,
Eperjesi, F., Ford, S., and Larøi, F. (2014). Visual hallucinations in the psychosis spectrum and comparative information from neurodegenerative disorders and eye disease. *Schizophrenia Bulletin*,
40(4), S233–45.

About the Authors

Peter Moseley is a Senior Research Fellow in Psychology at Northumbria University.
He is interested in linking phenomenology, cognition, and brain processes associated with voice-hearing.

Kaja Mitrenga is Assistant Professor in the Department of Psychology and the
Institute for Medical Humanities at Durham University. She is interested in cognitive processes associated with auditory and visual hallucinations.

9

Lost Agency and the Sense of Control

John Foxwell, Department of English Studies, Durham University

There would appear to be some variation in the extent to which we feel like we control our thoughts. On the one hand, there are thoughts that we might experience as being effortfully constructed, such as when we deliberate over a problem or make plans for the future. On the other hand, as the philosopher Harry Frankfurt suggests, there are some thoughts to which we appear to be 'mere passive bystanders', thoughts 'that we *find* occurring within us' (Frankfurt, 1988, p. 59). For instance, there are thoughts that appear to 'pop up' out of nowhere, thoughts that we struggle to rid ourselves of, sudden flashes of insight, unbidden images and memories, earworms, etc. There are also the descriptions provided by some writers and artists of the feeling that the work is emerging and developing outside of their control (such as when fictional characters are referred to as having 'minds of their own'). Finally, there are some forms of 'passive' thought which are highly distressing, such as those which psychologists term 'obsessive' and 'intrusive' thoughts: thoughts which are unwanted and difficult to control, and which interrupt ongoing activity (Rachman, 1981). At the very least, therefore, there would appear to be some difference between the *feeling* of control, or 'agency', experienced in relation to different kinds of thought.

Yet distinguishing between different kinds of thought in terms of control might present something of a conceptual problem when it comes to the experience of hearing voices. In the Voices in Psychosis study, almost all of the interview participants were directly asked how, if at all, the voices differed from their own thoughts. Across the forty interviews, the difference was attributed to a variety of features (e.g. the fact that the voices were spatially located, or that the voices were accompanied by additional physical/emotional sensations, or that the voices said things that the voice-hearer would never think). Yet the distinction that was sometimes made between voices and thoughts was in relation to the sense of agency:

> It's a, because it just feels like there's something, it's another person inside me as well, so it just feels like I haven't really got full control over, over everything . . . like if I've got to make a decision, is it really my decision I'm making now, or is it their input that's reflecting that decision? (Will)

John Foxwell, *Lost Agency and the Sense of Control* In: *Voices in Psychosis*. Edited by: Angela Woods, Ben Alderson-Day, and Charles Fernyhough, Oxford University Press. © John Foxwell 2022. DOI: 10.1093/oso/9780192898388.003.0009

[B]ecause it's not invited, it's not an invited thought, it can be completely impulsive... and there's no provoking the thought, it just comes out of nowhere, like a glitch in your own mind ... Whatever's being said, it's ... it's outside of your own conscious power, that's as best as I can describe. (Bill)

I'm one of them people that talk to themselves and that quite a bit, so I do just ramble and it is just a thing that I know I'm doing that. Whereas this is just ... sometimes I won't even be thinking, I'll just be like getting on with stuff. ... And it will happen. And it's like ... completely out of my control, like I haven't prompted myself to do that. (Page)

I can tell it's not my thoughts because it's like with my thoughts I can, I could intercept something, so when I'm thinking negative things, like oh you know you're a terrible person, things like that, I can think, oh this is, this is my thought and you know this is my thoughts telling me that, but when you hear it shouting, it's like you can't intercept, so my thoughts can't override it, if that makes sense. So it's like this constant channelling that you can't shut off, whereas with my thoughts, although I struggle to shut them off, I could change my thought pattern if I want to and I could make a conscious decision, but when that comes into your head, it's like you can't make a decision because it's very overpowering, if that makes sense? (Dan)

[Y]ou know that running commentary everyone's got in their head? ... It's sort of like that but sometimes I can notice it changes, and then I'm not in control of it anymore ... And I'll not realise it at the time until about five minutes into the whole thing, and I'm like, what's going on, this is ... I shouldn't, I wasn't thinking like this two minutes ago. (Brad)

One immediate complication that presents itself is that these voice-hearers appear to be talking about different senses of not being in control. Will, for instance, seems to be describing a more generalized lack of control which relates to the possibility of the voice's interference in his own decision-making. Bill and Page, however, appear to be referring to the feeling of not having actively produced the voice, while Dan (and Bill also) describe how the voice feels outside of their control when it is present. Lastly, in Brad's account, it is difficult to determine whether the loss of control is always retrospectively felt after recognizing the change in thought content, or if the change is sometimes felt immediately. A further complication is introduced when considering these interviews in their entirety, since participants sometimes referred to other kinds of lost or attenuated agency at a later point in the interview (e.g. Dan also describes moments when he feels 'possessed', in which 'it feels like there's someone like just controlling everything that you do', and Bill states that the voice 'chooses which mood it puts me in. It chooses how I act and how I live'). Finally, although a lack of control was the feature which these participants focused on when asked about the difference between thoughts and voices, the voices usually exhibited other features which would distinguish them from thoughts (for instance, Bill's most prominent voice often starts with a barking sound which turns into words, and sometimes the voices are accompanied by other sensations such as pain; Page hears a male voice which agrees with her negative thoughts, but also 'whispering voices' which seem to be located in physical space).

Nevertheless, the accounts of Bill, Page, and Dan suggest that there is a difference in the feeling of agency as it pertains to thoughts and to voices, and one which has a bearing on what it means to feel agency for thoughts more generally. Literary works by writers who heard voices or saw visions also gesture towards this immediate sense of disrupted agency, often resorting to formal or impressionist strategies to represent an aspect of the experience that seems difficult to express directly. What I will attempt to provide in this chapter is an account of how we might characterize the difference between voices and thoughts in terms of control, in a way that would still allow for a distinction to be drawn between thoughts that feel active and passive. After considering some of the theories of agency which appear within philosophy of mind, I suggest how these theories might be supplemented by ideas from ecological psychology which conceive of objects and events in terms of potential interactions.

The experience of agency is sometimes described by philosophers as being 'thin' or 'phenomenologically recessive'—it is usually part of the background of experience, and only rarely becomes the focus of conscious attention. Theories of agency thus often draw on examples from experiences that can occur in psychosis, which sometimes foreground aspects of the sense of agency that are usually so taken for granted that they pass unnoticed. For instance, we might not always be consciously aware of an action that we undertake automatically, such as adjusting our posture or scratching our nose. Yet the phenomenology of an automatic action appears to be very different from cases of 'alien control', where the individual feels that a part of their body is moving entirely of its own accord (or is being moved somehow by another agent). Similarly, although there are thoughts which might ordinarily be said to 'pop into' our minds, the phenomenology of what is termed 'thought insertion' appears very different, since the inserted thought is described as having been placed into the mind of the individual by another agent.[1]

The theories put forward to characterize and explain such experiences vary regarding the extent to which the phenomenology of agency is taken to reflect its causes. On the one hand, there are models which suggest that the sense of agency is essentially a matter of post hoc attribution—that is, we feel that we are the agent behind an action because certain aspects of our conscious experience match up in the appropriate way (even if we are not always correct in this self-attribution). For instance, George Graham and G. Lynn Stephens suggest that our sense of agency for our actions (including our thoughts) is dependent on whether their occurrence can be rationally explained in terms of our beliefs and desires (Graham and Stephens, 2000). Psychologist Daniel Wegner, meanwhile, suggests that the feeling of agency

---

[1] There is still an open debate over whether thought insertion and voice-hearing are fundamentally similar or different experiences (Wilkinson and Alderson-Day, 2016). While it is therefore possible that the account of agency disruption provided here might apply to thought insertion as well as to voices, a proper assessment of the issue goes beyond the scope of this chapter.

is a matter of 'apparent mental causation' (Wegner, 2005), an interpretation which arises when there is an appropriate matching of intention and outcome: when we mean to produce some sort of change in our environment, and that change happens in the right temporal window, we determine ourselves to be the agent behind the change.

On the other hand, there are the approaches which suggest that despite its apparent 'thinness', the sense of agency is many-faceted, comprising multiple senses and experiences which might be conceptually distinguished. For example, Elisabeth Pacherie proposes an extensive (though still 'non-exhaustive') list of possible distinctions that might be drawn between the different facets of the experience of agency (Pacherie, 2007, p. 6):

> awareness of a goal, awareness of an intention to act, awareness of initiation of action, awareness of movements, sense of activity, sense of mental effort, sense of physical effort, sense of control, experience of authorship, experience of intentionality, experience of purposiveness, experience of freedom, and experience of mental causation

Accounts which acknowledge the multiple aspects of the sense of agency rarely address all of these features (and even Pacherie only deals with some of them). However, as Shaun Gallagher suggests, the territory might be usefully divided up in terms of those aspects which are reflective (such as the attribution of agency, or agency 'judgements') and those which are 'pre-reflective' (i.e. which are an implicit part of conscious awareness but are not reflectively dwelt upon) (Gallagher, 2012). As examples of such pre-reflective aspects, Gallagher points towards what he terms the 'intentional aspect' (the perceptual monitoring of the effects our actions are having on the world) and the 'motor (or efferent) aspect' (the sense of causing or controlling bodily movement) (Gallagher, 2012, p. 22). Such pre-reflective aspects would provide a way of accounting for the different phenomenologies of alien control and automatic actions: although the latter can appear not to enter reflective consciousness at all and, in some cases, are too fine-grained to allow for specific intentions, they still do not feel palpably *non*-agentive (unlike cases of alien control).

However, in ordinary experience, not all aspects of agency are necessarily contributing to the sense of agency all of the time, and it is possible that not all contributories are equally weighted. As a result, we might feel some actions to be more or less agentive (Gallagher, 2012). For example, an action performed deliberately would be likely to feel more agentive than the same action performed automatically, since the former could involve various reflective aspects such as an awareness of intention and a sense of effort (e.g. changing gear while learning to drive, as opposed to changing gear as an experienced driver). Equally, in some cases, the sense of agency for an action might be so ambiguous in terms of its pre-reflective contributories that the matter positively requires a reflective judgement (e.g. when caught in a crowd, I might question the extent to which I am pushing or being pushed). Finally, the phenomenology of agency is by no means expected to be as clean and ordered as conceptual distinctions would suggest, being for the most part a 'holistic, qualitative, and ambiguous experience' (Gallagher, 2012, p. 29).

Nevertheless, at least some of the distinctions suggested by hybrid models of the sense of agency appear to be reflected in voice-hearers' descriptions of 'lost control', inasmuch as they appear to be describing different kinds of disruption in the sense of agency. Brad's sense of realizing that he is not in control of his thoughts seems closely connected with his reflective awareness of a change in their style and/or content, whereas Page and Bill appear to be describing a more immediate experience of lacking a sense of authorship for the voices, which arrive suddenly 'like a glitch in [the] mind' (Bill). However, the aspect of the sense of agency I wish to focus on here is related to the experience of the voice being 'outside of' the voice-hearer's control, as suggested by Bill's comment that the voice is 'outside of [his] own conscious power' and Dan's account of his inability to 'intercept' or 'shut off' the voices. Indeed, the way in which Dan explicitly contrasts the voices with 'anxious' and 'obsessive' thoughts is further suggestive of the specific sense of control that is at issue here. Although such obsessive thoughts are not accompanied by any deliberative intent, and although they are not necessarily explicable in terms of Dan's beliefs and desires, they differ in terms of Dan's sense of being able to inhibit or 'intercept' them. Note that this does not mean that Dan is always successful in interrupting obsessive and anxious thoughts, but merely that they present a potential for interaction which the voices do not—a potential which Dan suggests is part of what makes such obsessive thoughts identifiable *as* thoughts.

According to Gottfried Vosgerau and Martin Voss, the sense of control which we usually feel for our thoughts is essentially linked to the ability to inhibit them: 'thought suppression is certainly a very important way of thought control, and it might be the only one' (Vosgerau and Voss, 2014, p. 545). The kind of suppression described in their account is essentially reflective, since they distinguish it from the hypothetical ability 'to prevent a thought from being produced, such that it does not even come into existence' (Vosgerau and Voss, 2014, p. 545). In accordance with this distinction, they suggest that intrusive thoughts also lack a sense of control, given the resistance of such thoughts to suppression. However, I would suggest that since we would appear to ordinarily have a sense of control over thoughts even when we do *not* try to inhibit them, it is possible that the sense of control also involves a pre-reflective awareness of the *potential* for inhibiting a thought. In a similar vein, Terry Horgan and Shaun Nichols argue that part of the pre-reflective (or as they put it, 'zero-point') phenomenology of agency involves the experience of 'core-optionality': the experience of 'being able to refrain from so behaving' (Horgan and Nichols, 2016, p. 152). Importantly, core-optionality is still present even in those cases where refraining from a particular action would appear to be abhorrent or irrational to the subject (e.g. when presented with death or extreme pain as an alternative). Even acts arising from compulsion or addiction still have core-optionality. Though we might not want to assign full 'responsibility' to the subject, the possibility of not acting is still there—it is just unconscionable, since the potential consequences would appear as being too terrible to bear.

The sense of control might thus be characterized more generally (with regard to both physical and mental acts) as a pre-reflective sense of being able to interrupt the progress of *any* ongoing action. Like other kinds of pre-reflective awareness of possibility—such as our sense that what appears as a three-dimensional object has a back to it, without needing to actually rotate it all the way around—the possibility of inhibition does not necessarily need to be explored to feel that it pertains. In this regard, it might perhaps be more accurate to say that what is being described here is a sense of the thought's openness to being controlled—in other words, one of the possibilities afforded by the thought.

The concept of 'affordances' as it appears within ecological psychology is usually discussed in relation to objects, and relates to the potentials for interaction which are experienced as being offered by an object. A chair, for instance, affords sitting, and in having the properties it does, 'it should *look* sit-on-able'—that is, the affordance 'is perceived visually' (Gibson, 1966, p. 128), rather than requiring a reflective recognition of this action possibility. While thoughts are not objects in this sense (although in ordinary language, they are frequently referred to using object-metaphors), events are also said to present us with affordances (Gibson, 1966, p. 102), which allows for a slightly more intuitive application of the concept.

The advantage of conceptualizing thoughts in terms of affordances is that it allows for drawing an important distinction between being unable to 'control' intrusive thoughts and the voices which respondents describe as being 'outside' of their control. In the case of the former, the individual is presented with an experience which is recognizably thought-like insofar as it appears to afford the possibility of being inhibited, and in the way that thoughts are usually inhibited—it is just that actually accomplishing that inhibition is so incredibly difficult that it might never be attained. In the case of the latter, the individual is presented with an experience which appears to afford no possibility of being inhibited in the way that thoughts are usually inhibited. It therefore does not appear to be thought-like at all, or at least seems different enough from ordinary thought experiences to be described by the voice-hearer as a 'voice' (even if, as in some cases, it does not present any auditory properties). The difference might be characterized in terms of realizing that an action cannot be performed and having no sense that the action is even available. For instance, I might never succeed in climbing a particular mountain and ultimately (reflectively) decide that, for all practical purposes, it is impossible. The mountain might even seem so sheer and forbidding at first glance that its 'climbability' is at issue, such that I do not even try. Yet in neither case would the climbing of the mountain have presented itself to me as impossible in the same way that running through it or jumping over it would have done—affordances which are entirely absent in my experience of the mountain as a mountain.

In essence, it would appear that we are dealing with two subtly different senses of a 'lack of control'. On the one hand, there are experiences of (reflective) inhibition failing or as bound-to-fail, while on the other, there are experiences where the (pre-reflective) possibility of inhibition is altogether absent. I suggest that whatever other aspects of the sense of agency are or are not involved in passive thought experiences (e.g. lack or presence of authorship), the affordance of inhibition still makes such experiences recognizable as thoughts. Of course, while the absence of the possibility of inhibition might sometimes be a part of what distinguishes voices phenomenologically from thoughts, we should not be surprised that it is rarely referred to explicitly. Quite apart from the difficulty of characterizing these different senses of control in ordinary language, some voice-hearers state that the voices are indistinguishable from actual voices in their surroundings. In such cases, the absence of the pre-reflective sense of control is already implied, insofar as our ordinary experiences of the voices of other people also do not present as affording thought-like inhibition. However, given the heterogeneity of voice-hearing experiences, it is certainly possible that some voices do not differ from thoughts in terms of the sense of agency (or at least not in terms of this particular aspect of agency).

As with so many of the cornerstones of the phenomenology of everyday experience, pre-reflective aspects of the sense of agency are rarely noticed until they are in some way disrupted; as one respondent puts it, 'You don't realise . . . the advantage of being in control until suddenly it gets taken off you' (Olivia). It is therefore not surprising that the reports of voice-hearers should sometimes make us aware of fine-grained distinctions in experience which we might otherwise overlook. The particular distinction between different senses of control that has been considered here is—like so much of what is pre-reflective—understandably difficult to pin down in a meaningful way, which would potentially account for why it is rarely described in depth. After all, saying that the voice feels 'outside of' conscious control still describes the phenomenon as it appears—it is just that it fails to cover how this particular experience differs from other, less disturbing and troublesome experiences which could also be said to be outside of conscious control. It is at least possible that the analysis provided here explains why some voice-hearers, upon being asked how the voices differ from the rest of their thoughts, consider the 'lack of control' to be a significant distinguishing feature.

References

Frankfurt, H. (1988). *The Importance of What We Care About: Philosophical Essays*. Cambridge: Cambridge University Press.

Gallagher, S. (2012). Multiple aspects in the sense of agency. *New Ideas in Psychology*, 30(1), 15–31.

Gibson, J. J. (1966). *The Senses Considered as Perceptual Systems*. London: Allen and Unwin.

Graham, G., and Stephens, G. L. (2000). *When Self-Consciousness breaks: Alien Voices and Inserted Thoughts*. Cambridge, MA: MIT Press.

Horgan, T., and Nichols, S. (2016). The zero point and I. In: S. Miguens, G. Preyer, and C. B. Morando, eds. *Pre-reflective Consciousness: Sartre and Contemporary Philosophy of Mind*. Abingdon: Routledge, pp. 143–75.

Pacherie, E. (2007). The sense of control and the sense of agency. *Psyche: An Interdisciplinary Journal of Research on Consciousness*, 13(1). http://psyche.cs.monash.edu.au/ (accessed 25 October 2019).

Rachman, S. (1981). Part I. Unwanted intrusive cognitions. *Advances in Behaviour Research and Therapy*, 3(3), 89–99.

Vosgerau, G., and Voss, M. (2014). Authorship and control over thoughts. *Mind and Language*, 29(5), 534–65.

Wegner, D. M. (2005). Who is the controller of controlled processes? In: R. R. Hassin, J. S. Uleman, and J. A. Bargh, eds. *The New Unconscious*. Oxford: Oxford University Press, pp. 19–36.

Wilkinson, S., and Alderson-Day, B. (2016). Voices and thoughts in psychosis: an introduction. *Review of Philosophy and Psychology*, 7(3), 529–40.

About the Author

John Foxwell was a Postdoctoral Research and Engagement Fellow on Hearing the Voice, having completed his PhD with the project in 2018. His doctoral thesis examined hallucinatory experience in mid-twentieth-century fiction, focusing on how the phenomenology of such experience is conveyed through the manipulation of stylistic and narratological conventions. His postdoctoral research with the project dealt with the phenomenology of writers' experiences of their characters' voices, focusing particularly on the various similarities and differences that such experiences exhibited in comparison with voice-hearing and inner speech.

10

Pollution and Purity

Understanding Voices as Punishment for Un-Wholly Sins

Adam J. Powell, Department of Theology and Religion, Durham University

Early in the nineteenth century, a Native American leader of the Seneca people in north-eastern United States revived Iroquois religion after recounting a set of unusual visionary experiences he had during a period of acute illness. Relaying to his followers the religious messages he received from the supernatural visitors he saw, Handsome Lake told what was essentially a tale of purification, a transformation from sacrilegious alcoholic to restorer and reformer of tradition. He decried European influence on indigenous peoples—particularly the introduction of liquor—and preached a message of rigid moral probity. More importantly for present purposes, the most common account of Handsome Lake's story attributes his pre-vision illness to acts of defilement and impropriety, illuminating that intersection—in terms of cultural structures and meaning-making—where concepts of sacrality, order, punishment, and purity meet (Fadden, 1955, p. 345):

> He was like the rest of the Seneca people of that time. He loved the white man's firewater. When he was drunk, he did things that were not right, singing the sacred songs, the Harvest Song, the Great Feather Dance Song. He offended the Creator. Because he did such things he became very ill.

Here the appropriately timed singing of ritual songs is implicitly linked with social/cosmological order. In this way, Handsome Lake's illness is understood as a justified consequence of wrongdoing—not in terms of causing direct harm to others but, instead, in terms of acting contrary to sacred norms. Handsome Lake 'did things that were not right' in the eyes of the 'Creator' and was punished accordingly. His physical suffering was a function of his defilement of the 'sacred songs', sung not under the influence of proper piety, but under the influence of 'firewater'.

Handsome Lake is one example of the common human struggle to find order in the undesirable, to identify a logic that may successfully transform senseless suffering into purposeful punishment. This chapter suggests that the meaning-making processes operative in the Seneca histories of Handsome Lake are also evident in

Adam J. Powell, *Pollution and Purity* In: *Voices in Psychosis*. Edited by: Angela Woods, Ben Alderson-Day, and Charles Fernyhough, Oxford University Press. © Adam J. Powell 2022. DOI: 10.1093/oso/9780192898388.003.0010 the reports of those who, in the twenty-first century, understand their unusual and distressing visual and auditory experiences as 'punishments'. The notions of punishment invoked by participants in the Voices in Psychosis (VIP) study may serve at least three meaningful functions: (1) belief in a system of punishment implies an overriding existential order governing otherwise extraordinary experiences ('There is a definite reason for these experiences'); (2) feeling that one deserves punishment connects those experiences to a personal past ('I must have done something wrong'); and (3) receiving punishment locates the individual within stable impersonal sociocultural structures of purity and wholeness ('Some actions are simply wrong and punishment rectifies them').

Perhaps the most influential text on this relationship between wrongdoing, punishment, ritual, and the power of culture is anthropologist Mary Douglas's *Purity and Danger* (Douglas, 2002). Amidst a compelling argument for the underlying logic connecting seemingly arbitrary rules of taboo and ritual cleanliness across ancient, indigenous, and modern cultures, Douglas (2002, p. 140) introduces her concept of 'pollution' and offers a theoretical formula useful for structuring the present analysis:

> There ... are pollution powers which inhere in the structure of ideas itself and which punish a symbolic breaking of that which should be joined or joining of that which should be separate. It follows from this that pollution is a type of danger which is not likely to occur except where the lines of structure, cosmic or social, are clearly defined. A polluting person ... has developed some wrong condition or simply crossed some line which should not have been crossed and this displacement unleashes danger ...

This chapter will focus on interviews conducted with Dan and Ryan, two participants in the VIP study who suspect that they have crossed a dangerous line. Dan is identified as an 18-year-old male who reports both visual and auditory hallucinatory experiences and whose voice-hearing began seven years prior to his participation in the VIP study. Ryan is a 20-year-old male who began hearing voices less than one month before being interviewed. Like Dan, Ryan also reports having visual experiences as well as depression. Unlike Dan, Ryan reports his voices beginning during a traumatic period and associates them with a sense of fear. Both believe their unusual visual and auditory experiences are a sort of punishment. But why?

Is there a connection between Dan's and Ryan's appraisals of their experiences and potent cultural notions of anomaly and wholeness, pollution, and punishment? For present purposes, 'appraisal' refers to an individual's unique perception or evaluation of a specific event or experience that then determines or corresponds with a set of emotions and values. The subjectivity of an appraisal means that two or more individuals may have strikingly different responses to the same experience. In fact, many voice-hearers do not appraise their voices in the way that Dan and Ryan do. With that in mind, the following pages explore the question of whether, and to what extent, these two voice-hearers' individual experiences represent a sociocultural 'symbolic breaking of that which should be joined or joining of that which should be separate' which may have influenced their similar evaluations.

Psychologists Lucy Holt and Anna Tickle offer the important reminder that when it comes to voice-hearing, 'individuals may not necessarily hold a solitary framework of understanding, and imposing just one explanation could confuse' (Holt and Tickle, 2015, p. 261). Indeed, the pluralism and fluidity of modern life seems to provide a dizzying assortment of cultural paradigms from which individuals may construct meaning. By positing a possible role for just one of these paradigms—the 'pollution dangers' paradigm, to use Douglas' term—in voice-hearers' understandings of their voices as punishments, this chapter attempts to expand the range of sociocultural variables considered relevant to mental health beyond facts of family history and immediate social context.

Medical humanities scholar Angela Woods argues that diagnosis itself figures significantly in identity construction and meaning-making for those experiencing depression, hallucinatory experiences, and other psychological concerns, precisely because diagnoses 'insert [the diagnosed] into a cultural context that is beyond their control' (Woods, 2001, p. 105). With philosopher Sam Wilkinson, Woods suggests that it may be necessary to consider how 'appraisal' involves prior beliefs and expectations shaping psychotic experiences just as much as it entails retrospective interpretations of those experiences (Woods and Wilkinson, 2017, p. 891). With that in mind, perhaps cultural structures of pollution and punishment form part of a larger context and, as such, are also beyond individual control, constructing and construing voice-hearers' appraisals of their voices. What is more, those very structures ordering social existence may be mirrored by, or require, corresponding psychological/somatic order. Could a transgression in the former be perceived as a punishment in the latter?

Body as Culture, Wholeness as Holiness

Certainly for Douglas (2002, p. 2), 'dirt is essentially disorder', an explicit affirmation of continuity between the body and the social world: 'The body is a model which can stand for any bounded system . . . We cannot possibly interpret rituals [of pollution] unless we are prepared to see in the body a symbol of society, to see the powers and dangers credited to social structure reproduced in small on the human body' (Douglas, 2002, p. 142). Accordingly, Douglas alludes to anthropologist Alfred Radcliffe-Brown's structural functionalism as support for her conclusion that the punishments resulting from the breaking of pollution rules reveal underlying social values. More to the point, with the body as a microcosm of the sociocultural system, otherwise inexplicable and quite specific rules of taboo, impurity, or abomination come into focus as guarantors of more generalized order or wholeness.

Drawing on data gathered among several indigenous populations in sub-Saharan Africa—primarily the Nuer and Lele—as well as on the case of the ancient Israelites whose abomination rules are preserved in the biblical book of Leviticus, Douglas demonstrates the extent to which conceptions of pollution have often extended far beyond what twentieth- or twenty-first-century societies deem strictly necessary for proper hygiene. Indeed, her exposition of the Levitical code of cleanliness discusses both food and sex taboos among the Israelites in terms of 'hybrids and other confusions being abominated' (Douglas, 2002, p. 66). Along with failing to complete tasks, eating animals with confounding or anomalous attributes or engaging in sexual activity (such as incest or homosexuality) that did not fit with the socio-cultural categories of the Israelites resulted in uncleanness, a state quite apart from moral or legal failing. To be unclean was to be unholy was to be unworthy was to be in danger of punishment (Douglas, 2002, pp. 63–5).

It is important to recall that one of Douglas' primary purposes is to challenge the social Darwinism endemic to anthropology's early years. Thus, she utilizes data from various indigenous populations across the world to establish a cross-cultural comparison, all while insisting that modern cultures are hardly different. As communities seek cooperation and survival through the establishment of systems of exchange, social institutions, and communication, symbol-systems emerge to order and harmonize the widest possible set of experiences and exigencies. Religion, however defined, is often taken to be a particularly acute example of this; however, systems of ritual and classification permeate even so-called secular societies. If Douglas is correct that the body is culture in miniature, and if we accept her claim that pollution and prohibitions regarding individual behaviour put preferred social orders in relief (Douglas, 2002, p. 90), then it may be that one's interpretation of embodied experience points to predominant cultural structures, regardless of whether the latter is taken to be the product or reflection of either divine ordering or powerful social construction.

Voices as Punishment: Two Cases

In the context of voice-hearing, it should be noted that Douglas' theoretical connection between wholeness (symbolic and personal) and worthiness among the Israelites could have much wider applications. On the one hand, it has been proposed that voice-hearing itself causes an almost literal sense of fragmentation for those who seek treatment, as the voices combine with fractured social relationships and stigmatized diagnoses to destabilize a once unified identity (Powell, 2017, p. 111). On the other hand, although Dan and Ryan dismiss overtly religious interpretations of their voices, they do exhibit a strong commitment to the notion that the voices are 'deserved' punishments, presumably imposed by some sovereign arbiter of justice. In other words, a general splintering of the self resulting from psychosis and its identification seems to be, in these two instances, accompanied by a conviction that one is worthy of punishment, rather than of cultural approval.

Just as Handsome Lake retroactively attributes his illness to his socio-religious misdeeds and the Nuer cited by Douglas (2002, p. 166) assume an adulterous affair has occurred if the suspect's spouse becomes ill shortly after the alleged incident, so Dan and Ryan search for causal relationships in their experiences of voice-hearing. Dan, for example, notes that his first two hallucinatory occurrences followed intense bereavement, depression, stress, and religious reflection, but then, explicitly label-ling them as 'punishment', claims that the disparaging and distressing things said by those voices are 'what I deserve . . . they're just giving me a bit of like . . . tough love . . . so that I can make myself a better person, or because I've done something to deserve it'. With similar rationale, Ryan reports having become suicidal after being in a close romantic relationship with an individual who 'self-harmed . . . [and] talked a lot about suicide'. Eventually, he heard a voice say, 'today's the day' and placed items necessary for the suicide in an online shopping cart, but he never went through with the task. Distressing voices and visions began the following day, and while Ryan notes having first 'put [them] on to religion', he has concluded that that was 'just [him] trying to make sense of it . . . trying to figure out where they were from'. He now believes that the voices and the things he sees 'are there as a punishment'. When asked how convinced he is of this conclusion, Ryan responds, 'about 90' per cent.

Just as Holt and Tickle suggest, Dan and Ryan offer various interpretations of their hallucinatory experiences at various times. Ryan, for instance, has begun to see dark, shadowy figures quite regularly, and when he has nightmares, he believes those fig-ures cause the nightmares, rather than positing them as an outcome of, say, depres-sion or anxiety. Dan indicates that a difficult home life and a family history of mental illness likely explain much of his ordeal. However, both voice-hearers also describe themselves as being abnormal in some substantial way that implicitly justifies their psychological predicament. Ryan says he is not mentally ill but prefers being labelled an 'anomaly' because he 'shouldn't be here anymore'. At times, Dan also abandons a straightforward mental health argument about stress and family history, instead stating that he is 'different from other people' with a 'brain [that] works differently' and 'a special ability to be horrible'.

Strikingly, in Douglas' framework, anomalies and ambiguities, like the 'hybrid' acts and animals deemed unclean by the ancient Israelites, are 'abominated' and condemned by culture (Douglas, 2002, p. 66). In fact, she argues that pollution as a concept functions not just in promoting wholeness, but also in the gap between moral prescriptions and individual ambivalence, serving as a 'kind of impersonal punishment for wrongdoing' that accompanies situations inadequately linked with practical social sanctions (Douglas, 2002, p. 165). Inherent structures of pollution thus operate in the background of culture to uphold its broader order, since they ef-fect a self-regulating punishment in which the 'transgressor is himself held to be the victim of his own act' (Douglas, 2002, p. 165).

Following this understanding of pollution, one could expect Dan and Ryan to be-lieve themselves to have committed some act of cultural contamination, some sym-bolic wrongdoing of 'joining' or 'separating' cultural categories and structures, the outcome of which is dangerous voices.[1] In this sense, the structuralist's analysis is not necessarily different in its observations from the voice-hearer's appraisal, as both seek to identify the social mores deemed sacred enough to have generated a sense of both profanation and penance. Ryan seems to view his unwillingness to follow through with suicide as a sort of weakness, asserting that the voices 'are there solely as punishment for not being strong enough to take my life . . . I need to right what I did wrong, so I need to, at some point, take my life'. It seems plausible that the weakness Ryan notes, as well as his embracing of the language of 'anomaly' and wrongdoing when describing himself, results from some intuited sense that to plan or anticipate suicide, but not follow through, is to embody ambiguity and to take up residence in precisely that obscure space between culture's clear moral codes and individual uncertainty. Dan's circumstances also entail a connection between hallucinatory experiences and suicide, with the onset of highly distressing visual phenomena coinciding with hospitalization following a suicide attempt. However, Dan's voices had started earlier. At age fourteen, in a particularly troubling episode, Dan was reading his Bible and reflecting on his sexual orientation when a 'deep man's voice . . . aggressive and very loud' began to shout 'that [Dan] was going to be stoned, that [he] was going to hell, that [he] was a terrible person'. Perhaps by contemplating sex and suicide, Dan and Ryan confronted two cultural ideas with deep histories and contested boundaries that, despite lacking clear and effective social sanctions, shoulder a great deal of burden in society's efforts to order and to classify itself.

Joining (Sex)

In his *The History of Sexuality*, Michel Foucault joins Douglas in positing a sociocultural space between explicitly punishable acts and their tacitly permissible expressions, pointing to homosexuality as a striking historical example (Foucault, 1978, p. 102). In fact, Douglas (2002, p. 194) also dedicates much of her analysis to a discussion of sexual norms, stating that 'pollution fears seem to cluster round contradictions involving sex'. She notes, for example, that for the Lele, men and women occupy distinct hostile spheres, and sexual contact is thus governed by strict rules—outside of these bounds, contact is contamination (Douglas, 2002, p. 188). With that in mind, it is significant that Dan and Ryan join with others in the VIP study who report sexual confusions, conflicts, and outright violations in relationship to their voices. For example, several participants report hallucinatory experiences following sexual assault or amidst pubescent struggles with sexual orientation and gender identity, the latter entailing aggressive voices that yell homophobic language.

---

[1] NB. Holt and Tickle found that the stigma of voice-hearing caused their participants to fear being labelled 'bad' by others. Here, the voice-hearer seems to perceive deviance from society's norms as being potentially iniquitous in some way.

Indeed, in the light of the pollution model, perhaps homosexuality may be seen as a notable example of the 'symbolic joining of that which should be separate', bringing danger and the fear of punishment as a marginalized individual navigating the mixed messages and insufficient symbols of heteronormativity (Douglas, 2002, p. 140). Dan, for example, reports voices coming as a punishment in the aftermath of considering his own sexual orientation—voices that told him he would be stoned to death like transgressors in the Bible. Even Ryan, whose experiences appear less conspicuously linked to ideas around sexuality, recounts one persistent voice that relies upon a predominant cultural–linguistic repertoire when calling Ryan 'a faggot' and using 'a lot of homophobic' terms to signal the weakness or shame of not taking his own life. This, Ryan insists, is deserved. It seems that in these instances, the notion that distressing voices have come as punishment serves to superimpose order/justice/logic on what is often a matter of contradiction and ambiguity in and between religious faith, family life, public perception, and the lived realities of twenty-first-century British culture.

Separating (Suicide)

As shown in the example of Ryan's homophobic voice above, culture is also implicated in the tensions and anxieties associated with suicide. Psychologist Menno Boldt highlights, 'No one who kills him or herself does so without reference to the prevailing normative standards, values and attitudes of the culture to which he or she belongs' (Boldt, qtd. in Colucci and Lester, 2013, p. 25). As we have seen, Dan and Ryan relate suicidal thoughts and suicide attempts to the onset or intensification of both voices and visions. For Ryan, who says of his voices, 'they're solely a punishment, they weren't around before I deserved punishment', the notion that something about him is anomalous serves to join the punishment with a sense of the self as a pollution: 'I tell every doctor that I'm . . . an anomaly, an accident, something that shouldn't be here anymore'.

Suicide researchers have argued that the meaning of mental illness within a given context is inseparable from the metaphors used to describe it (Colucci and Lester, 2013, p. 31). Perhaps Ryan's description of himself as an 'accident' and an 'anomaly' that is being punished for failing to take his own life is as much indicative of a cultural meaning assigned to suicide as it is of Ryan's depressive mood. It is certainly plausible to see in suicide a symbolic division of the self. Self-killing violates the usual categorical separation of victim and assailant, subverting cultural ideals of personal wholeness, self-preservation, and self-esteem while stretching the domain of individual sovereignty. In Ryan's case, however, those boundaries and ideals are being transgressed continuously, as he feels caught in a state of limbo between desiring the act and acting on the desire. His notion of punishment, then, comes not from actual self-separation, but from the disquieting sociocultural territory he inhabits as one who sees suicide as a responsibility, even a necessity, but who nevertheless resists subversive action. Thus, as one component of the complex explanatory narrative offered by voice-hearers like Ryan or Dan, suicide may represent a breaking or testing of crucial sociocultural structures that, along with the symbolic joining of sexuality, contributes to an ultimate sense of voices and visions as completely justified punishments.

Therapies of Purification: Some Concluding Thoughts

To understand one's voices as punishment is to experience them as punishment. The symbolic codes, social structures, preferred emotions, and plausible values of one's culture control, create, and contain experience—both as event and interpretation. The separations and unifications that help generate such an explanation are powerful organizers whose function reaches above and beyond individual appraisal to demand conformity lest critical categories be muddled. Fortunately, Douglas' model does not end there; ordering structures of pollution are accompanied not only by intrinsic notions of punishment, but also by frameworks of purification and efforts at restitution.

Handsome Lake's voices and visions eventually led to both his physical and social recovery, providing a meaningful message that redeemed his wrongdoing and set him on the path to great socio-religious reforms in his community. Recalling William James' observation that the 'completest' religions are those capable of putting 'pessimistic elements' in their proper place, Douglas (2002, p. 200) highlights the 'paradox' of pollution: 'the search for purity is . . . an attempt to force experience into logical categories of non-contradiction'. However, 'the facts of existence are a chaotic jumble', and the body is like a garden, since 'if all the weeds are removed, the soil is impoverished' (Douglas, 2002, p. 201). Purification, Douglas says, is the process by which the soil is enriched with the compost generated by those pulled weeds.

Insomuch as the body represents or encompasses culture, purification rituals afford the opportunity for somatically righting cultural wrongs through a transposition of power. Punishment may maintain a sense of cause and effect, but it is frequently deemed insufficient precisely because its premise of orderliness is incongruent with experience and its discomfiting potential may appear haphazard, rather than regulatory. Within ritual frameworks, however, power shifts from the offended structures to the polluting force itself, as the pollution is integrated into its own purifying process. Returning to the Lele, Douglas describes the way in which their food taboos illustrate this power inversion. Hybrid animals, such as flying squirrels, do not fit the tribe's taxonomies and are considered unclean. However, those same 'abominations' are precisely the animals taken to be 'powerful sources of fertility' prepared for consumption in initiation ceremonies (Douglas, 2002, p. 206).

To ritualize the ambiguous and unify distinctions in this way is to confront the ordering of reality with the inadequacy of its own structures, rendering existing categorical distinctions (sane/insane, clean/unclean, healthy/unhealthy) impotent. This, as Douglas highlights, requires a strong sense of individual agency operative within a safe ritual space. For voice-hearers like Dan and Ryan, this may also represent a hope of renewal. The same culture that bestowed a belief in punishment also possesses therapeutic frameworks intended to 'purify', or redeem, voices. Various forms of relating therapy—including voice dialogue and AVATAR therapy—function as comparable rituals in which the pollution (persecutory voices) is separated out, not, ultimately, as a source of distress or a consequence of transgression, but as a powerful force to be addressed directly and fitted into a new framework of meaning. This, too, requires a strong sense of agency and the safety of a supported space.

Indeed, although individual voice-hearers may feel powerless against formidable structures demanding penance, the very presence of their voices—of these so-called anomalies and abnormalities—betrays the insufficiency of those structures as well as the unfinished business of humanity's reflection on its own existence. Therapies of purification offer potential redress for the 'punishment' inflicted by culture's imperfections and possess the means/impetus to transform pollution into a purifying agent and to put the 'pessimistic elements' of mental health in their proper place.

References

Colucci, E., and Lester, D., eds. (2013). *Suicide and Culture: Understanding the Context*. Göttingen: Hogrefe Publishing.

Douglas, M. (2002 [1966]). *Purity and Danger: An Analysis of Concepts of Pollution and Taboo*. London: Routledge.

Fadden, R. (1955). The visions of Handsome Lake. *Pennsylvania History*, 22(4), 341–58.

Foucault, M. (1978). *The History of Sexuality*, Vol. 1. Translated from French by R. Hurley. New York, NY: Pantheon Books.

Holt, L., and Tickle, A. (2015). 'Opening the curtains': how do voice hearers make sense of their voices? *Psychiatric Rehabilitation Journal*, 38(3), 256–62.

Powell, A. (2017). The hearing voices movement as postmodern religion-making: meaning, power, sacralisation, identity. *Implicit Religion*, 20(2), 105–26.

Woods, A. (2011). Memoir and the diagnosis of schizophrenia: reflections on *The Center Cannot Hold, Me, Myself, and Them*, and the 'Crumbling Twin Pillars' of Kraepelinian psychiatry. *Mental Health Review Journal*, 16(3), 102–6.

Woods, A., and Wilkinson, S. (2017). Appraising appraisals: role of belief in psychotic experiences. *The Lancet Psychiatry*, 4, 891–2.

About the Author

Adam J. Powell is a Research Associate in the Institute for Medical Humanities and the Department of Theology and Religion at Durham University, as well as Director of Research at the Institute for Faith and Resilience. His work primarily explores identity formation, mental health, and spiritual experiences among minority religions. He is the author of *Hans Mol and the Sociology of Religion* and *Irenaeus, Joseph Smith, and God-Making Heresy*.

PART THREE

APPROACHING EXPERIENCE

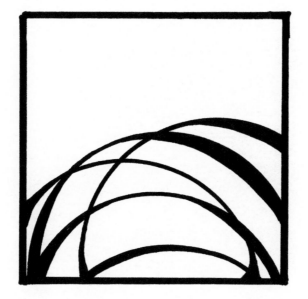

11

Voices in Psychosis

A Medieval Perspective

Hilary Powell, Department of English Studies, Durham University

Bringing the past into dialogue with the present is one of the central objectives of interdisciplinary scholars working in the medical humanities. But how do we strike up a conversation and, more importantly, how can we ensure that both sides hear and understand each other? For a scholar of medieval Latin, the gulf across which we speak is more than merely linguistic; we are separated by different frameworks of critical and epistemological thought. The invitation to respond, as a medievalist, to a collection of descriptive accounts of voice-hearing raises important questions not only about how interdisciplinary dialogues develop, but also about the perceived value of such conversations and to whom they might be valuable.

The collection comprises forty transcripts of phenomenological interviews conducted with users of Early Intervention in Psychosis services in the north of England. A medieval response to such reports might seem, at best, irrelevant and, at worst, a dangerous distortion of either medieval or modern experience. Yet the similarities between these transcripts and the stories found in medieval Latin hagiography are striking, and treated carefully, paying respect to their different cultural and historical contexts, the medieval parallels may open up new ways of thinking about the contemporary experience of hearing voices. Stories about the lives and miracles of saints were popular across the length and breadth of Christendom from the third century to the present day. My research focuses on texts written in Latin, in the British Isles, about British saints between the mid-eighth century and the end of the twelfth century. Over a hundred separate saints' lives and miracle collections have survived, with the average length in the region of 15,000 words. It is a large corpus and testifies to the significance of the genre. Hagiography was the major form of literary output during the eleventh and twelfth centuries, outstripping the production of historical and exegetical works, such as chronicles and biblical commentaries. The subjects of these hagiographical texts are largely male, and most feature an account of a period spent 'in the wilderness' when the saint lived alone either as a hermit or an anchorite, perfecting the art of prayer and enduring various feats of asceticism. Another hallmark of reclusion, however, was demonic temptation. Many of the texts contain accounts of the saints' clashes with 'Old Envier', the 'ancient foe', 'the deceiver', the devil,

Hilary Powell, *Voices in Psychosis* In: *Voices in Psychosis*. Edited by: Angela Woods, Ben Alderson-Day, and Charles Fernyhough, Oxford University Press. © Hilary Powell 2022. DOI: 10.1093/oso/9780192898388.003.0011

Satan himself. And it is in these accounts that we find the greatest overlap with the phenomenological accounts of psychotic episodes contained in the transcripts of the interviews conducted for the Voices in Psychosis study.

The interviews were conducted with people who had sought clinical help on account of hearing voices, but this was just one facet of their experience. Many of the voice-hearers interviewed also described a wide range of unusual visual, olfactory, and somaesthetic perceptions. At least two of the cohort of forty mention the smell of smoke, while several describe having difficulty breathing. Kate says it is as though there is a dead weight lying on her, choking the life out of her. Bill can feel his windpipe tightening and a burning sensation in his throat. Dan says he feels suffocated; he also describes feeling people holding onto his wrists. Menacing black shadows are often mentioned, watching, following, waiting. Dark silhouetted figures are glimpsed; for Yan, they are 'mooching through the window', while for Ian and Orla, they hover in doorways. Sean sees eerie black figures inching around the end of his bed. He says these figures are 'faceless', while Violet claims hers have 'holes for faces'. And nor are voices the only auditory components experienced. Dan hears crashes, explosions, people screaming, a heavy pounding. Gail describes having to 'tune in' to white noise. Other voice-hearers report hearing jumbled noises, knocks, clicks, echoes, and ringing. Leah describes it like a 'washer' or a 'tornado' that has picked up 'little bits and pieces' of people. Eric says something every similar, calling it a 'cacophony of like lots of bits of voices'. Bill describes his voice as a 'bark that speaks English', a sound no human can make.

The demonic foes plaguing the medieval recluses were described along similar lines. Godric, a twelfth-century hermit, saw demons emerge from the shadowy corners of his cell like pitch-black pygmies—they rose from the floor and burst through the cobbles. On another occasion, he saw two demons crouching at the foot of his bed (Reginald, 1845, pp. 104, 107, 164–5, 197, 225). Dunstan, two centuries earlier, saw a pitch-black shadow in the shape of a towering bear looming over him in a menacing way ('B', 2012, pp. 56–7). The somaesthetic experiences also exhibit close parallels—Bartholomew of Farne, a contemporary of Godric's, was almost asphyxiated as a demon entered his hermitage, seized him by the throat, and throttled him (Anon, 1882, p. 305), while a battery of ugly, disfigured demons bound the limbs of Guthlac, a mid-eighth-century hermit (Felix, 1985, pp. 102–3). The saints also heard non-human voices. Dunstan, like Bill, heard dogs barking, but Guthlac heard all sorts of animal voices—wolves howling, boars grunting, oxen lowing, and snakes hissing—not to mention the sounds of horses, stags, and ravens (Felix, 1985, pp. 114–17).

In Guthlac's case, the 'harsh and horrible shrieking' was designed to disturb or agitate the saint. Back in the twenty-first century, Sean persistently thought he overheard fraught and abusive arguments between the couple living in the flat above him and would turn up the TV in order to drown the couple out, becoming so agitated and threatened by the experience that he began to barricade himself in his flat and carry a knife. Voices are frequently intimidating and threaten physical injury: Alex's voices repeatedly tell him, 'we're going to kill you, we're going to beat you, break (?) your legs'. Medieval demons are no less menacing: the demons at Godric's bedside told him they'd come to cart him off to hell (Reginald, 1845, p. 311). Voice-hearers often accuse their voices of trying to draw their attention by whispering their name or talking about them very quietly in the third person. The devil employed similar tricks. An eleventh-century knight on his way to take monastic orders was stopped by the devil, who 'broke forth into a human cry at his side, uttering the words: "Cadulus, Cadulus, where are you going?" At these words the knight stopped, wishing to know who it was who had spoken', but there was no one there (Eadmer, 1962, pp. 42–3).

Being so sure that you have heard something that you go in search of it is a common experience among voice-hearers. Sean had the police visit the upstairs flat to confront the couple threatening him, only to find it was a taxi driver in his fifties, living alone. Dan and Alex persistently find themselves going to see if there's someone in the other room. Believing and acting upon the commands of her voices saw Leah give away all her belongings, board a train to London, and sleep rough for two weeks. She says that while having an episode, 'I can thoroughly believe that I'm being spoken to by archangels [Michael and Gabriel] and they're telling me to do something'. Matt's voices are even more dangerous; they tell him to stab people. Medieval demons did the same. Having pandered to his vanity and inflated his mind with arrogant thoughts, an evil spirit suggested to Beccel that if he were to kill his master Guthlac, he would inherit both the hermitage and the goodwill of kings and princes (Felix, 1985, pp. 110–13).

The voice-hearers often mention their voices exhorting them to self-harm. Ian's voice, a dark shadowy figure called Peter, tells him to hurt himself, to hang himself, to throw himself under a bus. In Eric's case, a woman urges him, albeit in soothing tones, to hurt himself, reassuring him that everything will be alright if he does. The medieval saints were also tormented by exhortations to extreme forms of asceticism—behaviours designed to mortify the body such as fasting or flagellation. In one instance, a devil pretending to be a hermit visited Godric at Finchale. He drew back his cloak to reveal putrid, ulcerous flesh, almost dissolving because of his punishing mortifications, and asked Godric, who stood appalled, to inspect his repulsive body. If Godric were a genuine hermit, boasted the imposter, he would be following his example (Reginald, 1845, pp. 164–5).

Voices and demons are presented as possessing the uncanny ability to seize on sensitive subjects. For Godric, it was his doubt about his performance as a hermit, while for Fred, it was his paranoia about his partner cheating on him. Fred persistently heard moaning and sexual noises while on the phone to his girlfriend, which made him so angry that he described this as a 'redness' building inside him. Barbed comments and ugly insults, meanwhile, are personally targeted. Bill's voice is often abusive. It swears at him, calls him names. Bill finds the insults 'humiliating' and 'disgusting'. Invited to elaborate on the specific words used, he replies, 'it sort of leans more towards my mental capability really', something he confesses he is 'still a little bit sensitive about'. Dan's voice targets his social and body image anxieties: 'you're pathetic, and you're so fat and disgusting and everyone hates you', 'you're such a pathetic failure'. Eric's voice victimizes him along similar lines: 'you're a shit human being, you need to lose weight', 'you're shit and you're fat'. Shit and fat are the taunts directed at Godric, over 800 years ago. 'You're no true hermit you fat peasant', jibed one demon, 'It's shit-heap you should be called not Godric! This Godric's the foulest peasant, the filthiest pigsty cleaner . . . you make a show of being holy but you're the most detestable of all humans'. Demons also jeered at his psalmody: 'Oi uncouth pile of shit! I know how psalms should be sung as well as you know how to croak them out with hisses!' (Reginald, 1845, pp. 234, 93). These remarks stung; the demons knew how to wound their medieval sufferers just as the voices exploit their voice-hearers' sensitivities.

The affective impact of the experience also bears striking similarities. The voice-hearers say it makes them feel worthless, angry, demotivated. Gail says it makes her doubt herself. It worsens their mental health: Alex overdosed in order to make the voices stop and excoriates—he picks at his face and scratches his skin with his nails. St Cuthbert saw a boy 'possessed' by a demon tearing at his skin, shouting and violently distressed (Anon, 1985, pp. 132–3), while Guthlac 'pierced with black venom' experienced despair, self-doubt, and extreme agitation (Felix, 1985, pp. 94–8).

There are clear correspondences between the phenomenological reports of psychotic experience related by early intervention service users and scenes of demonic temptation found in high medieval Latin hagiography. We cannot, of course, claim that the experiences are equivalent, only that the language used to describe these two experiences shows considerable and potentially interesting parallels. This point cannot be overemphasized. To suggest that voice-hearing and demonic temptation are connected in any way other than in the efforts made by sufferers to describe them far exceeds the available evidence. But the fact that we find such similarities is curious and justifies the comparison.

The congruity between these two experiences is not lost on voice-hearers; Bill says, 'It's definitely more demonic than anything else', and Leah talks about 'coughing up demons'. Several speak of an external malevolent force. Although uncomfortable with the word, Dan compares the experience to being 'possessed', 'like someone's put it [the voice] in my head'. Matt, whose voices tell him to stab people, says, 'people like directly come into my head'. Other voice-hearers recognize their personal agency. In speaking of hearing the voices of her grandmother and baby, Zara says, 'it's just me wanting to hear them'. Eric ascribes his voices to his 'overactive imagination', saying he needed 'a role model' and adding, 'Let's face it, they're a construct of my head'. But whether their preferred frame of interpretation is external or internal, their focus is firmly self-oriented. Eric chalked his voices up to *his* need to create a role model, a fault of *his* imagination. Bill, crediting his voice to an external agent, wonders why *he* was selected. The reasons, however construed, lie within them; that they are, in some way, personally at fault. Predictably enough, responsibility for coping with these voices is both individual and internalized. Bill dwells on how lonely it can be when you realize you're different from everyone else: 'you feel like a freak'. Sean, meanwhile, feels 'weak-minded' for hearing voices, as though he should have the mental strength to stand up to them but lacks it.

This personal dimension is markedly absent in the medieval material. Even when the experience occurs within the mind, the cause is external: the black venom which befouled Guthlac's mind came from a poisoned arrow of despair shot by the devil, the 'ancient foe of the human race' (Felix, 1985, pp. 94–5). According to the medieval Christian worldview, evil was an existent and operational force within the world. This not only provided a consistent explanation of external causation, but also removed any element of personal culpability. Since the devil was the 'foe of the *human race*', his attacks were indiscriminate; it was your fault only in the fact that you were human.

Early theorists of demonic operation believed that demons attacked humans by 'sprinkling harmful suggestions in us like grains of sand' (Cassian, 1997, p. 258). They were said to create imaginary visions which mingled with human thoughts and crowded out true sensory perceptions, leaving the human unable to distinguish between what was true and what was false. With one's judgemental capacity impaired, the mind fell into error—that is, sin—assenting to emotions (and ultimately behaviours) which, when in sound mind, it would normally reject. Demons induced humans to betray themselves by clouding their perception with false images, impairing their judgement and allowing those emotions 'concealed in the innermost recesses of the inner man' to be revealed, creating distance from God (Cassian, 1997, p. 258). Demons were haphazard in that they sprinkled all sorts of thoughts within us and then waited to see which hit the mark. As rejecting or assenting to thoughts was a matter of choice, an ethical decision, one was personally culpable. However, temptation was universal in that no human was exempt from demonic assault and there was no human who could not be tempted. John Cassian declared that it was 'impossible for the mind *not* to be troubled with thoughts . . . [for] no one, apart from Christ, our Lord and Saviour, has so stilled the wanderings of his mind . . . that he has never sinned' (Cassian, 1997, p. 799). All humans were tempted, and all humans sinned.

It is customary within the discipline of medieval history to see the protagonists of saints' lives as, well, saints, heroic figures conquering the forces of evil. But while we must not brush aside the trope of success, these texts are portraits of sinners, individuals plagued by demonic thoughts, whose perceptive powers are impaired and whose rational capacities are compromised. They are stories about endurance and suffering. Cuthbert was tortured by all manner of 'phantasmal temptations' who cast him headlong from a high rock and hurled stones as if to kill him. But although they never managed to mar his body by injury or his mind by fear, he never won a decisive victory. In his final days, alone and nursing a suppurating ulcer, he was persecuted by demons, and he said, 'as never before' (Bede, 1985, pp. 266–67). Saints' lives may be bravura examples of human fortitude, but they show the inherently human experience of living with demons. And, as Cuthbert demonstrates, living with demons was not the sign of someone being 'weak-minded' (as Sean puts it), but the very opposite. Far from being a 'freak' (to use Bill's term), the demonic sufferer was feted.

Let us return for a moment to the question of value and the perceived benefit of a dialogue between demonic suffering in the past and present-day psychotic experience. For some voice-hearers, learning that seemingly similar experiences were valorized and celebrated in the past may prove enriching and allow them to re-evaluate their relationship with their voices and their identity as voice-hearers. For others, this revelation may have little worth; it won't change their daily lives or transform their treatment. If this is the response of the medieval past to the phenomenological interviews of the present, how do we deflect the counter-response: 'Interesting . . . but so what?' How do we move beyond the superficial small talk of similarities and differences to a more satisfying and deeper engagement which can open up new perspectives and effect some real change?

For this to happen, we need total honesty, but, regrettably, the remoteness of the past often renders it inaccessible and opaque. The phenomenological interviews (represented here by the forty transcripts) were undertaken in one of the first large-scale, longitudinal studies seeking to gather empirical data about the qualia of voice-hearing, specifically in relation to psychotic experience. Open-ended questions by trained professionals encouraged the participants to dig deep to access and communicate in their own words the contents of their experience. The phenomenological interview, conducted without interruption, preconception, or judgement, remains one of the most robust methodologies for eliciting and examining lived experience. But it was not a research technique known in the Middle Ages.

While the medieval stories about demonic suffering claim to be bona fide accounts of veridical experience, they were rarely so. Authenticity was vouched for stories that were received at second-, third-, even fourth-hand. Godric's hagiographer Reginald took great pride in having Prior Roger as his source, a man who had met with, and spoken to, Godric and had even heard his confession. Few hagiographers were as lucky, but it is unlikely that they would have cared. Veracity was just a trope which belied the genre's carefully contrived and stylized nature. The stories of demonic suffering, like so many of the miracle narratives, exhibit evidence of formulaic pre-patterning in content, structure, and semantics. Among the animal voices designed to terrify Guthlac was a roaring lion, a howling wolf, and a hissing snake. Some 350 years later, an anchorite living in a cell on the Isle of Thanet was tormented in precisely the same way: a roaring lion, a howling wolf, and a hissing water-snake (Rollason, 1986, p. 208). It is impossible to know whether these similarities are the intentional result of intertextual borrowing or merely recurring habits of thought. An intermediate text, however, the Life of Oswald, appears to offer novelty on the same theme: bleating sheep, barking dogs, grunting pigs, and braying donkeys accompany a roaring lion (Byrhtferth, 2009, p. 48). Yet these animals are not without their own possible textual precursors. In this case, as the editors note, an early medieval text which circulated as Voces animantium featured the same animals speaking in the same voices.

These examples underscore the point that these stories of demonic suffering are not necessarily authentic accounts of lived experience, and reading them as though they were is misguided. Should their origins lie in veridical experience, that testimony is no longer recoverable, having been distorted by rhetoric, literary conventions, and audience expectations. Does this then make a mockery of our attempts to forge a dialogue between the past and the present? Should we bring our conversation to a close?

Although one side is speaking about veridical experience and the other most likely is not, there is, nevertheless, value still to be found in the conversation. Historicist readings of hagiography view the texts as historical *acts*, their significance lying in the political, cultural, and social circumstances of their production. Demonic stories exhibiting strong thematic and verbal affinities are dismissed as trite hagiographical filler, superfluous and secondary to the political content. But if we shift our perspective and view hagiography not as a historical *act*, but as a cultural *artefact*, we find new ways of reading these fictional, yet professedly truthful, stories. Foregrounding ideas of use and consumption turns the spotlight onto the communities who read them. Typically, these were tight-knit, closed communities of monks, whose lives revolved around obeying the monastic Rule and perfecting their spiritual practice. Saints' lives, if we recall, are not about saints, but tales with universal appeal and application. They are stories of spiritual struggle, of suffering and endurance. Written for an intimate audience of brethren, they held up a mirror to the monks' own experience, offering a reassuring, non-judgemental, and empathetic exploration of the perils and pitfalls of the spiritual life. They advised young monks of the sorts of experiences they might encounter—crises which would shake them to their very core and cause them to doubt their perception, their better judgement, and even themselves. Terrifying and overwhelming, these experiences were thought to potentially result in the monk feeling compelled to commit heinous acts of violence against himself and others, to behave in ways contrary to his self-interest, and to sin against God.

What these narratives show, however, is the normality of such experiences. Even the very best monks could suffer such afflictions. Experiencing demonic assaults was treated with compassion. Sufferers were encouraged to confide in older monks and to share the experience with younger members of the community (Reginald, 1845, pp. 357–8). Recovery was a collective responsibility, undertaken in a spirit of empathy and forgiveness, and in a mutual effort to further understanding. There are clear parallels here with contemporary approaches, particularly talking therapies and the groups set up through the Hearing Voices Network. The crucial difference, however, lies in group composition. Recovery groups are predicated on the premise that members share a similar experience. Stories about demonic suffering were shared among a far larger circle, beginning with the entire monastic communities and trickling down to the world at large. Demonic sufferers may have been few, but theirs was a tale which was heard and shared by many.

This brings us to an interesting point in our conversation. What would happen if the present embraced a more medieval approach by sharing the experiences of

voice-hearers more widely (i.e. beyond select groups of academics and the immediate voice-hearing networks)? And what if voice-hearers were listened to and
supported by all sectors of society? Such utopian thinking is not new. There are, of
course, plenty of mental health charities already working towards this goal of making
voice-hearing more visible in mainstream culture. But what this conversation has
done is to show how the past can validate and give greater voice to such approaches.
Sharing stories about demonic suffering may help patients with psychosis reconsider
their own experiences, but this only takes the conversation so far. Of far greater value
is what can be learnt about the processes and contexts through which these stories
were shared and the engagement of the wider community in their support and recovery. The response proffered by the medieval past is to ask how and with whom we
should be sharing our stories about voice-hearing in the present.

References

Anon (1882). *Vita Bartholomaei Farnensis.* In: T. Arnold, ed. *Symeonis Monachi Opera Omnia, Rolls
    Series.* 75(1). London, 295–325.
Anon (1985). *Vitae S. Cuthberti Anonymae.* In: B. Colgrave, ed. *Two Lives of Saint Cuthbert.*
    Cambridge: Cambridge University Press, pp. 60–139.
'B' (2012). *Vita S. Dunstani* by 'B'. In: M. Winterbottom and M. Lapidge, eds. *The Early Lives of St
    Dunstan.* Oxford: Clarendon Press, pp. 1–109.
Bede (1985). *Vita Sancti Cuthberti.* In: B. Colgrave, ed. *Two Lives of Saint Cuthbert.*
    Cambridge: Cambridge University Press, pp. 142–307.
Byrhtferth (2009). *Vita S. Oswaldi.* In: M. Lapidge, ed. *Byrhtferth of Ramsey, The Lives of St Oswald and
    St Ecgwine.* Oxford: Oxford University Press, pp. 1–203.
Cassian, J. (1997). *The Conferences.* Translated from Latin by B. O. P. Ramsey. New York,
    NY: Newman Press.
Eadmer (1962). *The Life of St Anselm, Archbishop of Canterbury by Eadmer.* Translated from Latin by R.
    W. Southern. Oxford: Clarendon Press.
Felix (1985). *Felix's Life of Saint Guthlac.* Translated from Latin by B. Colgrave. Cambridge: Cambridge
    University Press.
Reginald (1845). *Libellus de uita et miracula S. Godrici, heremitae de Finchale, auctore Reginaldo
    monacho Dunelmensi.* J. Stevenson, ed. London: J. Surtees Society Publications 20.
Rollason, D. W. (1986). Goscelin of Canterbury's account of the translation and miracles of St Mildrith
    (*BHL* 5961/4). *Mediaeval Studies,* 48, 139–210.

About the Author

Hilary Powell is a medievalist who has worked on several Wellcome-funded projects in the medical humanities, including Hearing the Voice. Her interests lie in
the intellectual and cultural praxis of monasticism, particularly the cognitive and
affective preparation for prayer. Her recent publications include essays exploring
daydreaming through the medieval trope of the demon and critical engage-
ments with the concept of mind-wandering as it is framed within the cognitive
neurosciences.

12

Conspiration in the Archive

Sense-Making and the Research Interview Methodology

Tehseen Noorani, Department of Anthropology, Durham University

Reading the archive of transcripts generated by the Voices in Psychosis (VIP) study, it is tempting to try to map the genesis, nature, navigation, and (self-)governance of voice-hearing experiences. Any findings thereby generated would be central to important ethical imperatives, such as believing people's testimonies and taking their experiences seriously. These are long-standing demands of those with lived experience of mental distress whose agency and experiences continue to be marginalized and denied. Yet the transcripts, which are rich and layered with cascading content slipping back and forth between experiential accounts and adverse life events, are resistant to 'phenomenological reductions' (Moustakas, 1994) that bracket away life events to reveal experiences in and of themselves. At the same time, reducing interviewee responses to ordered chronologies of life events that shape ongoing experiences, as one might in formulation approaches (Johnstone, 2017), requires simplifying what interviewees often express as confused or unknown. What other approaches might honour these transcripts as they are?

It is commonplace across the psychological sciences today to consider memory as more reconstruction than recollection, and thus, in delimited ways, to accept that interviewees are engaged in creative processes. In reading the transcripts, I wonder if and how participants are engaging in processes of recall shaped by their interaction with the interviewer and the context of the interview. Such an approach is useful for highlighting collaborative and relational aspects of the research process. It is also risky: focusing on the processes by which knowledge is always being (re)made has recently come under fire for seeding claims to 'post-truth' and a renewed relativism with political agendas (Kofman, 2018). What could it mean to mine this archive for insights without reducing what we find to the power of force or the force of power?

In what follows, I approach transcripts as tracing how interviewers and interviewees *conspire*—that is, learn to work together, and to breathe together, across the multiple divides that separate them. This is not to suggest that the interviews should have been conducted differently. Instead it is to suggest that the reporting of experiences here reveals something about *experiences of reporting*. In particular, it casts light upon interview methodologies that are keen to generate data and wider

Tehseen Noorani, *Conspiration in the Archive* In: *Voices in Psychosis*. Edited by: Angela Woods, Ben Alderson-Day, and Charles Fernyhough, Oxford University Press. © Tehseen Noorani 2022. DOI: 10.1093/oso/9780192898388.003.0012 contexts of scientific reductionism, stigma, and taboo. It is also to take insight from, and recapitulate, attempts at understanding psychosis or madness itself as a relational phenomenon (see Seikkula and Olson, 2003).

Therapeutic Conspirations

Conspirators must first learn to trust one another. The interviews reveal the building of trust and rapport through initial instructions, encouragements, reassurances, and recognition from the interviewer that the interviewees are engaged in a tricky and perhaps impossible labour. In response to Dan's apology that his descriptions may not make sense, the interviewer insists early on that 'none of this has to make sense', and 'we really appreciate you having a go at this'. Often the interviewee acknowledges—and the interviewer affirms—how hard it is to describe the experiences, further building trust:

BILL: It's quite hard to explain because I'm quite new at describing it to somebody
     else . . .
INTERVIEWER: Yeah, yeah! I can imagine it's hard to describe.
BILL: Yeah.

Such exchanges reveal both participant and interviewer seeking to be witnessed and witnessing each other. At times, we are also reminded that both the interviewer and interviewee are negotiating the possibility of voices being present who may be less than keen about the interview itself. Early on, for instance, Xander says of an angry male voice:

Xander: [R]ight now he's telling me to pick up one of them paintbrushes and just
                throw it at your head! (laughs)
Interviewer: OK!
Xander: Obviously I'm not going to but . . . (both laugh)

Soon after this, Xander introduces the interviewer to Roxy as a 'protector' voice. In the newly formed collective of the interviewee, their voices, and the interviewer, could we read Roxy as protecting not only Xander, but also the interviewer from the angry voice?

Trust and rapport are central to the process by which the interviewers, as also researchers, are seeking data from which to generate and refine their knowledge base of concepts and constructs. Yet all this must be done in the time span of standalone interviews. Exchanges risk being transactional, born not only of the restricted parameters of the encounter, but also of social mores urging agreement. Across the transcripts, we gain a sense of the interviewers resisting the temptation to find adequate data to populate pre-existing categories, starting with the presumed 'basics' of how many voices participants hear, when, why, and how they are heard, and who they may be or correspond to. The open-ended style of questions helps but is ultimately bound by expediency and politeness—two forces of conspiration that could be attenuated through more extended or iterated research methods (see Rabinow, 1977 for an example of such approaches in relation to ethnography).

Despite being a 'research study', and not a therapeutic intervention, the interviewees also appear to gain from conspiring. Not only do the interviews provide a framework for bearing witness, but the interviewees often appreciate the event of the interview itself, sometimes reporting having minimal social contact, including rarely leaving their homes. Moreover, in endeavouring to document the phenomenon of voice-hearing in its intimate experiential, contextual, and historical specificity, we can see moments where the interviewees' own understandings of their voice-hearing deepen. When Anthony is asked how he feels towards his voices, he remarks, 'I've never been asked that before actually.' When the interviewer notes to Gail in reference to her hearing the voices of bullies from her school days, 'I guess that you know maybe there might be things that link for you', the moment feels poignant, and Gail hesitates, appearing to vacillate between her already stated conclusion that the voices are the result of an isolated brain illness and a lurking suspicion, prompted by the dialogue, that they may connect with her past. Neil stops his interviewer mid-sentence at the beginning of their interview to ask whether telepathy is actually possible. At the end of their interview, Kate implores the interviewer to send her any information on research into voices being caused by allergic responses, hoping the interviewer might help her avoid hours of pointless Googling. And Bill is happy to say at the end of his interview that his answers will be important if they help others, promising to go away and study his voice and come back with more information at the one-year follow-up. Giving the lie to any clear-cut distinction between research study and therapeutic intervention, these interactions represent so many ways of finding and making meaning together.

In Search of Narrative

At the beginning of the interviews, the interviewers offer examples of what voice-hearing can be like:

> for some people [voices] might involve sound, for example, but for others it might feel like, just like someone or something's communicating with you. Ehm, some people have described them a bit like loud thoughts, other people have described them a bit like feeling like telepathy. (From interview with Emma)

As the interviews unfold, the interviewers regularly reiterate and summarize participant responses, seeking confirmation. We may expect what is discussed earlier on in interviews to shape later descriptions, but does this extend to the specifics of the voices being discussed? When Will explains that one of his voices Louise sounds 'old talking', his interviewer suggests that she may not be from this era. Will seems intrigued, remarking that he has never considered it before. Later, when asked what she wears, Will refers to a 'Victorian-y' petticoat dress.

Amidst a social expectation of coherence, some of the most layered narratives are generated around contradictions and confusions, elaborating, rather than resolving, them. Every time the interviewer is ready to pin down Alex's experience, he foregrounds awareness of his own paranoia and hence *double-awareness* (see Bleuler, 1950) about whether these are 'just' voices in his head, or whether a group of three acquaintances he had known for fifteen odd years and fell out with a month and a half ago have, in fact, put cameras in his house and perhaps even chipped him 'like a dog'. The mysteries deepen over the interview, as Alex explains that he and his wife have been getting threatening messages on social media—in which case how could it be all in his head?

Near the end of the interviews, the interviewees are asked why they think they are hearing voices. At first, many say that they don't know, but breathing into the silence, they begin to muse and therein to experiment. Are the questions then sparking speculations, inviting us to read in the transcripts the activity of phenomenological stabilization—what Karen Barad has called 'intra-action' (Barad, 2007)—within the interview space? Consistency across responses at different times in the interview—standardly an indication of how sure-footed recollections are—equally may indicate path dependencies, following where an open experimentation leads. If, then, we associate coherence in narratives with the veridical description of one's experiences, what space do we leave for spinning a really good yarn, in co-production with those one engages with? Leah's relationship to her voices is elusive to the interviewer, indicated by the confusions and apologies on behalf of the interviewer trying to get a handle on her experiences. Might we be inspired by her description of her voices as being 'in cahoots' with one another, to consider them as also approaching the interviewer the same way, improvisationally, inviting the interviewer into new co-productions? If so, even if we want to designate Leah's experience as an outlier, somehow more extreme than the rest, this may not imply that it is less phenomenologically stabilized.

Perhaps instead, Leah's interview reveals another enduring kind of experience for which the narrative-seeking research interview could be damaging, a failure to connect, a frustration of her desires to co-create in preference of a search for consistency that echoes the long-standing confessional technologies (Foucault, 1981) underpinning modern therapeutics. While the therapeutic effects of seeking narration may convince us that it is the fragmentary nature of things that makes them traumatizing, this ignores both the meaningfulness and the possibilities lying with the fragment (see Gumbs, 2018). That which is beyond language, or cannot faithfully be expressed in terms of language, requires being performed or otherwise indexed. Yan, for instance, uses imagery—'it's not 3D or anything ... like stained glass ... you know like you can look through stained glass can't you and stuff through the picture'—while

Anthony uses colours—'I do also have kind of flashes of colour as well, which I've never been able to figure out. . . . If I'm having a particularly kind of, what I'd say was anxious day, that's when the colours are a bit more kind of prominent, and they just blur out everything'. These more mysterious qualities of experience risk being hidden by the easy search for narrative (see Jones, 2018). With Leah, signs appear to be not causally connected, but image-driven. Towards the end of the interview, she summarizes how she knows when the voice of Michael is present: because 'it's like aliens'. The opacity of the referent matches the opacity of that which needs explicating, and the interviewer has to move on.

Looking for Absences

Studying those who hear voices requires a commitment to hearing what most of us usually cannot. Can we extend this ethos to how we approach the interview transcripts themselves? Speculating about backgrounded and excluded phenomena is necessarily risky. We might open ourselves to hearing things that aren't there—or at least, not in the way that we think they are.

Such phenomena include what is not asked about or disclosed, but somehow still marked in the transcripts. Many of the descriptions of the onset or changing activity of voices are spatially demarcated. Carl reports getting paranoid in public, which affects how distressing his voices are, while Gail describes having had a 'complete breakdown' in the supermarket. Jade's voices belong to criminals and police officers outside her house, threatening the integrity of her home, while Kate is troubled by voices from the alleyway behind the wall to which the television is affixed. Conversely, when Hugh goes to the doctor's surgery, the hospital, or the library, his voices stop. This is suggestive of an opportunity to learn about the role of space and the negative effects of stigma, which are usually considered secondary to the primary phenomena located 'within' the person. What gets ignored when we keep returning to focus on the relationship of voice-hearers and their voices, bolting on context as supplemental? And what would be the implications for research that centred the effects of libraries, hospitals, and doctor's surgeries on voices?

A second example of a conspicuous absence concerns that which threatens to destabilize the trust that enables the interview to proceed. In conspiring together, interviewer and interviewee must make implicit pacts about whether and how to sit within discomfort to maintain their connection and keep the interview going. What, then, of that which is considered taboo? While interviewers explicitly ask whether participants understand their voices in spiritual terms, the question packages it up with religion, and many interviewees respond only to the latter, saying that they are not religious. Some play off the idiom of 'I'm not religious but . . .', ending their responses by trailing off or even with a counter-question because, well, if others were to ask, 'what do you say to that?' (Kate). But turning the question back on the interviewer is not going to lead anywhere in this style of interviewing, where priming would be a reason to invalidate participant responses. It might be better understood as the sharing of a public secret: that to believe in spirituality is to risk looking like a 'fruit loop' (Kate).

And yet spiritual tropes abound. For example, when Xander is asked if his experiences are religious or spiritual in some way, he responds only that they are not religious. Later in his interview, he describes a curious special skill he has, arising at dusk when walking along the road, to float above the road as the cars pass by under him. He then immediately dismisses it, saying, 'I don't know why that would be a special ability, it just sounds idiotic!' (laughs), and the interviewer moves on. Yan initially responds in the same way as Xander, saying, 'I'm not really religious or . . . anything like that', but later notes how people can act as a phone mast, and of broader affinities between the spiritual and the technological, evoking the notion of the individual's brain as a receiver, rather than a generator, of consciousness:

YAN: Everyone's like a phone mast aren't they, sort of . . . you know if you grab your phone, the signal goes up, doesn't it?
INTERVIEWER: Yeah.
YAN: Because it starts using you, so . . . it just doesn't seem that improbable that everybody could be like a . . . sort of phone.
INTERVIEWER: Yeah.
YAN: You know and you can just tap straight into their head if you had the right number.
INTERVIEWER: The right tech, yeah.
YAN: Yeah.
INTERVIEWER: And was that . . . around when it [your voices] started when you were thinking about that? Or is that, so you're still kind of wondering about that as a possibility now or . . .?
YAN: Oh I'm still wondering about that.

Despite all denying that they are spiritual, Gail says that she has a feeling that the voices are watching her and wanting to punish her for something she doesn't know about; Orla's main voice can predict the future which 'freaks us out a little bit', and, as noted above, Neil wonders throughout the interview whether telepathy is possible. Are we to understand these as all merely rhetorical statements? Interviewer and interviewee conspire, wandering past tunnels that they seem to agree are better left unexplored.

Conclusion

Embracing the interviews as events in their own right, my overarching objective has been to highlight how we can approach the gathering of data about voice-hearing as an active, creative, co-produced, and socially situated enterprise whose endurance must constantly be renegotiated. This analysis troubles several common assumptions about the interview format: that it transparently represents what knowers know, that knowledge about the self is straightforwardly accessible, and that the continuity of experience is recalled, rather than worked out together.

References

Barad, K. (2007). *Meeting the Universe Halfway: Quantum Physics and the Entanglement of Matter and Meaning*. Durham, NC: Duke University Press.

Foucault, M. (1981). *The History of Sexuality, Volume 1: The Will to Knowledge*. London: Penguin.

Gumbs, A. P. (2018). *M Archive: After the End of the World*. Durham, NC: Duke University Press.

Johnstone, L. (2017). Psychological formulation as an alternative to psychiatric diagnosis. *Journal of Humanistic Psychology*, 58(1), 30–46.

Jones, N. (2018). Powers and seductions of personification. In: N. Jones. *Personification Across Disciplines*. https://vimeo.com/296837250 (accessed 10 October 2020).

Kofman, A. (2018). Bruno Latour, the post-truth philosopher, mounts a defense of science. *New York Times Magazine*. https://www.nytimes.com/2018/10/25/magazine/bruno-latour-post-truth-philosopher-science.html (accessed 10 October 2020).

Moustakas, C. E. (1994). *Phenomenological Research Methods*. Thousand Oaks, CA: Sage Publications, Inc.

Rabinow, P. (1977). *Reflections on Fieldwork in Morocco*. London: University of California Press.

Seikkula, J., and Olson, M. E. (2003). The open dialogue approach to acute psychosis: its poetics and micropolitics. *Family Process*, 42(3), 403–18.

About the Author

Tehseen Noorani is a Senior Lecturer in clinical and community psychology at the University of East London. His research focuses on the resurgence of psychedelic science in the West and its implications for understandings of psychopathology, psychiatry, and mental health care. He was a lead organizer of the 2021 conference *Psychedelics, Madness, & Awakening: Harm Reduction and Future Visions*, accessible at: http://www.psychedelicsmadnessawakening.com.

13

Reading for Departure

Narrative Theory and Phenomenological Interviews on Hallucinations

Marco Bernini, Department of English Studies, Durham University

Within psychology, phenomenology, and philosophy of mind, the term 'mindreading' is used to describe a variety of cognitive processes we deploy to make sense of other people's minds via outer behaviours. This process, however, has little to do with the proper act of reading. Although some recent work in psychology and cognitive narratology suggests that reading literature might help train our mindreading skills, real people differ from literary characters in important ways: they are embodied and largely concealed subjectivities, and their minds are not transparently readable in the same way most fictional minds are. Mindreading in the sciences rather stands for a broader, primarily non-linguistic and multimodal interpretive activity. As such, scientific literature on social cognition has resisted borrowing from narrative theory and cognitive literary studies concepts or frameworks used to analyse the activity of reading narrative artefacts, fictional minds, and literary storyworlds.

Written reports of phenomenological interviews, on the other hand, are proper, albeit peculiar, texts about real minds. Actually, we can say that mindreading and the reading of reported minds are almost complementary processes. The reason for which we need phenomenological interviews (i.e. reading minds), in fact, is partly to compensate for the outer inaccessibility (i.e. mindreading) of some phenomenological states or experiences. This compensatory need becomes even more acute with hallucinatory experiences such as hearing voices or feeling shadowy or diaphanous presences, because here the intersubjective anchor of a shared outer reality between the feeling subject and the mindreading interpreter risks getting rickety, misty, or lost.

Within the psychological and social sciences, written reports such as these are mostly analysed to identify patterns that could fit a model or coded for quantitative or qualitative analysis, rather than treated as (more or less narrative) texts to be read. Drawing narrative theory into conversation with scientific understandings of hallucinatory experiences, this essay will consider instead a set of problems in the readerly dimension of phenomenological interviews. What kind of interpretive dispositions do we, as readers, bring to these qualitative reports? How can narrative theory help illuminate our relationship to forms of storytelling which often seem to

Marco Bernini, *Reading for Departure* In: *Voices in Psychosis*. Edited by: Angela Woods, Ben Alderson-Day, and Charles Fernyhough, Oxford University Press. © Marco Bernini 2022. DOI: 10.1093/oso/9780192898388.003.0013 surface out of confused or inconsistent pre-verbal and pre-narrative experiences? What kind of active, yet tensive, relation exists between the background world of readers and the reported world of the voice-hearer? What is the readerly role played by the interviewing frame in shielding us from, or ushering us into, the storyworld (e.g. the world emerging out of the reporting activity) of the voice-hearer? Adapting key concepts from classic and post-classic narrative theory, this chapter sets out a novel interdisciplinary approach to phenomenological interviews on hallucinations. As well as arguing that the narratological toolbox can help us understand the interpretive dynamics underlying the reading of interview transcripts (reading minds), it will suggest that a readerly conceptualization of phenomenological interviews might have something to offer back to our direct encounters in the intersubjective, embodied, and non-textual social world (mindreading).

When examining the textual structure of the transcripts of phenomenological interviews, we might first want to consider the function of the interviewing frame. If we think of these transcripts as nested narrative architectures, the interviewing threshold would be the first narrative level we encounter, with the interviewer and the interviewee facing each other on the doorstep of the interviewee's story and storyworld that is about to emerge or be disclosed. The classic narratological concepts of 'frame narrative' and 'narrative embedding' capture some important aspects of this threshold zone and its ontological and functional relationship with the voice-hearer's reported world. In narratology, a narrative frame is usually a shorter narrative prelude or ancillary scaffolding (level 1) which serves to introduce the main reported events of a story (the embedded narrative on level 2). Narrative frames are part of the stereotypical conventions of artefactual storytelling, and they have been modulated according to different historical periods, genres, or media (e.g. Boccaccio's *Decameron*, Henry James' *The Turn of the Screw*, Woody Allen's *Melinda and Melinda*, and David Lynch's *Inland Empire*). Joseph Conrad's *Heart of Darkness*, for instance, is a standard example of how a narrative frame is usually constituted by characters talking to each other (here on a boat on the Thames), followed by one of them beginning to talk about a more or less distant past (the embedded, primary narrative of Marlowe's journey in colonial Congo), then circularly returning back to the initial framing situation at the end of the novel.

Phenomenological interviews have their own framing conventions. Each of the phenomenological interviews in the Voices in Psychosis (VIP) study begins with small variations on the same formulaic introduction to what is about to take place ('For this interview I'm going to be asking some questions . . .'; 'Quite a few questions are going to be about hearing voices . . .'; 'People sometimes worry about this topic, do you have any concerns, is it OK to ask some questions about it?'). However, even when the interviewing frame gradually starts to fall into the background as the first experiential windows open onto the interviewee's storyworld, it never becomes entirely marginalized or forgotten (as it does, for instance, in Conrad's novel). This is quite unlike artefactual frame narratives. As Monika Fludernik points out, 'usually in the setting of a frame narrative the framing primary story is quite marginal in relation to the embedded story, which takes up most of the text. Hence, indeed, the term *frame* narration, since the framing situation of storytelling merely serves to bracket the "real" story and mirrors the reader's gradual access to the story proper' (Fludernik, 1996, p. 257). By contrast, the interviewing frame stands in a constant, resilient, and recursive tension with the storyworld of the interviewee.

For interviews about unusual or hallucinatory experiences, this tension can be perceived by the reader as ontological (that is, related to the nature, laws, possibilities, and impossibilities of a world). Through the answers of the interviewee in the conversational frame, we access a world that is rife with impossible or unnatural events (more on this soon), a world that departs in many fundamental aspects from our own. The role of the interviewer in this respect is manifold. While working within the frame as the prompter for guided introspection, constantly trying to unlatch new experiential windows by moving the interviewee's retrospective attention to different phenomenological nuances of their storyworld (the embedded world), the interviewer is also the implicit bearer of a non-hallucinatory perceptual worldview to which we recursively align as readers (in the framing world). Far from being forgotten or marginalized, the interviewing frame is a world we are continuously brought back to by the interviewer (even by neutral phatic signals such as a 'Yeah'), after briefer or longer immersions into an embedded world often logically and ontologically remote from ours. It is with a hybrid sense of comfort and disruption that our readerly mind keeps its feet anchored in what we consider to be the real parameters of perception and cognition. To understand the relationship between the world of the frame (the interviewer's and reader's) and the hallucinated world of the interviewee therefore means to understand our inclination to share or to resist experiences that depart from our own in some radical way.

Once again, narrative theory might help us reflect on what kind of disposition we bring when moving between the world of the frame and the perceptually and informationally more noisy world of the interviewee. In literary narratives, the textual presentation of a storyworld is always incomplete, yet our mind makes a lot of conscious and unconscious inferences to compensate for these gaps. For example, even if a text does not tell us that the law of gravity is present or that human beings are made of flesh and breathe air, unless told otherwise, we assume this to be the case. This readerly principle, which spares a lot of cognitive effort for both writers and readers, is what Marie-Laure Ryan has called the 'principle of minimal departure', an inferential disposition which 'enjoins readers to construct fictional worlds as the closest possible to their model of reality, amending this model only when it is overruled by the text' (Ryan, 2012, p. 376). When facing the embedded storyworld disclosed by voice-hearers, we similarly bring a model of our own world to guide our inferences. From the outset of many of the interviews, however, we face the need to depart from this model to accommodate events and perceptions that, in our own world, would be logically and ontologically impossible. Even the simpler reports of voices heard in the absence of any embodied speaker require an update of our model of reality, towards an experiential recentring in the new possibilities offered by the interviewee's storyworld. For instance, when Dan, one of the VIP participants, tells us that 'sometimes it sounds like it's somebody maybe within the same room as me, or sat next to me, but when I look around it's like they are not there, but I swear like I can hear it', we are now accommodating the possibility that, in the voice-hearer's world, voices that feel physically present can nonetheless be disembodied.

One of the key factors that makes phenomenological interviews challenging reading experiences is that this kind of updating of a reality model keeps happening all the time, in a constant renewal of possibilities and perceptual events which, for many of us, does not fit our own everyday experiences of the world. In addition, in spite of some internal consistencies within a single interview and storyworld (e.g. recurring religious or personified voices or visions), there is a high degree of variation across the forty transcripts. In some of these embedded worlds, there are talking animals (e.g. Olivia describes a mouse toy that 'I've had that since I was a little kid and I used to call her Mrs Mouse, and she's got a really soft, calming voice'), in others religious presences and visions (e.g. the Archangel Michael in Leah's storyworld); some of them have guiding disembodied voices, others tormenting, many both. Each readerly plunge into all of these embedded worlds, however, requires a significant departure from what is for many people a standard model of reality. How does our mind negotiate these impossible storyworlds? Turning to narratology, we can conceptualize and critically evaluate further these dynamic readerly adjustments.

If the embedded hallucinatory storyworlds of the interviewees were artefactual creations, in fact, they would be the objects of a recent branch of narratology called 'unnatural narratology', which deals with 'physically, logically, or humanly impossible scenarios and events. That is to say, the represented scenarios or events have to be impossible according to the known laws governing the physical world, accepted principles of logic (such as the principle of non-contradiction), or standard human limitations of knowledge or ability' (Alber et al., 2013, p. 102). A central contribution of unnatural narratology is to have reflected on the strategies whereby we 'naturalize' such impossible storyworlds in order to make sense of, or reduce, their strangeness. The concept of 'naturalization' originally comes from narrative theorist Jonathan Culler, who coined it to describe how readers tend to tame unfamiliar or impossible elements in a storyworld because 'the strange . . . must be recuperated or naturalized, brought within our ken, if we do not want to remain gaping before monumental inscriptions' (Culler, 1975, p. 134). Because they abound in unusual experiences that depart from shared models of reality, the VIP interviews therefore radically call for readerly naturalization.

Take, for example, Olivia talking about the occurrence of unnaturally disembodied voices which destabilize her environment and transform people into shadows ('it looks like the room's shaking or people can be shadowed out when

I start hallucinating'), or Leah's reporting of voice-hearing experiences accompanied by the vision of a huge wing protecting her on the quayside (a 'massive like black . . . like eagle wing or something like that, it was absolutely huge. And it kinda came round the side of us like that, and kinda . . . as if it kinda hugged us'). Within the available naturalizing strategies proposed by unnatural narratology, such hallucinatory events might be familiarized by what Jan Alber calls 'subjectification' (Alber, 2012, p. 377; for a similar concept, see Ryan's idea of 'mentalism', 2012) or 'reading as internal states', whereby we attribute these impossible elements to an altered state of mind. As Alber puts it, through subjectification 'some impossible elements can simply be explained as parts of internal states (of characters or narrators) such as dreams, fantasies, visions, or hallucinations. This reading strategy is the only one that actually *naturalizes* the unnatural insofar as it reveals the ostensibly impossible to be something entirely natural, namely nothing but an element of somebody's interiority' (Alber, 2016, p. 51). In other words, naturalization of hallucinatory states works against the feeling of departure, so that instead of having to postulate a different world where unnatural events are actually possible, we can treat hallucinatory experiences as happening in the world as we know it, where it is indeed possible that someone is *just* hallucinating.

Even literary storyworlds, however, sometimes resist this interpretive strategy (e.g. Beckett's or Agota Kristof's trilogies) because of an unresolved ontological ambiguity between a single world (with perceptual and physical laws that only some characters might perceive as altered) and what Ryan has called the 'many-worlds' (Ryan, 2012, p. 377) readerly disposition (i.e. accepting multiple possible realities as overlapping or being compossible). To say that the VIP interviews are entirely 'natural' (in a narratological sense) experiences in/of a single world, because they reflect someone's interior altered states, however, is a far less innocent manoeuvre than naturalizing ambiguities or uncertainty in literary impossible storyworlds, no matter how much it facilitates our illusion of understanding. If we want to understand the experiential qualities of hallucinatory or unusual states (or become better aware of the difficulty of so doing), in fact, there might be good reasons to reject a unified view of a single world shared between the interviewer (or reader) and the interviewees in favour of a pluralistic approach where the feeling of departure into unexplored new worlds should not be abandoned or disavowed.

Similarly to naturalization of impossible storyworlds, the subjectification of the interviewees' experiences (i.e. impossible worlds are still impossible, but what is possible is that they are hallucinating an altered reality) is intended mainly to reduce the unnatural to the natural, transforming a possible clash of worlds into a categorizing harmony (i.e. in the only possible world, I consent to believe there can be people hallucinating). In the clinical domain, we can think of naturalization by subjectification as the instrument of diagnosis, and diagnostic manuals as the sediment of diachronic naturalizing processes. While this might be a valuable, even necessary heuristic tool for clinical treatment, the purpose of phenomenological interviews is rather to access what is like for a subject to live in *their* world (the only world they know or come to know). A diagnostic naturalization of unnatural states or events is therefore opposed to an openness to radical phenomenological departures. The former needs to preserve a single world to be operationally effective, but the latter equally needs to resist categorization to allow a maximum of experiential displacement into another person's reality, outside of the reassuring threshold of the interviewing frame. Regardless of our need to accommodate alien experiences in the only world in which we end up living, feeling, perceiving, and thinking, this reduces the experiential import of phenomenological windows into other worlds (worlds *felt* as possible and as other) and the significant efforts made by the interviewees to keep them open.

Traces of the tension between (and of the will to bridge) two different worlds are painstakingly evident in the voice-hearers' hypertrophic use of analogical or metaphorical connectors such as 'it's like', 'as if', 'sort of', or 'kinda'. In narratological terms, these clauses can be considered as introducing what Dorrit Cohn has called 'psycho-analogies' (Cohn, 1978, pp. 41–4): analogical images that either a narrator or a character uses to approximate mental experiences that elude linguistic or narrative reports (e.g. Musil's 'the world was as pleasantly cool as a bed in which one stays behind alone' (qtd. in Cohn, 1978, p. 42)). Psycho-analogies are common currency in literature and even everyday conversations whenever there is a need to share mental experiences with someone else, and are among the linguistic devices used to open a bridge between different experiential realities. The ubiquitous, iterative presence of psycho-analogical formulas in the VIP interviews signals the opacity felt by the interviewees when it comes to sharing those experiences, as if the analogical mode were the only oblique scalpel available to penetrate retrospectively into the leaden surface of non-linguistic, highly sensorial, and unnatural events. In this respect, psycho-analogies are tentative bridges between people sharing inaccessible or distant experiences (here the interviewer's and the interviewee's experiential worlds). On the other hand, however, we can never be entirely sure whether the analogical correlative is entirely metaphorical, or rather some actual experiential event that happened in the interviewee's 'impossible' world (where impossibility, however, is a quality projected by interpreters, not felt by the subjects).

Take, for instance, Leah's report of hallucinatory events feeling to her like a magnetizing tornado ('So me own voices and the things that I thought other people around us, their little bits and pieces, and that went into a cycle. Like a tornado, you know, when it picks stuff up like this?'). As readers, we cannot be sure whether Leah is referring to feeling *as if* voices picking up the contents of their emissions from several external and internal sources, or whether the experience is phenomenologically closer to an *actual* tornado (e.g. with noise, strong wind, a felt threat of possible physical injuries, and so on). If we take the naturalizing option of subjectivizing this report as an altered mental state, we might be more inclined to make fewer efforts to explore these phenomenological ambiguities as possible actual experiences of an unfamiliar world. We might just end up reading this as the strange event of a hallucinating mind in an otherwise natural world. By contrast, if we resist this naturalizing temptation, we are forced to simulate what would be like to live in a world where suddenly disembodied voices take on the shape, strength, and unpredictable behaviours of hurricanes, physically threatening to carry us away.

Following Caracciolo's model of reading fictional consciousnesses as a complementary mixture of attribution of states from the outside of a character's viewpoint (which he calls 'consciousness-attribution') and the inner enacting of their experiences (which he calls 'consciousness-enactment') (Caracciolo, 2014, pp. 115–32), we can think of our readerly options with phenomenological interviews as an interpretive crossing. If we are content simply to *attribute* hallucinatory events to mental malfunctioning (via subjectification), we will end up with a diagnostic distance that integrates the unnatural into our world. If, instead, we are open to *enacted immersions* into the interviewees' worlds of new possibilities and experiential qualities (via departure), we might get challenged by the unfamiliar, thus getting closer to a reality where multiple worlds might be the norm. Only then might we realize how these worlds can be immersively explored or defended, even at the cost of getting lost in the unknown (a feeling that people with hallucinations are experientially forced to endure themselves).

Even if we are willing to undertake enactive departures into hallucinatory worlds, however, the risk of naturalizing egocentric biases are not easily dispelled. As Monika Fludernik persuasively argues, we tend to process unnatural storyworlds by simply concocting a blending or alteration of our cognitive parameters of reality with the different, diminished, or augmented versions proposed by the text (Fludernik, 2010). For instance, if we read Olivia's statement that hearing voices 'feels like you're driving in your car, by yourself and then somehow two people have just got in the back', we might resort to, and then just blend, our experience of being alone in a car driving with that of being in a car with people talking in the back. This blending might allow us to simulate an enactive experience of this hallucinatory event. However, it would still be far too close to our model of reality because we never experienced what it was like to undergo this experience as an actual perception in a world where such things become possible, even likely, events. Enacting by blending could be a starting point, but we need to be aware of the radical departure that these phenomenologically distant worlds are calling us to perform.

As is evident from the very unfortunate conceptual baggage of words such as 'disability' or 'illness', we tend to prepare our encounters with sufferers in terms of a diminished version of what we know. In his foundational article on the difficulty of accessing experiences other than our own, Thomas Nagel famously took the radically distant example of a bat to show how objective scientific knowledge of another being's cognitive apparatus (sonar and echolocation) will not give us subjective, phenomenological knowledge of what it is like to be a bat (Nagel, 1974). In his article, Nagel hints at how inter-species phenomenological bridges might be just as difficult as interpersonal ones, because whenever someone tries to enter another person's worldview, they are 'restricted to the resources of [their] own mind, and those resources are inadequate to the task. I cannot perform it either by imagining additions to my present experience, or by imagining segments gradually subtracted from it, or by imagining some combination of additions, subtractions, and modification' (Nagel, 1974, p. 439).

Narrative theorists, however, are likely right in suggesting that subtracting or blending are the key strategies we deploy when, as readers, we face impossible storyworlds such as the ones hosting hallucinatory events. Reflecting on our naturalizing inclinations as readers of mind (on paper), though, might change our attitude also as mindreaders in our social encounters (in life, both with sufferers living in different worlds and with others in general as experiential bearers of individual worldviews). Phenomenological interviews are precious texts in this respect. They can become pedagogical tools teaching us an interpretive stance that I would call a 'reading for departure': or how to resist intuitive naturalization of unfamiliar experiences so as to be open to a pluralistic view of the human ecosystem as a rich multitude of many worlds, each with its own idiosyncratic and original possibilities or impossibilities. We might also discover that, by radically departing from what we know, we might end up recognizing (experientially, rather than diagnostically) elements of the unnatural in us. This is within the scope of the ongoing quest in psychology for a phenomenological continuum between clinical and non-clinical experiences (e.g. Alderson-Day et al., 2017). This continuum, however, should not conceal ontological gaps (gaps lived as ontological); it should rather foster an acceptance of gaping before monumentally complex inscriptions that we should not translate, but actively experience as powerfully challenging our phenomenological alphabet.

References

Alber, J. (2016). *Unnatural Narrative: Impossible Worlds in Fiction and Drama*. London: University of Nebraska Press.

Alber, J., Iversen, S., Nielsen, H. S., and Richardson, B. (2013). What really is unnatural narratology? *Story Worlds: A Journal of Narrative Studies*, 5(1), 101–18.

Alderson-Day, B., Lima, C. F., Evans, S., Krishnan, S., Shanmugalingam, P., Fernyhough, C., and Scott, S. K. (2017). Distinct processing of ambiguous speech in people with non-clinical auditory verbal hallucinations. *Brain*, 140(9), 2475–89.

Caracciolo, M. (2014). *The Experientiality of Narrative: An Enactivist Approach*. Berlin: De Gruyter.

Cohn, D. C., and Cohn, D. (1978). *Transparent Minds: Narrative Modes for Presenting Consciousness in Fiction*. Princeton, NJ: Princeton University Press.

Culler, J. (1975). *Structuralist Poetics: Structuralism, Linguistics and the Study of Literature*. New York, NY: Routledge.

Fludernik, M. (1996). *Towards a 'Natural' Narratology*. London: Routledge.

Fludernik, M. (2010). Naturalizing the unnatural: a view from blending theory. *Journal of Literary Semantics*, 39(1), 1–21.

Nagel, T. (1974). What is it like to be a bat? *The Philosophical Review*, 83(4), 435–50.

Ryan, M. (2012). Impossible worlds. In: J. Bray, A. Gibbons, and B. McHale, eds. *The Routledge Companion to Experimental Literature*. New York, NY: Routledge, pp. 368–79.

About the Author

Marco Bernini is Assistant Professor in Cognitive Literary Studies at Durham University and formerly a Hearing the Voice Postdoctoral Research Fellow. A narratologist interested in literature and cognition—notably the narrative representation of consciousness and altered, liminal, or opaque mental states—his monograph on Samuel Beckett *Mind, Models, and Exploratory Narratives* is forthcoming with Oxford University Press in 2021.

14

Relating to Leah's Voices

Angela Woods, Institute for Medical Humanities and Department of English Studies, Durham University

2017. Two people are speaking in a hostel in the North of England:

INTERVIEWER: [C]ould you try to describe to me some of the voice or voice-like experiences you've had recently?
LEAH: Do you want actual examples or do you want a summary?
INTERVIEWER: Ehm, a bit of both. Maybe start with a summary and give me some examples.
LEAH: Ehm . . . I hear ehm actual people's voices.
INTERVIEWER: OK.
LEAH: Or things that I deem to be specific people.

Many things are established within the first few seconds of this conversation: an acknowledgement of the challenges ('try to describe') of articulating, identifying, and categorizing voices ('or voice-like experiences'); recognition that there are choices to be made in their representation ('actual examples' or 'a summary'); and a sense that difficulties arising in the register of communication might reflect underlying ambiguities within experience itself. Is the distinction between hearing 'actual people's voices' and 'things that I deem to be specific people' one of identity or ontology? Is it a question of who these people are, or a question of whether they are people at all?

* * *

1907. The patients of an esteemed psychiatrist report hearing (Kraepelin, 1981):

'resonant voices', 'organ voices', 'voices of conscience', 'voices which do not speak with words', 'false voices', 'abortive voices', an 'inner feeling in the soul', an 'inward voice in the thoughts', voices 'between hearing and foreboding', 'the brain talk', 'voices in the whole body', 'murmurings and natural spirit-voices', 'underground voices from the air', 'whispering voices from the whole of mankind', 'voices of spirits which are quite near', 'telephone gossip', 'good voices', 'double speech', the 'voice trial', an 'apparatus for reading thoughts'.

Angela Woods, *Relating to Leah's Voices* In: *Voices in Psychosis*. Edited by: Angela Woods, Ben Alderson-Day, and Charles Fernyhough, Oxford University Press. © Angela Woods 2022. DOI: 10.1093/oso/9780192898388.003.0014

These statements offer tantalizing insights into the spatiality of voices: voices which are at once of the earth and of the air, ethereal, outside but close by; voices which come from an affective and spiritual interior; and voices which are robustly corporeal—lodged in the organs, permeating the whole of the body, emanating from the brain. Extended cognition is materialized in the voice as invasive prosthesis, surveying from without the sovereign space of the mind, and in the voices that crackle with the electric chatter of telephone gossip. While some voices speak softly and of great mysteries, others speak without words at all, and others still play out the dramas and dynamics of judgement: good, false, and abortive voices; the weightiness, repetition (or is it duplicity?) of 'double speech'; the voices of conscience raising the question of who or what is on trial.

Anonymized and unattributed, yet preserved for posterity in one of the most influential textbooks of clinical psychiatry, these quotations direct our attention to embodied metaphor, affective resonance, and relational consequence. Voices here have an agency in and beyond the psyche: they address, judge, mock, and talk among themselves; they construe a subject, interpolating the voice-hearer as seer, scoundrel, patient, saint. From their vantage point, contemporary accounts of auditory verbal hallucination—as the false perception of auditory stimulus—can only seem flat and narrow.

* * *

2017. Leah's description of the voices she hears builds in layers over the course of the interview. She hears the Archangel Michael and knows that Gabriel, too, is present, even though he does not speak and she has not seen him. She hears the voices of three lads and one woman with whom she used to be close, her grandmother, who recently died, and the tormenting voice of a long-dead uncle. She hears Loki, a black angel, who was sent to her by a gypsy. Coming from the realms of the living and the dead, of the intimate and the celestial, these voices are distinctive in their speech, tone, manner, and mode of appearance. Yet they are also so difficult to parse that the simple question of how many voices Leah hears is returned to five separate times over the course of the conversation.

* * *

1989. In an event that will not be repeated by any other leading scientific psychiatry journal, *Schizophrenia Bulletin* publishes a special issue on the subjective experience of schizophrenia. Two articles offer novel empirical investigations of the ways voice-hearers relate to their voices. In the first, Lorna Benjamin utilizes her Structural Analysis of Social Behaviour questionnaire to demonstrate across a sample of thirty psychiatric inpatients 'the existence of a well-articulated, interpersonally complementary and a sometimes friendly, sometimes hostile relationship with the auditory hallucination' (Benjamin, 1989, p. 306). Although routinely ignored within clinical practice, the way patients relate to their voices has, she argues, a major bearing on the quality and course of their illness experience. In the second article by Marius Romme and Alexandre (Sandra) Escher, 'an experiment is described in which people with auditory hallucinations were brought into contact with each other' (Romme and Escher, 1989, p. 215). The contact begins with a television programme in which a patient talks with her psychiatrist (Romme) about her voices. Four hundred and fifty voice-hearers call into the programme and are sent questionnaires about their experiences; twenty participate in a follow-up interview and are invited to speak at the first congress of voice-hearers, which 300 people attend. Synthesizing these data, Romme and Escher's article identifies distinct phases in the experience of hearing voices, reflects upon the ways different explanatory frameworks configure the relation between voice and self, and concludes, somewhat controversially, by encouraging clinicians 'to consider helping the individual communicate with the voices' as well as seek out other voice-hearers (Romme and Escher, 1989, p. 215). Benjamin's and Romme and Escher's articles suggest that, far from being the meaningless symptom of an underlying disease process, the experience of hearing voices is full of subjective meaning. More precisely, they argue that the meaning of voice-hearing should be sought more in the relationship people have with, and to, their voices, rather than in an inventory of the properties, qualities, or characteristics of the voice itself. Over the course of the 1990s and into the early 2000s, feeding on, and into, debates about the relationship between dissociation, trauma, and psychosis, voice-hearers' relationships with their voices have become the site of increasing attention and intervention. Observing that 'beliefs about voice omnipotence (i.e. the perceived power of voices) and voice intent (i.e. perceived malevolent or benevolent intentions of voices) can explain the way that voices are responded to, acted on, and complied with' (Strauss et al., 2018, p. 95), clinical psychologists working in the cognitive tradition have focused on the practices and effects of appraisal. Romme and Escher's Maastricht approach to accepting and making sense of voices provides practical tools for profiling voices as a first step towards understanding their role in a person's life, and has inspired many working in the International Hearing Voices Movement. The Talking with Voices and Voice Dialogue approaches actively support voice-hearers to have respectful exchanges with their voices, and Relating and AVATAR therapies likewise advance techniques for changing the nature of the interpersonal relationship between a person and their distressing voice (Deamer and Hayward, 2018; Ward et al., 2020). A diverse body of evidence—ranging from the randomized controlled trial to the circulation of recovery narratives—speaks to the benefits to voice-hearers of shifting from a policy of eradication to one of improved relation.

* * *

1987. A terrifying vision from childhood:

[A] little girl's leg in a calliper, in the back garden of me mam and dad's old house, and it was whirring round on a, like a rotisserie, like you would do a hog roast. . . . It was going round on a rotisserie like that. And it was all in grey. And that was like something I saw that wasn't actually there, do you know what I mean, it wasn't physically there. But I saw that and I . . . I had a really bad problem with that house, they had to move out that house for me. . . . Because I was having such bad . . . screaming at night and nightmares and stuff like that. (Leah)

Seen, but not heard. A dismembered limb, visceral, vulnerable, stripped of identity and turning with rhythmic menace. 'I think it was him that sent us the images when I saw the little girl's leg in the back garden', Leah says towards the end of the interview—'him' being an uncle, 'accused, when I was a bairn, he was accused of fiddling with me when I was little'. She can remember sitting on his knee, being taken to the Wizard of Oz. That is all she can remember. But she knows that her uncle was taken out by his brothers, that there was an accident, and that he never came back. And she knows that as an adult, his voice has returned to torment, to accuse her. 'So I've tried', she says, 'all I can say here, look, I was a child, I don't know what happened, I don't know what, you shouldn't be punishing me for it, it's not my fault you're dead, I didn't kill you'. He does not listen to her.

* * *

2018. In the North East of England, academics, clinicians, and activists gather for an international conference on *Personification Across Disciplines*. We ask: How are voices like people? Do voices have intentions, traits, agency, emotions, and mental states?

The panel on 'Relating to Distressing Voices' crackles with the energy and electricity of deeply committed clinicians arguing the case for their therapeutic approaches. Within this context, although much is made of the differences between AVATAR therapy, Talking with Voices, and Relating therapy, particularly with regard to the use of specialist or everyday technologies, their shared emphasis on the therapeutic utility of personification is striking. Voices become amenable to relational therapies to the extent that they are experienced, recognized, represented, or even produced as persons—persons who are or who will be responsive to the behaviour and beliefs of the voice-hearer. The relational framework effects a double domestication of experiences which are elsewhere considered exemplary of all that is unusual, un-understandable, or frankly bizarre about psychosis. The voice is a person, but s/he is a person of tactically limited psychological complexity. The personified voices of relating therapies are stripped of their raging ids, capricious and contradictory personalities, and supernatural talents, permitted only to inhabit spaces of empathetic understanding and positive transformation.

At the same conference, Ben Alderson-Day, Peter Moseley, and I present preliminary findings from the Voice in Psychosis study. Our analysis is in dialogue with Sam

Wilkinson and Vaughan Bell's account of voice-hearing as being not primarily an auditory or perceptual experience, but a representation of agency that can take one of four forms (Wilkinson and Bell, 2016, pp. 107–8):

1. Absent or functionally absent agency
2. Agency without individualization
3. Internally individualized identity (anonymous 'incognito voices' or those given purely internally generated names)
4. Externally individualized identity (whether fictional or real).

While there is an intuitive appeal about these distinctions, my paper draws out two areas of unease. The first concerns the relationship between agents and agency. According to Wilkinson and Bell, 'We represent something as an agent when we represent it as having an informational and a motivational profile (or perspective) . . . to represent something as an agent is to ascribe it beliefs and desires' (Wilkinson and Bell, 2016, p. 111). Agency, by contrast, can be thought of as a capacity for action, for exerting power. Wilkinson and Bell appear committed to the idea that agency is something wielded by agents, and, further, that the more detailed or complex the agent profile, the greater its capacities for action. Hence, when they 'start with the lowest level of agent representation, namely, an absence of it, and work our way up to the richest agent representations in AVHs' (Wilkinson and Bell, 2016, p. 106), it is implied that the progression from 'low' to 'rich' agent representation is also a steady accumulation or increase of agency, and that the flow is typically one-way, rather than multidirectional.

In what ways are minimally personified voices 'less' consequential or distressing than voices with externally individualized identity? Is it possible to conceive of degrees or qualities of agency being independent of the agentive qualities of the entity? While some 'richly' personified agents are indeed also extremely agentic, voice-hearers also report opaque or non-human agents which intervene, disrupt, and unsettle; unidentified voices which are present and active presences; and soundless voices whose agency is felt independent of any recognizably sensory experience. By contrast, voices which have known or externally real counterparts are sometimes reported as having comparatively minimal influence. It might be important, then, to disentangle agents and agency, personification and power, and not to make any fixed assumptions about the relationship between the characterful qualities of voices and their effects on and for the voice-hearer. As Nev Jones, in her keynote presentation 'Powers and Seductions of Personification', puts it, we need urgently to identify resources which 'would allow us to grapple with discontinuous forms of agency, with agents that jump or leap unpredictably from one modality to another, that are not stable, energy that circulates outside what we might describe as a circuit of persons and/or egos' (Jones, 2018).

* * *

2017. Leah describes her voices and 'voice-like experiences'. Clicks in each ear are the way certain voices signal their presence and command her attention. A healing, tingling sensation accompanies the angel's voice; the gypsy 'comes in bubbles'; Loki's low, slow, gruff voice speaks through her gut and her bowels. Shadows, 'shadows of like angels and stuff', guide her towards safety. The huge, eagle-like wings of the Archangel Michael envelop her; swooping down one night, they 'moved us off the quayside, and told us that somebody had been raped there and they got us moved off'. Homeless in a distant city, at the peak of her crisis, 'Jesus was in the water, and all the racism was in the water', and Leah finds herself 'coughing up demons . . . expelling it out'. Then there are the moments when no such action or demarcation can reinstate the boundaries between inside and outside, me and not me:

> [W]hen I was, when I was really bad with it, I heard it through me heart. . . . It was through me heart, where they were coming from, it was as if me heart was like a speaker. . . . And I could hear these things echoing and it would pick up other people's vibrations and other people's thoughts. And that was like a big washer, and that were ongoing, this whirring washer as well. . . . So me own voices and then things that I thought other people around us, their little bits and pieces, and that went into a cycle. Like a tornado, you know when it picks stuff up like this? . . . And that would just like echo throughout us to the point where I would have to split and just run away from wherever I was, because the people, the telly and the radio and you hear stuff, it picks that up as well. . . . Ah, so bad.

Voice—irreducible to the auditory, the linguistic, or the characterful—becomes vision, becomes sensation, becomes lodged in the body just as its referents multiply, proliferate, and collapse.

To the speaker that is your heart, what kind of relation is possible?

* * *

1972. In their anarchic *Anti-Oedipus: Capitalism and Schizophrenia*, Deleuze and Guattari sketch a liberatory account of madness pitched against the psychoanalytic fixation on psychosexual development. 'How does one dare reduce to the paternal theme a delirium so rich, so differentiated, so "divine" as the Judge's . . .?' they ask (Deleuze and Guattari, 1982, p. 56). The Judge in question is Daniel Paul Schreber, whose *Memoirs of My Nervous Illness* have sustained over a century of often passionate and contested analysis, dissection, and debate (Woods, 2011). For Deleuze and Guattari, Schreber's madness is the best evidence that before 'being crushed in the psychiatric and psychoanalytic treadmill', 'all delirium possesses a world-historical, political, and racial content, mixing and sweeping along races, cultures, continents, and kingdoms' (Deleuze and Guattari, 1982, pp. 274, 88). This is 'not mere metaphor' (Deleuze and Guattari, 1982, p. 2). When Schreber describes inhabiting a world of 'fleeting-improvised-men', being persecuted by God's rays, tormented by incessant voices, and slowly transformed into a woman (Deleuze and Guattari, 1982, pp. 2, 19):

> Nothing here is representative; rather, it is all life and lived experience: the actual, lived emotion of having breasts does not resemble breasts, it does not represent them…Nothing but bands of intensity, potentials, thresholds, and gradients. A harrowing, emotionally overwhelming experience, which brings the schizo as close as possible to matter, to a burning, living centre of matter.

Psychosis is not about depth, knots, psychic secrets. The symptom is not a hieroglyph; its antecedents, contents, and consequences go far beyond Oedipal drama. *Anti-Oedipus* insists instead on the fragment; its commitment is to a kaleidoscope of moving parts traversed by desire, history, and capital. Out for a stroll with 'sunbeams in his ass' (Deleuze and Guattari, 1982, p. 2), Deleuze and Guattari's celebratory 'schizo' reads as an utterly fantastical figure, impossible to reconcile with the frightened, homeless woman moved along a dangerous quayside by the shadowy wings of an archangel. So is there a way of acknowledging the fragment—its agency, its irreducibility—without risking a hermeneutic violence to the person?

To Leah, and the speaker that is her heart, what kind of relation is possible?

References

Benjamin, L. S. (1989). Is chronicity a function of the relationship between the person and the auditory hallucination? *Schizophrenia Bulletin*, 15(2), 291–310.

Deamer, F., and Hayward, M. (2018). Relating to the speaker behind the voice: what is changing? *Frontiers in Psychology*, 9. https://www.frontiersin.org/articles/10.3389/fpsyg.2018.00011/full

Deleuze, G., and Guattari, F. (1982). *Anti-Oedipus: Capitalism and Schizophrenia*. New York, NY: Viking Press.

Jones, N. (2018). Powers and seductions of personification. In: N. Jones, ed. *Personification Across Disciplines*. https://vimeo.com/296837250 (accessed 17 November 2020).

Kraepelin, E. (1981). *Clinical Psychiatry*. New York, NY: Scholars' Facsimiles & Reprints.

Romme, M., and Escher, A. (1989). Hearing Voices. *Schizophrenia Bulletin*, 15(2), 209–16.

Strauss, C., Hugdahl, K., Waters, F., Hayward, M., Bless, J., Falkenberg, L., Kråkvik, B., Asbjørnsen, A., Johnsen, E., Sinkeviciute, I., Kroken, R., Løberg, E., and Thomas, N. (2018). The beliefs about voices questionnaire—revised: a factor structure from 450 participants. *Psychiatry Research*, 259, 95–103.

Ward, T., Rus-Calafell, M., Ramadhan, Z., Soumelidou, O., Fornells-Ambrojo, M., Garety, P., and Craig, T. K. J. (2020). AVATAR therapy for distressing voices: a comprehensive account of therapeutic targets. *Schizophrenia Bulletin*, 46(5), 1038–44.

Wilkinson, S., and Bell, V. (2016). The representation of agents in auditory verbal hallucinations. *Mind and Language*, 31(1), 104–26.

Woods, A. (2011). *The Sublime Object of Psychiatry: Schizophrenia in Clinical and Cultural Theory*. Oxford: Oxford University Press.

About the Author

Angela Woods is a Professor of Medical Humanities at Durham University and the Co-Director of Hearing the Voice. Her work in the critical medical humanities focuses on psychosis and narrative.

PART FOUR
LOCATING VOICES IN LANGUAGE

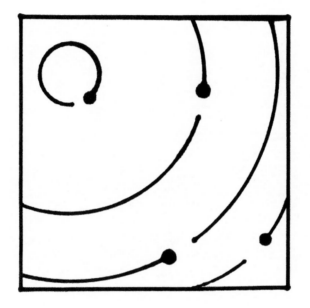

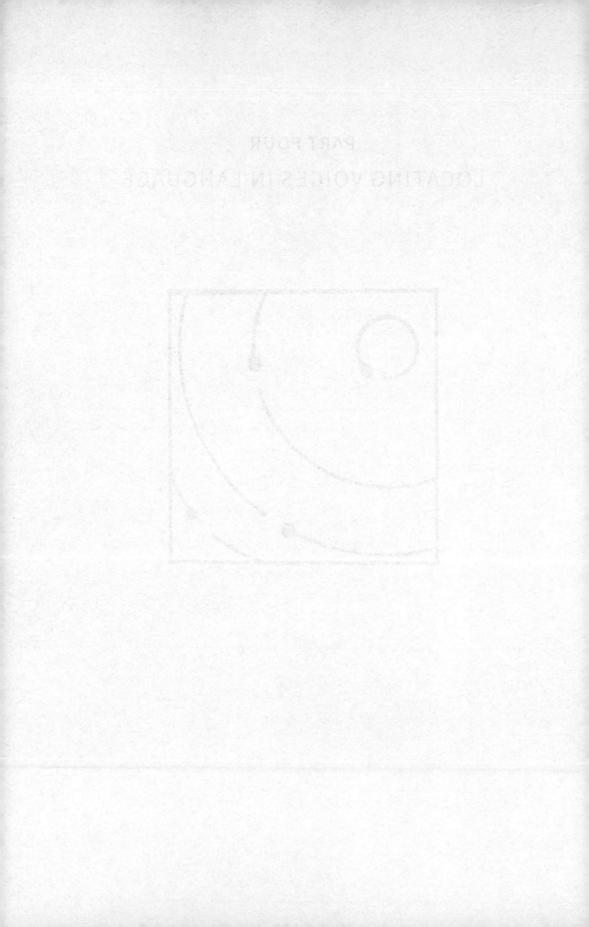

15

The Phenomenology of Voice-Hearing and Two Concepts of Voice

Sam Wilkinson, Department of Philosophy, University of Exeter

Joel Krueger, Department of Philosophy, University of Exeter

What has struck us both about the Voices in Psychosis (VIP) interview transcripts is that the experiences reported in them that are called 'voices' are, first, hugely varied, and, second, do not all happily fall under the label 'auditory verbal hallucination' (AVH).[1] Accordingly, a more phenomenologically sensitive engagement with detailed first-person reports (of which these transcripts are exemplary) is needed. In this context, phenomenology can be helpful in several ways. For one thing, it can help develop a more accurate description of the individual's experience—i.e. one that preserves the integrity of both their experience *as lived* as well as their subsequent reports *about* that experience—which, in turn, can serve as a tool for cultivating a kind of empathy (Ratcliffe, 2012). Additionally, although phenomenology is generally not concerned with providing an account of underlying cognitive, neural, or biological processes, it can nevertheless assist with developing such accounts. For example, it can assist the development of neurocognitive and biosocial models of voice-hearing—which *are* primarily concerned with causal–mechanistic explanations—both by providing an explanatory target for such models and by assisting the evaluation of existing models against the experiences as described in first-person reports such as these (McCarthy-Jones et al., 2013).

Phenomenology starts with open-ended questions such as: 'What is it like for an individual to be in a certain mental state, such as hearing a voice?' and 'What is the meaning of that experience for the individual?' This phenomenological orientation is apparent in the consistent way the interviews in these transcripts begin. First, the interviewer acknowledges that voices 'can mean lots of different things' to different people, from something that 'might involve sound', to the feeling 'that someone or something is communicating with you', to something akin to 'a form of telepathy or loud thoughts'. This is an acknowledgement to the individual being interviewed that voice-hearing is a rich and experientially diverse kind of experience, and that they should describe the experience as it happens *for them*. This experiential diversity is

---

[1] The label of AVH has been criticized by many (e.g. Slade and Bentall, 1988), including contributors to this volume.

Sam Wilkinson and Joel Krueger, *The Phenomenology of Voice-Hearing and Two Concepts of Voice* In: *Voices in Psychosis.*
Edited by: Angela Woods, Ben Alderson-Day, and Charles Fernyhough, Oxford University Press. © Sam Wilkinson and Joel Krueger 2022.
DOI: 10.1093/oso/9780192898388.003.0015

also tacitly acknowledged by the open-endedness of the very first question—'Could you try to describe to me some of the voices or voice-like experiences you've been having?'—along with an encouragement 'to use your own terms, your own language' in providing these descriptions.

Inspired by these transcripts—and as a way of gesturing towards a more nuanced phenomenological characterization of voice-hearing—we want to acknowledge the rich diversity of experiences found in these reports by isolating at least two things that 'voice' seems to mean in this context. We say 'at least' because we do not suggest that these two concepts are in any way exhaustive. However, notice that we do not need them to be. If the category of things called 'voices' in clinical contexts actually picks out a number of distinct phenomena (two, three, or four, etc.), then we should be mindful of that plurality in general and wary of using the term 'auditory verbal hallucination' in particular. A commitment to phenomenological sensitivity should breed this kind of caution.

Before we embark on this brief project, a word about method. We are an analytic philosopher and a phenomenologist, and so we will proceed by conceptual and phenomenological analysis. How do these things fit together? Talking about experience is a strange phenomenon, since it involves using a public tool to get at something very private. The public tool—language—is a rather blunt and coarse-grained instrument for capturing the precise nature of a given experiential episode, such as, for instance, the character and structure of hearing voices versus more general features of audition as a distinct perceptual modality. As long as it is not actively misleading, any given description of experience rules out a large number of possibilities about what that experience might be like. However, it does not rule out *all* of the possibilities; it does not narrow them down to one. In such a situation, the description is accurate, but inevitably too coarse-grained. In light of this relationship between the language used to talk about experience and the experience itself, we proceed in two steps:

Step 1. The conceptual analysis of 'voice' will pick out two different things that could be meant by 'voice'. This is coarse-grained.

Step 2. The phenomenological analysis then elaborates on the precise possible nature of the experience in question.

In principle, then, the coarse-grained conceptual categories further subdivide phenomenologically. Little wonder thinking of voices as a unified phenomenon is misleading!

Two Concepts of Voice

Concept 1

Let us begin with the concept that is closest to that of 'auditory verbal hallucination'. This concept picks out a particular auditory quality of experience, namely, a speech-like quality. This is the sense of 'voice' you might find in the utterance: 'This synthesizer has a "voice" setting.' Note how there are two further subtle ambiguities here. 'Voice', with this focus on auditory quality (pointing out that it *sounds* like a human voice, rather than, say, a violin or a klaxon), can refer to the subjective experience or the environmental stimulus (the speech sound, the pressure ripples in the air). It can also refer to someone's capacity or disposition to produce a sound with a particular quality: the statement 'She has a beautiful singing voice' holds true even when the person is not singing. So, 'voice' in this sense, with its auditory qualitative focus, can take a subjective or objective flavour and can also pick out something actual or dispositional.

Many speakers in these transcripts seem to use this sense of voice. Alex, for instance, talks explicitly about the 'pitch and tone' of his voices, and says, for example, that the voices he hears are like 'like someone's whispering in your ear [. . .] Except it's that, it's not necessarily at a whisper's volume'. There is also explicit mention of the location of the sound and how that varies: 'Sometimes it can be as if they're sitting right next to you or standing alongside you. And then other times, I could be in another room and think it's coming from a different room.' What is interesting here is that, despite variations in volume, location, and felt proximity of the voices, Alex consistently experiences these voices *as voices*. In other words, he does not confuse them with other auditory stimuli, despite the fact, he says, that they are often hard to hear. Moreover, while Alex's descriptions contain some mention of the thematic *content* of the voices—i.e. what they say to him (threats, insults, etc.)—the bulk of his report focuses on the speech-like qualities of these voices and how, despite a variety of ways these qualities are presented to him, he nevertheless experiences these qualities *as speech-like*. Often, he tells us, he is unable to understand the voices. However, he still recognizes the voices by their speech-like qualities: 'It's just slight distinctive differences in the voices, like in the pitch and the tone.'

Similarly, Bill consistently describes hearing voices that start like 'a bark' or 'a shout or a noise, you know like someone that is more just ehm like a bang on the table or something like that, sort of . . . but more of a vocal version of that'. However, Bill does not confuse these voices with a bang on a table or genuine barking. He tells us that 'it's similar to a dog bark but it's not entirely a dog bark'—again, because the voices manifest experientially with a distinctive auditory quality that identifies them as voices. Like Alex, Bill spends some time describing what the voices say. However, most of his focus is on qualities of his experience of the voice, independent of this content. Again, these qualities are what appear to be most phenomenologically salient.

When we say that this concept of 'voice' picks out a particular 'auditory quality', there are two different ways in which this can be interpreted: as rich or sparse. This issue is related to an ongoing debate in philosophy of perception about whether the content of perceptual experience can ever be rich, namely, can ever go beyond the 'low-level properties' that are thought of as basic to that sensory modality. For vision, the question is whether all we ever really see are colour, shape, and shade, or whether we literally see trees, or even, with relevant expertise, *oak* trees (Siegel, 2006). For audition, the question is whether what we experience goes beyond loudness, pitch, and timbre. Without going into the technicalities of this debate, we certainly intend a rich interpretation of 'auditory quality' here. We intend it to include properties that go well beyond the 'low-level properties' and include the experience of, for instance, personhood, feminity, aggression, and so on. One might think that allowing this richness risks collapsing Concept 1 into Concept 2, which we are about to introduce, but this would be to misunderstand the two concepts. However rich we take auditory experience to be, when we use 'voice' to express Concept 2, we are not picking out the auditory aspects of an experience at all (even though the experience may well be an auditory one).

Concept 2

The second concept that 'voice' can express picks out, not so much an auditory quality of a sound (however richly this is conceived), but a particular agent: what Felicity Deamer and colleagues (Deamer and Hayward, 2018; Deamer and Wilkinson, 2015) have called the 'speaker behind the voice'. This concept is intrinsically related to the experience of something with its own perspective and agency, and goes beyond the superficially auditory. (Indeed, not only does this build onto the auditory experience, it also sometimes circumvents it altogether, as in the case of soundless voices (Wilkinson, 2019).) Often, it involves the binding of this agentive experience into a singular agent representation persisting over time (see Wilkinson and Bell, 2016). This is the sense of 'voice' that is very commonly used in the context of hearing voices. Indeed, it is implicit in a question that is so often asked of voice-hearers: 'How many voices do you hear?' This question is asking the voice-hearer *how many re-identifiable agents are represented over time* across several experiential episodes. The question makes no sense otherwise. It is not a question about the qualitative variety of some relatively two-dimensional auditory experience. Indeed, it is not even a question about the variety of what is said (i.e. its thematic or semantic content), or even about the qualitative personality of the represented agents. The personality of a 'voice', in this sense that picks out the identity of an agent, can change over time. Voices can shift from being nice to nasty. Personality traits are features of these voices, but they are not definitive of them. The question 'How many voices do you hear?' is one about specific individual identities. In many of the VIP transcripts, the voices have personality traits, but these do not appear fully bound to clearly re-identifiable individuals. The question of how many voices are heard by these voice-hearers is therefore not answerable, since although they hear voices in both the speech–sound and agentive sense, the voice-as-agent is transient and untrackable. In some of the transcripts, however, the agents can be tracked, and hence counted.

We find an example of this second concept of voice in Dan's transcript, when he says that 'over the last couple of months I've sort of been hearing I think up to seven different voices'. Of phenomenological interest here is the fact that Dan experiences these voices as individuated by their spatial continuity (i.e. where each of these voices originate from, respectively, within his inner psychoacoustic landscape). Sometimes, he says, 'when it's inside the head, [it's] very, very loud and it's like it consumes all the space around you, and you feel like you're kind of suffocating in it'. At other times, the voices are externally located, but very close by (e.g. 'it's like it's pounding right in your ear, it's like it's, they're talking right into your ear'), or even more spatially remote ('sometimes it sounds like it's somebody maybe within the same room as me, or sat next to me'). Other voice-hearers in these transcripts seem to individuate their voices by personality trait (e.g. Sean individuates one of his voices as an angry person).

The take-home message from this is that the grounds on which is built the singular representation that constitutes the voice (Concept 2) as a persisting entity over time can vary enormously, as can the 'depth' of agency represented in the experience (Wilkinson and Bell, 2016). These grounds, however, cannot constitute the singular representation itself. For example, one of Dan's voices, though originally bound to a singular representation on the basis of location, could, in principle, move location. Similarly, Sean's angry voice might cheer up. Note that there must be this singular representation, however sparse, in order to enable enough continuity over time to allow the voice-hearer to judge that (or even wonder whether) *this* voice, heard now, is the same as *that* voice, heard yesterday.

A Paradox in Voice-Hearing

There is one final phenomenological feature of these transcripts that we would like to mention—a feature that further highlights the experiential complexity of voice-hearing, while also reaffirming the need to remain committed to preserving this complexity in our descriptions and analyses. This complexity can be seen by highlighting what appears to be a kind of tension, or contradiction, running through many of the transcripts. In short, the experience of hearing voices is described as being both like *and* unlike voices heard in everyday life (often simultaneously).

On the one hand, the voices are regularly described as having an experiential profile like voices heard in everyday life. They have auditory qualities and speech-like properties that everyday voices have: they have thematic or expressive content that is often directed towards the hearer (sometimes positive and affirming, although more often negative and distressing), and they are bound to distinct owners in that they are tied to re-identifiable agents over time. On the other hand, even though voices share these qualities with everyday voices, they also present other qualities that further complicate their phenomenological profile, and are thus often experienced as radically *unlike* everyday voices in some important ways. This can be seen in the way that some of the participants describe the experience of voice-hearing as being clearer, or somehow more pronounced, than the experience of perceiving a voice in everyday life. In other words, the voice is experientially manifest with an intensity that can be overwhelming. Of course, similar experiences can happen when hearing voices in everyday life, such as when the ambient vocal noise at a pub or party becomes too much and one flees outside for an auditory break. However, unlike the pub and party cases, these participants are describing experiences of voices that seem to em-anate from *within*; their overwhelming character comes not from a relentless pen-etration of sounds coming in through one's ears (although some have this quality, which further complicates things), but rather from the way in which they bubble up from within one's inner psychoacoustic landscape. Accordingly, these experience can seem 'more real than reality' (Karlsson, 2008) because the voice is not felt to have an external origin. Whereas voices from the external world are mediated by a variety of factors (the speaker's body, occlusion by other ambient noise, etc.) that specify their felt character, many of the voices in these reports lack this public character.

The phenomenological lesson, then, is that many of the voice-hearing experiences described in these transcripts seem to have a peculiar form of directedness, or what phenomenologists call 'intentionality' (Ratcliffe, 2017, p. 91). The voices are expe-rienced, on the one hand, as somehow less real because they are not rooted in the public world; yet, on the other hand, they are also felt to be more real *for precisely this reason*. The hearer cannot distance themselves from the voice, which is why they are often perceived as having extraordinary power over the hearer (Chadwick and Birchwood, 1994) and compel hearers to feel as though they lack the agency to rein-terpret or repudiate their negative appraisals.

There is much more that could be said about these transcripts, of course. But the takeaway message is simple: voice-hearing in psychosis is complex, both conceptu-ally and phenomenologically, in ways that far exceed the standard technical term 'auditory verbal hallucination'. Acknowledging this complexity can help us refine our descriptions, deepen our understanding, and, ideally, develop a more empathetic stance towards voice-hearers and their rich variety of voice-hearing experiences.

References

Chadwick, P., and Birchwood, M. J. (1994). The omnipotence of voices: a cognitive approach to audi-tory hallucinations. *British Journal of Psychiatry*, 164, 190–201.

Deamer, F., and Hayward, M. (2018). Relating to the speaker behind the voice: what is changing? *Frontiers in Psychology*, 9.

Deamer, F., and Wilkinson, S. (2015). The speaker behind the voice: therapeutic practice from the per-spective of pragmatic theory. *Frontiers in Psychology*, 6.

Karlsson, L.-B. (2008). 'More real than reality': a study of voice hearing. *International Journal of Social Welfare*, 17(4), 365–73.

McCarthy-Jones, S., Krueger, J., Larøi, F., Broome, M., and Fernyhough, C. (2013). Stop, look, listen: the need for philosophical phenomenological perspectives on auditory verbal hallucinations. *Frontiers in Human Neuroscience*, 7(127), 1–9.

Ratcliffe, M. (2012). Phenomenology as a form of empathy. *Inquiry: A Journal of Medical Care Organization, Provision and Financing*, 55(5), 473–95.

Ratcliffe, M. (2017). *Real Hallucinations: Psychiatric Illness, Intentionality, and the Interpersonal World.* Cambridge, MA: MIT Press.

Siegel, S. (2006). Subject and object in the contents of visual experience. *Philosophical Review*, 115(3), 355–88.

Slade, P. D., and Bentall, R. P. (1988). *Sensory Deception: A Scientific Analysis of Hallucination.* London: Croom Helm.

Wilkinson, S. (2019). Hearing soundless voices. *Philosophy, Psychiatry and Psychology*, 26(3), 27–34.

Wilkinson, S., and Bell, V. (2016). The representation of agents in auditory verbal hallucinations. *Mind and Language*, 31(1), 104–26.

About the Authors

Sam Wilkinson is a Senior Lecturer in Philosophy at the University of Exeter. As a Postdoctoral Research Fellow on Hearing the Voice, he was the project's resident conceptual hygienist but also worked on predictive processing and the experience of agency.

Joel Krueger is an Associate Professor in Philosophy at the University of Exeter and a former Postdoctoral Research Fellow on Hearing the Voice. He works on various issues in phenomenology, philosophy of mind, and cognitive science, especially on topics in embodied and extended cognition, emotions, and psychopathology.

16

Bridging the Gap in Common Ground When Talking about Voices

Felicity Deamer, Institute of Forensic Linguistics, Aston University

Despite the negative impact of voice-hearing often being bound up in what is said, there has been a distinct lack of attention paid to exploring the linguistic content of voices and/or the language voice-hearers use to describe their experiences. In this chapter, I will take a close look at how voice-hearers in the Voices in Psychosis (VIP) transcripts use language non-literally in order to convey their complex experiences, and what that might tell us about the nature of voice-hearing experiences, as well as about the function of different forms of figurative language.

The topic of figurative language is a vast area of debate and theorizing, with many different accounts of what is involved. For my purposes here, it suffices to say that figurative language is a way of talking about something (the primary subject/topic or tenor) by using words or phrases that do not typically, conventionally, or literally refer to that thing (the secondary subject or vehicle).

Although they are often treated as synonyms, I take 'figurative language' to be a slightly narrower category than 'non-literal language'. In other words, all instances of figurative language are instances of non-literal language, but not vice versa. Metaphors and similes are both instances of figurative language, and hence also of non-literal language. However, hyperbole (exaggeration) and approximation are non-literal, but they are not fully figurative in my sense (they could be described as 'loose use', or 'less than literal'). An understanding of figurative language requires a more complicated and lateral inference than simply understanding that someone is overstating for effect (hyperbole) or drawing a close approximation. That is, in part, why figurative language is so widely used in literature: it is a more adventurous use of language. It is more open to communicative failure, or to being interpreted differently by different people, but the pay-off can be great, with metaphors having the potential to yield rich and open-ended interpretations.

Figurative Language and Experiences

In recent decades, a great deal of attention has been given to exploring the role that figurative language plays in our understanding of experiences. For example, Lakoff (1987)

Felicity Deamer, *Bridging the Gap in Common Ground When Talking about Voices* In: *Voices in Psychosis*. Edited by: Angela Woods, Ben Alderson-Day, and Charles Fernyhough, Oxford University Press. © Felicity Deamer 2022. DOI: 10.1093/oso/9780192898388.003.0016 argues that metaphors should not be thought of as literary or communicative devices, but as a reflection of the way in which we think about the world and experience it. Levin (1988) argues that metaphors tend to be produced while speakers are experiencing extraordinary events and emotions because 'ordinary' language is not an adequate tool for the description of complex experiences and the expression of one's emotional response to such experiences. He suggests that one can at best 'approximate to such expression by means of deviant sentences' (Levin, 1988, p. xiii). Levin argues that just as the scientist uses metaphorical language to conceive of states of affairs previously unthought of, so must an individual who attempts to conceive of a reality or an emotion that is unlike any that they have encountered before or heard described before.

Metaphor and Mental Health

Figurative language is often used to explore emotion in psychotherapy, and advocates of these methods argue that a 'figurative mode of expression' is essential in understanding emotional distress. In fact, the overt and intentional use of non-literal language in the therapeutic context largely came about due to the 'rich and disturbingly imaginative metaphoric articulations' generated spontaneously by service users (Pollio et al., 1977, p. 104).

Charteris-Black (2012) argues that metaphors not only play an important role in communicating emotional intensity, but also expose the concepts underlying people's experiences. The prevalence of uses of containment metaphors by people reflecting on their experiences of depression (e.g. being trapped, coming out, pouring out, escaping, releasing) suggests that such metaphors are not just tools for expression, but are also fundamental to the lived experience of depression.

Attention has also been given to the use of metaphor by people experiencing psychosis. For example, Rhodes and Jakes (2004) examined first-person accounts of how participants with delusions remember the formation of their beliefs. They concluded that during the onset of early psychotic episodes, the attempts of individuals to make sense of their experiences lead them to think in 'figurative terms' which amplified the process of the formation of their delusions. They do not claim that delusional statements *are* metaphors. Instead, their point is that 'a delusional statement is a literal statement about aspects of the world or the self which [gets] transformed by metaphor' (Rhodes and Jakes, 2004, p. 15). Likewise, Parnas et al. (2005) argue that metaphors are commonplace in the language of people with psychosis, particularly when describing perceptual experiences and mental states which are hard to articulate in other terms.

Distribution of Tropes in the Transcripts

A recent study found that 'metaphorical' language is routinely used by voice-hearers with schizophrenia diagnoses, enabling them to frame their unusual experiences in different ways, and determining the power dynamic between the hearer and their voice (Demjen et al., 2019). Given this, it is at first striking to find (as a result of a specific analysis for the purposes of this chapter) that there are very few instances of metaphor in the VIP transcripts.

Below is a breakdown of the non-literal language use within a representative subset of ten of the transcripts (which were randomly selected) (see Table 16.1). The transcripts were manually scanned for instances of metaphor (any metaphorical use that was not deemed highly conventionalized/idiomatic), simile, approximation, and highly conventionalized metaphor (e.g. 'I was imagining all these dark situations' (Gail)).

What can this distribution of non-literal language use tell us about these voice-hearers' experiences, as well as the process they undergo in trying to express them? How can an analysis of the function, as well as the production and comprehension, of metaphor and simile shed light on the relative absence of non-conventionalized metaphor in these transcripts?

Metaphor versus Simile

First it is worth unpacking what we mean by metaphor. The Demjen et al. (2019) study worked with a very broad notion of metaphoricity, and as such, they included any use of a term in a less-than-literal way (including similes) in their analysis. Their coarse-grained approach, though valid for some purposes, does not differentiate between tropes, and hence does not allow you to reflect on how different tropes have different conditions of appropriateness. A number of studies have attempted to shed light on the contexts and/or conditions in which different kinds of metaphor and simile might be more or less appropriate, such as when highlighting variability between two things under comparison, creating a particular effect, referring to an abstract rather than a concrete idea, or expressing a novel or conventional idea (Bowdle and Gentner, 2005).

Josie O'Donoghue argues that metaphors are less likely to be used in a context in which the vehicle term is not familiar to the interlocutor as 'the hearer expects [a metaphor] to be easily interpretable in a fixed conventional sense' (O'Donoghue, 2009); an obvious point of comparison is made emphatically. However, it is because of the simile's focus on aspects of likeness between the topic and vehicle that a relevant reading is facilitated. If there is no well-understood vehicle concept to appeal

Table 16.1 Use of non-literal language in the transcripts

Approximations	Similes	Metaphors	Highly conventionalized metaphors/idioms
76	30	3	53

to (as in 'How is your new housemate?' 'He is a bluebottle'), the use of the metaphor form suggests that there is a particular understood, specific meaning (a sort of slang) of which the hearer is just not aware. If, on the other hand, the simile form (e.g. 'He is like a bluebottle') is used, the hearer would be much more likely to think (in the moment) of specific ways in which someone might be likened to the vehicle (a bluebottle) and would then have no problem coming up with possible intended meanings (e.g. 'He buzzes around the house making lots of noise and irritating me'). O'Donoghue (2009, p. 129) argues that the fact that simile invites comparison as an explicit, quite conscious process, and 'that the form encourages contemplation of the precise terms of comparison' means that simile can, in the right context (particularly where novel descriptions are necessary or desired), lead to the arrival at a more precise and sophisticated meaning than metaphor, which might merely reinforce emphatically an already clear point. This line of reasoning is relevant to the VIP transcripts but requires some elaboration below.

Grounding and Communication

It has long been appreciated that when two individuals communicate, they need to have a large suite of common beliefs and common assumptions, which is sometimes collectively referred to as *common ground*. Grounding is vital for all aspects of communication, whether referring to things that are currently perceived or being discussed *in absentia*, or when talking about different kinds of things. The central point is that in order to talk about something, the person you are talking to needs to know what you are talking about. This is underpinned by a plethora of conditions, including (but not exhausted by) linguistic competence, conceptual understanding, shared knowledge, and beliefs and assumptions. This is known as conversational grounding. Different failures in conversational grounding result in different failures of communication.

Conversational Grounding for Voices

How is common ground established for voices? Voices are clearly private experiences, rather than public objects, and so one might think initially that grounding is bound to be difficult. However, we do often talk about subjective experiences such as pains, emotions, perceptions, and so on. So, conversational grounding is achievable for experiences, and it pays to reflect on how it is achieved in the best case. Two related features of these commonly talked-about experiences highlight how this grounding is achieved, and how it is harder to achieve in the case of voices.

The first is an assumption of phenomenological similarity. We can talk about our experiences with others because we know (or perhaps assume) that they have had similar experiences to a greater or lesser extent. The second, which plays a role in generating the knowledge (or assumption) that constitutes the first, is that we know what sorts of experiences are undergone in certain contexts. Experience of colour is a canonical case in point. I do not know what it is like to see red through your eyes, but I do know that the experience we call 'red' is the experience we both get when we look at ripe tomatoes or London buses. Similarly, I do not know if your fear feels exactly the same as mine, but I do know the sorts of contexts in which it occurs and the sorts of reactions it elicits.

Do voices allow for: (1) an assumption of phenomenological similarity; and (2) generalization with regard to the contexts in which they tend to occur? In relation to the second question, I would argue that regardless of the phenomenology of a particular voice-hearing experience, the context in which it occurs is one that a third party (e.g. interviewer) may or may not be able to fully track or understand, given that they themselves will likely have never experienced such a contextual trigger. So, what about the assumption of phenomenological similarity?

Contrary to what the term auditory verbal hallucination (AVH) might suggest, voice-hearing is often not exactly like hearing a voice in the everyday sense. Phenomenological surveys suggest that voice-hearing experiences vary widely from person to person, and some lack explicitly auditory properties altogether (Woods et al., 2015). So, our voice-hearers find themselves in a challenging communicative predicament, since there is something complicated to be explained: an experience that is hard to pin down, and that the interlocutor has never experienced, in terms of both phenomenology and context of occurrence.

Explaining the Trope Distribution in the Transcripts

The main thing to explain is the relative lack of metaphor in these transcripts. This divides into two very distinct dimensions. One involves the lack of metaphor relative to simile and approximation. The other involves the lack of metaphor for voices relative to the abundant use of metaphor for talking about other mental health experiences such as depression (Charteris-Black, 2012).

Metaphor versus Simile and Approximation

Our interviewees are not typically trying to explain an extreme version of an experience their interviewer will be familiar with. Rather, they find themselves attempting to describe something that they know is likely to be qualitatively unfamiliar to the interviewer. They are attempting to invite the interviewer to look to another concept or experience to provide a likeness, or to provide something with striking similarities, which will tell them something about the experience. The distribution of trope in these transcripts seems to reflect precisely this.

As O'Donoghue suggests, metaphor requires a significant degree of common ground. I want to go further, though, and argue that this is not just with respect to the vehicle being introduced as a point of comparison. Metaphor lends itself to contexts in which the topic being described is one which the speaker knows to be familiar to their interlocutor—even if only vaguely. Metaphor functions as an embellishment of existing common ground, on existing experience and awareness of the topic under discussion. It allows the speaker to emphatically express an analogy that is obvious to both interlocutors. This may be as a way of communicating just how salient or striking the point of comparison is (e.g. 'This life *is* a prison') or in order to put a valance on the analogy (e.g. 'My sadness is suffocating'). When there is not enough common ground to embellish, simile is preferred; it allows the speaker to establish a point of comparison with something familiar, to point their interlocutor explicitly in the direction of something they know well, endorsing the conscious search for salient features that the experience might share with the familiar concept or experience. In other words, similes are more likely to be used than metaphors in these interviews, in which voice-hearers are drawing comparisons as a means to inform their interlocutor of the nature of something unusual and unfamiliar.

This hypothesis fits with the abundance of approximations we see in the transcripts. In this context, similes are on a spectrum with approximations; both are attempts to pin down and describe features of voice-hearing experiences literally and accurately by drawing their interlocutor's attention to familiar ideas and experiences.

One important point of clarification is in order at this point. We do see in these transcripts some significant examples of highly conventionalized/idiomatic metaphors (e.g. 'My mind is playing tricks on us' (Fred); 'You're battling your own sanity' (Bill); 'these things are revolving around in my head' (Gail); 'I'll just kinda zone out' (Grace)). Such conventionalized metaphors are typically used to emphatically express an obvious comparison, and as such have been incorporated into our everyday lexicon (e.g. 'memory fading'; 'something being drowned out'; 'mind wandering'). That is why these conventionalized metaphors are sometimes called 'lexicalized' metaphors. It is important to see that, in the most important respects, these metaphors are not truly metaphors, except in an etymological sense. When used, the intention is not to express one thing in terms of another: it is simply, as one does with straightforward literal language use, to use the word with a meaning that the interlocutor will recognize (e.g. 'Thanks so much—you're an angel!'). Likewise, when understood, there is no process of inference from the literal to the intended meaning. The interlocutor does not first understand the word literally, and then work out from the context that it is intended non-literally: the colloquial meaning is understood directly. We could say that the interlocutor is just presented with a word that has two (or more) meanings, one of which has its history in the metaphorical but has now become literal (like 'chair leg'). It is because we are in the business of examining the context that elicits the metaphorical mode of use on the part of the speaker that words used in this way appear *not* to be 'metaphorical'. Indeed, many people use lexicalized metaphors without realizing, or needing to realize, that they are, histori-cally speaking, metaphors.

Metaphor Use for Voices Compared with Depression

Metaphors are often used to describe and to help process extreme instances of common experiences and emotions, such as anxiety and depression (Charteris-Black, 2012; Lakoff, 1987). In these instances, metaphors are particularly well suited since there is plenty of relevant common ground, but there is a degree of 'ex-tremeness' that the speaker is at pains to convey to the interlocutor (often conveyed through 'hyperbolic metaphors').

In contrast, voice-hearers are not just trying to describe something to their in-terlocutor that falls along a familiar dimension, but is simply an extreme example of it: they are, for the most part, trying to describe something that is qualitatively unfamiliar. Interviewees are attempting to bridge this gap in common ground (with respect to their voice-hearing experiences) by using simile (e.g. 'Like a banging on the wall' (Carl); 'More like a whisper' (Ulrik); 'Like when someone runs their hand up a curtain' (Kate)) and approximation instead (e.g. 'I'd say it's similar to a dog bark but it's not entirely a dog bark' (Bill); 'I'd hear mainly like sexual noises, like moaning' (Fred); 'I've been hearing like a child or a baby crying, like screeching crying' (Orla)).

There has been a general tendency to assume that metaphors are commonly used to express extreme or unusual experiences, and, by extension, a wide spectrum of experiences in the context of mental health conditions. This tendency seems to be misguided, since different kinds of unusual experiences are conducive to being ex-pressed through the medium of different tropes. An awareness of this more nuanced picture could be of benefit during clinical encounters.

References

Bowdle, B., and Gentner, D. (2005). The career of metaphor. *Psychological Review*, 112(1), 193–216.

Charteris-Black, J. (2012). Shattering the bell jar: metaphor, gender and depression. *Metaphor and Symbol*, 27(3), 199–216.

Demjén, Z., Marszalek, A., Semino, E., and Varese, F. (2019). Metaphor framing and distress in lived-experience accounts of voice-hearing. *Psychosis*, 11(1), 16–27.

Lakoff, G. (1987). A cognitive theory of metaphor. *Philosophical Review*, 96(4), 589–94.

Levin, S. (1988). *Metaphoric Worlds: Conceptions of a Romantic Nature*. New Haven, CT: Yale University Press.

O'Donoghue, J. (2009). Is a metaphor (like) a simile? Differences in meaning, effect and processing. *UCL Working Papers in Linguistics*, 21, 281–91.

Parnas, J., Møller, P., Kircher, T., Thalbitzer, J., Jannson, L., Handest, P., and Zahavi, D. (2005). EASE: Examination of Anomalous Self-Experience. *Psychopathology*, 38(5), 236–58.

Pollio, H. R., Barlow, J. M., Fine, H. J., and Pollio, M. R. (1977). *Psychology and the Poetics of Growth: Figurative Language in Psychology, Psychotherapy and Education*. Hillsdale, NJ: Lawrence Erlbaum.

Rhodes, J., and Jakes, S. (2004). The contribution of metaphor and metonymy to delusions. *Psychology and Psychotherapy: Theory, Research and Practice*, 77(1), 1–17.

Woods, A., Jones, N., Alderson-Day, B., Callard, F., and Fernyhough, C. (2015). Experiences of hearing voices: analysis of a novel phenomenological survey. *The Lancet Psychiatry*, 2(4), 323–31.

About the Author

Felicity Deamer is a Lecturer in Forensic Linguistics at Aston University where she is working at the intersection of Linguistics, Forensics, and Mental Health. Between 2013 and 2019, she was based at Durham University as a Research Fellow on the Language and Mental Health and Hearing the Voice projects, using insights from linguistics to inform our understanding of voice-hearing and therapeutic interventions.

17

Silences in First-Person Accounts of Voice-Hearing

A Linguistic Approach

Elena Semino, Department of Linguistics and English Language, Lancaster University

Luke Collins, Department of Linguistics and English Language, Lancaster University

Zsófia Demjén, Centre for Applied Linguistics, University College London

The phenomenon of voice-hearing involves an individual's perception of speech that others cannot hear—a personal 'non-silence' in the context of an interpersonal 'silence'. It is, in fact, among the key diagnostic criteria for psychosis. Discussions of voice-hearing therefore naturally focus on the characteristics of that private non-silence: what the voices say, how often, and to whom; whether and how the voice-hearer responds; and so on. Yet, even in a context that is defined by perceptions of speech, silences continue to exist. In this chapter, we focus on references to silence in first-person accounts of voice-hearing drawn from interviews with forty voice-hearers with a diagnosis of psychosis—the Voices in Psychosis (VIP) interviews. All interviewees were using the Early Intervention in Psychosis services provided by the UK's National Health Service in the North East of England in 2017–2018. The interviews contain frequent references to speech not occurring, as in: 'I didn't want to tell mum and dad' and 'I can't talk back to the computer [voice]' (Dan). These references are part of the broader phenomenon of negation (e.g. *didn't* and *can't*), which, as we show below, is a distinctive linguistic characteristic of interviewees' responses.

In the study of communication, both silence and negation matter. Silence among potential interlocutors is always meaningful. It is not a mere absence of sound or speech, but rather a multifaceted and interpretable communicative act, potentially indicating, for example, compliance or resistance, the inability to express oneself, the decision and freedom to refrain from speaking, and so on (Jaworski, 1993). Therefore, silence has implications for social relationships and potential asymmetries of power and control. As such, references to silence in the interviews can inform our understanding of the experience of voice-hearing, since as Bell (2013,

Elena Semino, Luke Collins, and Zsófia Demjén, *Silences in First-Person Accounts of Voice-Hearing* In: *Voices in Psychosis*. Edited by: Angela Woods, Ben Alderson-Day, and Charles Fernyhough, Oxford University Press. © Elena Semino, Luke Collins, and Zsófia Demjén 2022. DOI: 10.1093/oso/9780192898388.003.0017

p. 1) asserts, 'hallucinated voices have a social identity with clear interpersonal relevance' and 'are primarily experienced as social actors the hearers can relate to and interact with'.

Negation—the ability of language to express what is not—is both one of the universal and one of the most complex phenomena in language(s) (Horn, 2010). The forms and functions of negation can vary greatly, but often negation will expose a rupture with what is expected: out of the infinite number of things that are not the case, we usually choose to explicitly mention only those that need to be ruled out in a specific context, often because they may otherwise be believed to be the case. For this reason, negation is always a marked choice; it stands out and invites questions (Roitman, 2017). Like silence, negation also has implications for social power dynamics: in a particular context of communication, interlocutors may vary in terms of their ability and power to refuse, reject, or refute (Roitman, 2017, drawing on others).

In this chapter, we are particularly concerned with the implications of references to silence for the phenomenology of voice-hearing and for the portrayal of the relationships that the voice-hearer has with friends and family, and with the voices themselves.

A Linguistic Approach to the VIP interviews: Negation, Verbs of Speech, and Silence

As linguists, we began our analysis of the interviews by asking the question: what words are particularly distinctive of voice-hearers' contributions to the interviews? To answer this, we employed a technique from the field of corpus linguistics known as a 'keyness analysis' (McEnery and Hardie, 2011). This involved using specialized software to compare the word frequencies in the interviews (excluding the interviewer's questions) with the word frequencies in a set of oral history interviews collected as part of the British National Corpus (Aston and Burnard, 1998).[1] This data set was similar enough to our interviews to make the comparison meaningful (as opposed to, for example, using a collection of news reports), but different enough to allow us to consider what is linguistically 'special' about the participants' reporting of their voice-hearing experiences. The analysis generated a rank-ordered list of words that are 'overused' to a statistically significant extent in the VIP interviews, as compared with the oral history interviews.[2] In corpus linguistics, these words are known as 'keywords'.

As is often the case with this kind of analysis, the top keywords in the VIP interviews include some predictable findings (e.g. *voice* and *voices*), as well as some less

---

[1] The British National Corpus provides 777,132 words of interview data, compared with 153,989 words from the interviews with voice-hearers. The specialized software used in our analysis can be found at: https://ucrel-wmatrix4.lancaster.ac.uk/wmatrix4.html.

[2] We combined a measure of effect size, LogRatio, with a measure of statistical significance often used in corpus linguistics, Log Likelihood. The LogRatio values were 0.71 for *n't* and 1.32 for *not*. Log Likelihood was set at a level that corresponds to $p < 0.0001$.

predictable ones. Among the latter were the words *not* and *n't*, i.e. the two main written realizations of the adverb for negation in English. In combination, they occur 4653 times in the interviews, and both are among the top 25 keywords.

In the VIP interviews, *not* and *n't* (henceforth referred to simply as *not*) are used to negate a wide range of states of affairs. While some instances of negation occur in answer to yes/no questions from the interviewer (e.g. 'Can you always understand what's being said?'), most do not. *Not* was more often used to negate certain (expected) characteristics of the voices (e.g. 'at first it wasn't so much aggressive'), beliefs of voice-hearers ('I don't believe in ghosts and spirits'), and their emotional reactions ('I didn't get angry'). In 248 cases, however, *not* was followed by a verb related to speech. Given the focus on communication from, about, and with voices in the interviews, we decided to concentrate on these. Depending on the choice of verb and surrounding expressions, different aspects of communication were negated, such as manner of speaking (e.g. 'They don't talk as loudly as they did then'), topic ('They haven't been talking about us at all'), and addressee ('They don't talk to me'). We also identified a substantial minority of cases where *not* was used to negate the occurrence of speech itself, resulting in different kinds of 'silence'.[3]

Four Types of Silences in the Experience of Voice-Hearing

By examining all cases where *not* was used by interviewees to negate the occurrence of speech, we identified four main types of 'silences', which differ depending on who is silent and how/why: (1) *silent voices*; (2) *voice-hearer silent about the voices*; (3) *voice-hearer silenced by the voices*; and (4) *voice-hearer silent with the voices*. These types of silences are all, in different ways, highly meaningful in the experiences of interviewees, and tell us something about how the participants' social relationships are affected by their voice-hearing experiences. More specifically, what we call *silent voices* are a particular aspect of the phenomenology of voice-hearing, whereas the other three types are all related to aspects of voice-hearers' interactions with the voices and with other people.

Silent Voices

Studies of voice-hearing have shown that 'hallucinated voices are usually experienced as having identities and making coherent communicative speech acts' (Bell, 2013, p. 1). However, the data show that, in some cases, *not* is used to negate the occurrence of speech on the part of the entities that are referred to throughout the interviews as 'voices'. This results in what we oxymoronically call *Silent voices*.

---

[3] Forms of the words 'silent/silence' occurred only four times in the interviews.

For example, while talking about his experience of hearing the voices of absent relatives, Hugh mentions an uncle in particular:[4]

Extract 1

HUGH: [M]e Uncle's just, just there . . .
INTERVIEWER: Right.
HUGH: . . . not moving, he's just there, in a prayer stance . . . Ehm, and that's comfort.
   So like me neighbour said he'd be freaking out, and I said, no, I could see him . . .
INTERVIEWER: Yeah.
HUGH: . . . but *he didn't say anything.*

Another interviewee, Xander, says that he hears three voices and, as the interview progresses, describes one of them as 'the quiet one'. When asked directly about whether he would 'ever have a conversation with the quiet voice', he replies:

Extract 2

Xander: I would, but at times because he doesn't speak, it's hard to know if he's there.

Both cases exemplify an aspect of the phenomenology of voice-hearing that undermines the use of the term 'voice' itself, namely the experience of the presence of a personified agent who could potentially speak but does not, or not always (see Alderson-Day and Fernyhough, 2016). The silence that results from non-speaking voices can be experienced in different ways. In Extract 1, Hugh describes the silent presence of his uncle as 'comfort' and reports himself as contradicting his neighbour's imagined reaction of 'freaking out' in that situation. In Extract 2, Xander seems to present the fact that one of the voices does not always speak as a missed opportunity for social interaction with that voice. In both cases, however, the silence is meaningful, both as an experience in the moment and to reiterate that the entities labelled as 'voices' are not always perceived to 'speak'. In contrast, in the three other types of silence, it is the voice-hearer's speech that is being negated.

Voice-Hearer Silent about the Voices

Some of the instances of negated speech occurred as part of interview questions on whether voice-hearers talk about their voices with people in their lives. Ryan, for example, says:

---

[4] Relevant sections have been italicized for emphasis.

Extract 3

RYAN: [W]hen I do, they do get upset. So it is, it's quite a difficult thing to do, unless I sugar coat it quite a lot and then they can, they can sort of comprehend it but I find it easier just *not to talk about it.*

In response to similar questions, Xander mentions that he has talked about the voices with his mother and sister, but also adds:

Extract 4

XANDER: [W]ith my dad, *I don't really talk to him about it,* just like, it's always been like that with my dad. . . . with my gran and my granddad, *I don't talk to them about it,* because I don't want them to worry.

Here the negation of speech activities does not result in prototypical silence in the sense of a total absence of the sound of speaking, but rather in a form of self-censorship that constitutes a social kind of silence: the absence of communication about the voices in interactional contexts where such communication is, in principle, possible, and arguably even desirable.

The reasons for this kind of silence highlight both the sensitivity of voice-hearing as a topic and how closely intertwined the voice-hearing experience is with the person's most intimate social relationships. As a topic, the experience of voice-hearing is, to some extent, 'untellable' (Jaworski, 1993): it is hard to express ('I sugar coat it quite a lot and then they can, they can sort of comprehend it'); it is private and subjective, and therefore not suitable for people with whom communication is not usually particularly intimate ('it's always been like that with my dad'); and it is potentially upsetting for people with whom mutual relationships are more intimate and caring ('they do get upset and I don't want them to worry').

This kind of silence therefore reflects differences in the voice-hearer's existing relationships with other people, and in the ways in which these relationships are, in turn, affected by the voice-hearer's decision to share the experience of voice-hearing or not. While the underlying self-censorship is driven by the wish to protect others, as well as by one's own public image, it also obviously deprives the voice-hearer of the empathy and support that they could otherwise potentially receive from people in their lives. The detrimental effects of 'self-silencing' have been reported as affecting interpersonal relationships with respect to various health complaints (Jack, 1991).

Voice-Hearer Silenced by the Voices

In other cases, it is the voices that are presented as preventing hearers from engaging with others in their social environment. Ian, for example, says that his voice 'tells us *not to talk* to people' and that he 'hardly see[s] friends now'. Similarly, Will quotes his own voice as telling him:

Extract 5

WILL: *Don't talk* to that person because they don't like you, or *don't . . . ehm . . . speak* to them because you don't, you can't trust them.

In the previous types of silence, we saw how hearers are isolated through their own reluctance to discuss their voices, as a difficult or 'upsetting' topic. Here, the voice-hearers are discouraged from engaging with others altogether, despite their desire to do so. In the example above, Will both receives explicit instruction not to talk to someone and reports a more implicit form of oppression in which his confidence is undermined and the voice creates distrust ('you can't trust them'). In addition, in Extract 6, although the voice does not explicitly forbid talking to others, the name-calling that Carl experiences from the voices affects his participation in conversations with other people:

Extract 6

CARL: When I'm talking to people and that, and . . . *I don't want to talk* because I feel embarrassed.

Whether or not voice-hearing itself is experienced as distressing, this particular type of oppressive relationship with voices—where the voices prevent people from leading their lives as they would wish to—is known to cause distress (Varese et al., 2017).

Voice-Hearer Silent with the Voices

The final type of silence consists of cases where the voice-hearer does not 'respond' or 'talk back' in the voice-hearing situation, even though the voice is speaking. This group includes examples such as:

Extract 7

DAN: I *can't talk* back to the computer one. . . . That's never happened.

Extract 8

HUGH: And during the day I *don't respond* . . . to it, well I *try not to respond* to it anyway. . . . I'm just hearing it and doing that thing of putting it in the box . . . to deal with later. Because that's the only way I can deal with it.

In these cases, not responding to the voices is potentially a strategy that people have adopted, a kind of coping mechanism, as Hugh says. It is an exercise of power on the part of the voice-hearer. However, the voice-hearer's lack of response is hedged using the modal verb *can't* (Extract 7) and the semi-modal *try* (Extract 8). These, once again, suggest a potential thwarting of the voice-hearer's ability to behave in a way that they wish to. *Can't* suggests a lack of ability where the ability might be welcome, while *try* implies unsuccessful attempts at doing something, in this case not responding to the voices. This becomes clearer in the following examples.

Extract 9

ALEX: On a night time I *try not to talk* back. . . . Ehm, so sometimes if I try to ignore them, I mean I don't actually get to ignore them.

Extract 10

ZARA: I *don't want to answer* them. . . . Because at first I was saying, I would say, hello, and then people would say, there's nobody there.

These examples appear to be the converse of those where the voice-hearer is silenced by their voices. Here the voices force the hearer into non-silence, when the person would otherwise wish to remain quiet. Being prevented from staying silent has similar implications for the ability to live the life one wishes to, as in the case of being silenced by the voices, but a different aspect of the person's potential coping mechanism is affected. Above, the voices limit social engagement, and therefore social support, while here they interfere with the person's ability to exert control through refusing to engage with the voices. This is especially important as voice-hearers sometimes report that speaking back to the voice does not help the situation, but 'just sort of happens because it can be so overwhelming' (Dan).

Our discussion of the last three types of silences—between voice-hearers and their support network of family and friends (*Voice-hearer silent about the voices*), and between voice-hearers and their voices (*Voice-hearer silenced by the voices*; *Voice-hearer silent with the voices*)—emphasizes the importance of dialogue in the voice-hearing experience, which is consistent with a range of therapies for psychosis (Avdi et al., 2015). As Avdi et al. (2015, pp. 330–1) explain:

> through dialogue . . . the family or network's psychological resources are mobilized, and participants regain their voice and assume positions of increased agency with regard to the symptoms. Dialogue is considered to allow strong emotions to be expressed, new words for difficult experiences to be jointly created, and new understandings to emerge.

Our analysis has drawn attention to the ways in which voice-hearers are inhibited from participating in dialogue (e.g. because the 'voice' does not speak, or because the voice warns them against doing so) or set out to reduce their distress by not engaging in dialogue with the voice, and how this reflects their level of agency. This can have consequences for voice-hearers' engagement with (dialogically informed) therapies and their ongoing relationships with their voices.

Conclusion

In this chapter, we have described how a (computer-aided) linguistic analysis of the forty VIP interviews first drew our attention to negation as a distinctive feature of interviewees' contributions, and then enabled us to identify the more specific phenomenon of references to silence via the negation of speech verbs. We have distinguished between four different types of silences and shown that, as has been observed in other contexts, they amount to much more than the absence of sound and speech: depending on who is silent, with whom, and why, silences can reveal phenomenological nuances, as well as pressures and power asymmetries in the relationships that interviewees have with their voices and with important people in their lives. These can, in turn, reflect or lead to distress. In this sense, references to silence deserve as much attention as references to the perception and/or occurrence of speech in accounts of the lived experience of voice-hearing.

References

Alderson-Day, B., and Fernyhough, C. (2016). Auditory verbal hallucinations: social but how? *Journal of Consciousness Studies*, 23(7–8), 163–94.

Aston, G., and Burnard, L. (1998). *The BNC Handbook: Exploring the British National Corpus with SARA*. Edinburgh: Edinburgh University Press.

Avdi, E., Lerou, V., and Seikkula, J. (2015). Dialogical features, therapist responsiveness, and agency in a therapy for psychosis. *Journal of Constructivist Psychology*, 28(4), 329–41.

Bell, V. (2013). A community of one: social cognition and auditory verbal hallucinations. *PLoS Biology*, 11(12), e1001723.

Horn, L. R. (2010). *The Expression of Negation*. New York, NY: Walter de Gruyter.

Jack, D. C. (1991). *Silencing the Self: Women and Depression*. Cambridge, MA: Harvard University Press.

Jaworski, A. (1993). *The Power of Silence: Social and Pragmatic Perspectives*. London: Sage Publications.

McEnery, T., and Hardie, A. (2011). *Corpus Linguistics: Theory, Methods and Practice*. Cambridge: Cambridge University Press.

Roitman, M. (2017). *The Pragmatics of Negation. Negative Meanings, Uses and Discursive Functions*. Amsterdam: Benjamins.

Varese, F., Mansell, W., and Tai, S. J. (2017). What is distressing about auditory verbal hallucinations? The contribution of goal interference and goal facilitation. *Psychology and Psychotherapy: Theory, Research and Practice*, 90(4), 720–34.

About the Authors

Elena Semino is Professor in the Department of Linguistics and English Language at Lancaster University and Director of the ESRC Centre for Corpus Approaches to Social Science. She applies qualitative and quantitative linguistic methods to texts concerned with the lived experience of illness. She has a specific interest in the language used in first-person accounts of psychosis and voice-hearing.

Luke Collins is a Senior Research Associate in the Centre for Corpus Approaches to Social Science at Lancaster University. His research interests lie in the linguistic representations of mental health and illness in clinical contexts. Using methods in corpus linguistics, he examines patterns in the reported user experiences of clinical interventions to assess their impact.

Zsófia Demjén is Associate Professor of Applied Linguistics at University College London. She explores the implications of how language is used to describe experiences of illness, including in contexts associated with cancer, depression, and 'psychosis'. She recently led a project investigating the extent to which implicit power relationships in the language people use to talk about their voices can predict their likely level of distress.

PART FIVE
SPATIAL AND RELATIONAL DIMENSIONS

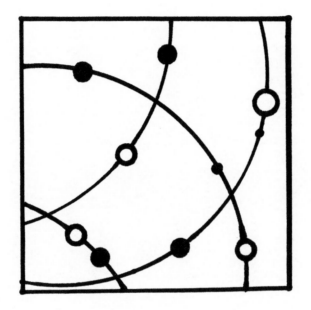

PART FIVE

SPATIAL AND RELATIONAL DIMENSIONS

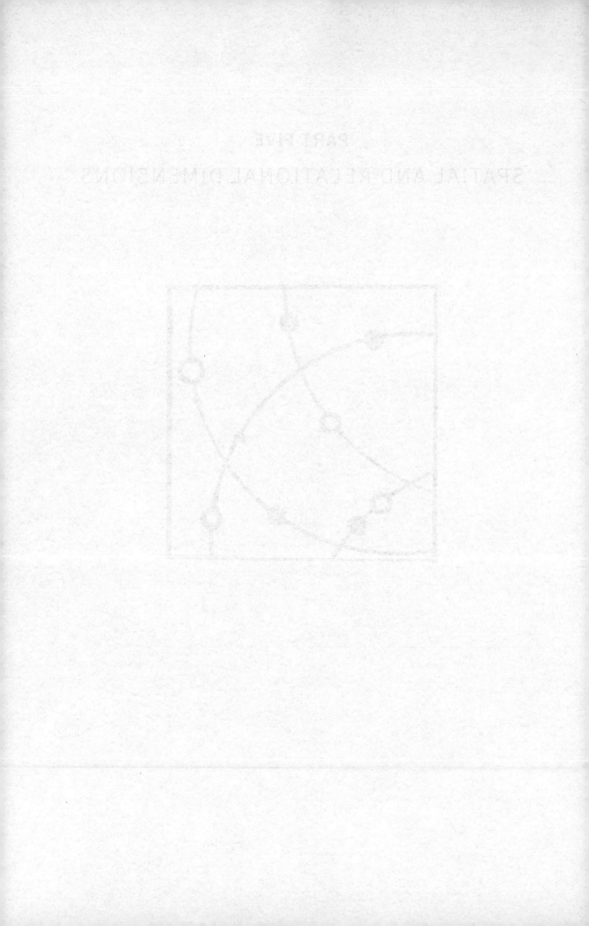

18

Household Ghosts and Personified Presences

Peter Garratt, Department of English Studies, Durham University

Some people describe hearing voices that feel thickened by history, voices located in or projected from a point recognizably in the past. Voices out of time. There are several such examples in the Voices in Psychosis interviews. Here is Will, for instance, describing one of his familiar voices 'Lucy':

> Oh yeah, I know what she looks like. She's about 5'4"....And she's got long black hair but it always covers her eyes, I can never see her eyes....And she's got like this like cream, like petti dress, like you know a petticoat dress on, it seems Victorian-y.

Lucy is richly personified, along multiple axes. Besides this strong visual imagery, her presence is associated with tactile and olfactory sensations, including a distinctive smell that Will describes as old and musty (like the Beamish Museum or 'Vikings') which often presages her appearance. He can reach out and touch her hair, which is long and black and conceals her face, as she sits before him—a sensation that once left Will unsure whether or not he had 'made a friend'. The quality of historicity accretes in these multisensory textures of Will's experience. Even though at times he feels Lucy's presence without any such imagery—she can go unseen and unheard, yet definitely be there—he still refers to her 'tangible' nature and repeatedly cites feelings of embodied proximity ('it's always like as if someone was sat next to me'). At the same time, Lucy has 'demonic' attributes. Intimate and remote, dominant yet evasive, touchable while also withdrawing: this is a voice clothed literally in the past, in 'Victorian-y' dress, at once inside and outside history, adrift, like some mysterious dream figure or a Victorian ghost.

Ghosts inhabit their own time and anticipatory structure: a ghost's surprise is, after all, uncannily expected. Their characteristic of returning, however it might strain the cordial bond of host and guest, makes possible certain kinds of spectral sociability. Certainly in classic Victorian ghost stories—still an important source of attitudes towards ghosts—supernatural encounters tend to be framed by this 'strange act of hospitality' (Thurston, 2012), as returning spirits turn up in houses, hotels, lodgings, parlours, and bedrooms, sometimes mutedly or with cryptic intent, but usually to

Peter Garratt, *Household Ghosts and Personified Presences* In: *Voices in Psychosis*. Edited by: Angela Woods, Ben Alderson-Day, and Charles Fernyhough, Oxford University Press. © Peter Garratt 2022. DOI: 10.1093/oso/9780192898388.003.0018 perturb a self made strange by the unchosen offices of witness and host. The sequence of ghosts that attend Scrooge in his chamber in Charles Dickens's *A Christmas Carol* (1843) is only the most famous example of this Victorian urge to domesticate hauntings, evacuating the ghost from its traditional locales of the abbey, castle, and ruin, all staples of eighteenth-century gothic literature, and making it literally at home. Household ghosts featured in *Household Words*, Dickens's weekly magazine. Many other distinguished nineteenth-century writers, from Elizabeth Gaskell to Thomas Hardy, turned their hand to a variant of the English ghost story in which haunting happens amidst everyday objects and surroundings. The late-Victorian master of the genre M. R. James raised the hearthside narrative of strange hospitality into an art form, with tales such as *The Haunted Dolls' House* (1923).

Will's interview, by illustrating how historicity enters into voice personification, invites some larger questions. How did Victorian ghosts, and the literary and cultural frameworks that made them legible, intersect with understandings of what it meant to hear voices? How were these phenomena related? And how might answering that question matter today, by yielding fresh perspectives on voices in psychosis or by enriching our understandings of the sort of language used to describe them?

Popular writers, including Dickens, were sometimes prone to depicting voices in the head as symptoms of disordered or diseased selves. Years before publishing his first ghost story, Dickens had written 'The Drunkard's Death', a fictional narrative from his early miscellaneous volume *Sketches by Boz* (1836) about an alcoholic's inexorable descent into penury and squalor, featuring bouts of psychosis (the term psychosis is not used, though it appeared in British psychiatry texts from around 1870). In the slim plot, the protagonist selfishly flees the deathbed of his wife, abandons his family, and later neglects his acutely ill daughter and unwittingly hands over his fugitive son to the authorities for hanging. All lives are ruined. At the end of the story, now destitute, weary, and guilt-ridden, he stands on the edge of the Thames, by Waterloo Bridge, in extremis (Dickens, 1995, p. 565):

> The tide was in, and the water flowed at his feet. The rain had ceased, the wind was lulled, and all was, for the moment, still and quiet—so quiet that the slightest sound on the opposite bank, even the rippling of the water against the barges that were moored there, was distinctly audible to his ear. The stream stole languidly and sluggishly on. Strange and fantastic forms rose to the surface, and beckoned him to approach; dark gleaming eyes peered from the water, and seemed to mock his hesitation, while hollow murmurs from behind, urged him onwards. He retreated a few paces, took a short run, desperate leap, and plunged into the river.

Hallucinations drive this final scene of the story to its tragic climax. The man drowns, and days later his 'disfigured' corpse is discovered downriver: 'Unrecognizable and unpitied, it was borne to the grave; and there it has long since mouldered away!' (Dickens, 1995, p. 566). The mind disintegrates, followed swiftly by the body. Strikingly, Dickens plays on the ear's susceptibility to impressions of sound: the momentary near-silence, the noise of rippling water, the 'hollow murmurs' the man hears from behind, which conspire with the ghoulish mocking faces that appear out of the river and urge him to leap—all of these details narrate an intense auditory world. Hearing conspiring malevolent voices testifies to a fully collapsing psyche. In narrative terms, there is no way back, no retrievable moral self, once this has happened. Voices betoken insanity. He ends up in the drink, in both senses of the word.

But even in this short story of an alcoholic suicide, Dickens's writing manages to open up subtly different kinds of voice experiences, not just overpowering torment. A last twist hints at this. Plunged into the Thames, the protagonist instantly yearns to live, not die. As he flails around helplessly in the current, these destructive whispers and murmurs cease, as if purified by water, and a familiar voice takes their place: that of his late son William, whom he betrayed, who swore vengefully to return at the hour of the father's death and 'cry for judgment' against him before God. Now, sinking under the water, 'the curse of his son rang in his ears' (Dickens, 1995, p. 565). The intrusion of this distinct voice, reviving words originally spoken aloud and reliving them as an involuntary echo, only deepens the pathos of the scene. Whether a product of memory, conscience, a fearful imagination, or mishearing— or even a sincere message from beyond the grave—this voice is not just a symptom of a deranged state. If anything, it pulls a fraying self back towards meaning and recognition, binding the past to the present, by compelling the drunkard to face his own misdeeds. The curse of the wayward son crystallizes the sins of the father. In sharpening that pattern of meaning, this voice at the very end of the narrative builds upon earlier suggestions of sensory disturbance and reverie. While wandering the streets, the man has a consoling vision in which his dead children are resurrected before him, like tactile ghosts, and their presences can keenly be heard as well as felt: 'voices long since hushed in death sounded in his ears like the music of village bells' (Dickens, 1995, p. 564). Later, lying in a filthy doorway and unable to sleep, he has the vivid sense of being back inside a tavern full of bonhomie and ready gratification: 'The well-known shout of drunken mirth sounded in his ear, the glass was at his lips, the board was covered with choice rich food'. As the narrator says, 'illusion was reality itself' (Dickens, 1995, p. 564). Such finely observed moments of hearing other voices—first as music, then as hubbub—capture understandable human longings that spring from the pain of social exile and its correlative feeling, shame.

One could think about this as Dickens creating an emotional landscape out of unbidden voices, anticipating the way his full-length novels liberally include human noise and the jabber and tics of characterful speech. Accents and phrases matter so fundamentally to Dickens that reading him partly becomes a practice of listening, of tuning in or overhearing. Examples are legion, from 'umble Uriah Heap to the mangled idiom of Mrs Gamp, the red-nosed nurse from *Martin Chuzzlewit* (1844). Marked vocal effects are everywhere, yet voices do more than simply add to the comic energy and wider textual *jouissance* of Dickens's worlds. They are also linked to the pervasive sense of agency within those worlds, the tendency of the physical environment to seem oddly alive and alert—a quality described by *Fraser's Magazine*, in

1857, as Dickens's habit of 'giving to inanimate things the attributes of life' (Forsyth, 1857, p. 262) and identified by later critics as his hallucinatory style (Van Ghent, 1950). From *Sketches by Boz* onwards, agency in Dickens is something that flows beyond the boundaries of individual personality and spreads out into the atmosphere of the novels. Voices emanating from unusual places belong to this larger attribution of person-like qualities to impersonal things.

Towards the end of *Great Expectations* (1861), for instance, Pip spends a terrible night in a cheap hotel in Covent Garden known as the Hummums. In the dark, everything emits noise (Dickens, 2008, p. 335):

> What a doleful night! How anxious, how dismal, how long! When I had lain awake a little while, those extraordinary voices with which silence teems, began to make themselves audible. The closet whispered, the fireplace sighed, the little washing stand ticked, and one guitar string played occasionally in the chest of drawers.

Pip's sense of self has recently been shattered by the revelation that Miss Havisham is not his secret benefactor as he long supposed—in his eyes, she appears a 'spectral figure' (Dickens, 2008, p. 334)—and now, discovering that he has been living in the wrong plot, Pip must refashion the entire narrative of his identity. Acute distress and personal threat both deepen the sense of crisis: he has just parted from Estella, whom he loves, seemingly for good, only to discover a note from the legal clerk Wemmick warning him not to return home. In the darkness of the dreary hotel room, the quiet of night becomes audible, and rich with acoustic texture. It crowds with 'night fancies and night-noises' (Dickens, 2008, p. 335) that whisper out of the furniture as if from a secret realm of animate matter—a roar lying on the other side of silence, to borrow a phrase from his fellow Victorian novelist George Eliot. It is no coincidence that this happens just as Pip feels existentially hollowed out, having lost his guiding star Estella, who intends to marry the brute Bentley Drummle, for it accords with the general tendency in Dickens for agency to leach into the life of physical things, away from human actors.

The Hummums episode rekindles a child's fear of the dark, in fact. As a response to the invisible otherness of night, hearing 'voices' in the room very briefly recasts Pip as the scared infant, indeed the boy he was at the start of the novel, as if his narrative instinctively gropes for its own origins at the onset of crisis. In Chapter 2, young Pip had lain awake at night 'in mortal terror' (Dickens, 2008, p. 14), too afraid to sleep, so this is an act of unconscious mimicry on his part. The whispering wardrobe and sighing fireplace are proxies for a haunting past. If fears about an unsafe world connect these distant points in *Great Expectations*, Pip's personifying is certainly not delirious or pathological at this fretful moment. The voices give a kind of shape to swirling anxieties over who or what he truly is—the proper parameters of his personhood—and yet they only exaggerate ordinary habits of perception, which in other contexts could have more positive effects, as Dickens's writing shows. A fanciful attitude can gently humanize the environment or even conjure companionable presences. Master Humphrey, the narrator of *Master Humphrey's Clock*, a serial begun by Dickens in 1840, would be one example: his old clock has morphed into a trusted friend in the corner of his room, its familiar chimes a kindly voice for Humphrey to interact with—'a cheerful watcher at his chamber door' (Dickens, 2012, p. 60), as Dickens explained to his friend John Forster. Elsewhere, characterful objects in passages of narrative description can leap out for attention by being carriers of active verbs, as in 'Meditations in Monmouth Street', from *Sketches by Boz*, in which the observing gaze falls upon clothes for sale in a shop window that rise up and walk (Dickens, 1995, p. 98):

> We have gone on speculating in this way, until whole rows of coats have started from their pegs, and buttoned up, of their own accord, round the waists of imaginary wearers; lines of trousers have jumped down to meet them; waistcoats have almost burst with anxiety to put themselves on; and half an acre of shoes have suddenly found feet to fit them, and gone stumping down the street with a noise which has fairly awakened us from our pleasant reverie.

This is noisy personification realized as urban enchantment. It remains faintly ghostly, too, like a whirl of phantom limbs, for these are second-hand clothes and once the property of the dead.

The impression Dickens creates is that there are no sharp distinctions between fanciful thoughts, reverie, everyday errors of the senses, and delusions or hallucinations. Gradations of experience are minutely subtle. This was a perspective that overlapped with the views of prominent late nineteenth-century scientists and pseudoscientists. The end of the Victorian period saw the first studies of hallucinations in the general population, carried out by leading lights of the Society for Psychical Research. *Phantasms of the Living* (1886), a compendious two-volume study by Edmund Gurney, Frederic Myers, and Frank Podmore, was based on data collected from over 5000 respondents, while a much larger study, begun in the late 1880s, with a sample size of 17,000, was published as a *Report on the Census of Hallucinations* in 1894. In the latter study, almost 10% of the Victorian public surveyed reported having had at least one hallucination in their lifetime, including hearing a voice in the absence of any external cause. To read these studies is to be impressed by the sheer labour of evidence-gathering they represent—statistical analysis, tables, and commentary on method abound, interspersed with liberal use of first-person testimonies—but, equally, they struggle to disentangle hallucinations cleanly from experientially similar phenomena, such as felt presences, waking dreams, hypnagogia, visions, or illusions. Healthy people reported having all such experiences, the studies illustrate.

A decade earlier, the scientific psychologist James Sully had made much the same point in his study *Illusions* (1881): 'if it is clearly made out that there are hallucinations in the strict sense, that is to say, false perceptions which are wholly due to internal causes, it must be conceded that illusion shades off into hallucination by steps which it is impossible for science to mark' (Sully, 1891, p. 12). Sully was similarly interested in how common it was to see and hear absent things, rather than in hallucinations as symptoms of insanity. And there were earlier advocates of this approach who were much closer to Dickens's orbit. Less well known than Sully's work is a short personal essay published by Dickens in *Household Words*, in February 1857, entitled 'My Ghosts'. Its anonymous author was probably John Robertson, a Scottish writer and journalist who lived on the fringes of mid-Victorian literary London. The 'ghosts' of his title turn out to have been hallucinatory states stretching back into a difficult, abusive childhood. 'I am a haunted man,' he declares, possibly with a glancing reference to Dickens's Christmas ghost story of that name from 1848, 'descended from haunted mothers' (Anon, 1857, p. 165). The essay is a somewhat portentous example of Victorian self-help, in one sense. As an infant, he suffered at the hands of female nurses, one of whom gave him night terrors; he would be punished and confined to a garret room; he went on to stammer, finding learning and literacy a challenge; he was treated as a delinquent and incurable type. Later, while studying at university, he was humiliated during a public examination when the 'sway of my ghostly mother asserted itself once more' (Anon, 1857, p. 168). These experiences of 'dreaming awake'—which he associates with a paralysed will—have led him to attribute his suffering to an acquired nervous disorder. But, in a remarkable final pivot, 'My Ghosts' explains how the author has consciously invented new voices to neutralize the negative ones (Anon, 1857, p. 168):

> Wherever I reside I find out the ancient residences of remarkable persons the memory of whom is fitted to increase the love of truth and justice. Portraits and descriptions enable me to recall from the dark of the past, the dead of distant days. Whenever I visit the towns in which they have lived, I call upon my ghosts more assiduously than upon my friends. I see them as they have lived. Knowing from their writings their thoughts, I freely discuss with them their opinions. Laugh at me as you may, it is to the device of voluntarily creating such good ghosts, that I owe my emancipation from the hideous phantoms which enslaved my childhood.

This practice he dubs 'ghost-making', an improvised therapy for managing distressing voices and visions, 'combating ghosts by ghosts' (Anon, 1857, p. 168). Examples of these ghost-voices include Shakespeare and Isaac Newton, both representatives of enlightened genius—and now imagined companionable presences. If this is coloured by a Victorian faith in the efficacy of isolated willpower, and by a Dickensian interest in the vulnerable child, neither point should divert attention from the 'strange hospitality' that links psychosis and haunting in this eccentric autobiographical narrative, as it does in fiction of the same period.

One could interpret a much-loved Dickens ghost story like 'The Signalman' (1866) along similar lines. In that story, an apparition at the mouth of a railway tunnel is the occasion for an intense connection between two men, a narrator who trespasses onto a branch line and a solitary signalman who anxiously welcomes him, to tell his tale of being haunted. A bond of guest and host is efficiently formed, paralleling the supernatural one, and immediately made strange by the narrator's unknowing repetition of the ghost's bellowed words 'Halloa! Below there!'. They are pulled curiously together, in a story about unexpected human contact and impulsive, even mildly furtive, male sociability. The ghost-mimicking narrator is himself a kind of companionable presence, an uncanny guest stripped of obvious social ties who politely imposes himself on the signalman at the start of the story, only to become his confidant. Trust binds them in temporary intimacy, which allows the tale to be told, though the source of that trust goes unexplained. Why is their bond so easily formed, so unencumbered? No account is given; it remains as mysterious as the spectre itself. In the end, like interlocking enigmas, acts of haunting and befriending in the 'The Signalman' come to resemble each other, even though the action happens away from the hospitable home.

Dickens frames the hearing of ghostly voices using this elaborate double structure without recourse to gothicized clichés of terror or madness. By the time he wrote 'The Signalman', literary narratives fed a wider appetite for encountering ghosts and, in a looping fashion, fed on it too, well before Freud, Janet, and the new theories of dissociation, and before the 'popular belief that visual [and auditory] hallucinations are uncommon in the general population and are probably prominent symptoms of major mental disorder' (McCorristine, 2010, p. 215). For this reason, the period's writing and culture valuably demonstrate that voices in psychosis and fictional voices can be a window on how we understand ghostly presences, whether as intimations of otherness or as richly personified companions—or what the signalman simply calls 'that someone else'. That someone else might involve a multifaceted sense of otherness, as the Voices in Psychosis interviews suggest: a crowding or clamour, a feeling of voices being 'like they're in the room' (Xander) or 'banging on [the] wall' (Carl), a 'static-y feeling' of there being 'someone there but you can't see them, but you know they're there' (Emma). For Will, his 'Victorian-y' voice Lucy sits and talks beside him. These transcripts, and others, carry the sense of something spectre-like beyond the self. The nineteenth century regarded such encounters differently. The complexity of earlier attitudes towards ghosts—and the variety in Dickens's imaginative use of voices—highlights how deeply culturally informed, and even strangely hospitable, this encounter could be.

References

Anon (1857). My Ghosts. *Household Words*, 15, 165–8.

Dickens, C. (1995 [1836]). *Sketches by Boz*, ed. D. Walder. London: Penguin.

Dickens, C. (2008 [1861]). *Great Expectations*, ed. M. Cardwell. Oxford: Oxford World's Classics.

Dickens, C. (2012). *The Selected Letters of Charles Dickens*, ed. J. Hartley. New York, NY: Oxford University Press.

Forsyth, W. (1857). Literary style. *Fraser's Magazine*, 55, 249–64.

McCorristine, S. (2010). *Spectres of the Self: Thinking about Ghosts and Ghost-Seeing in England, 1750–1920*. Cambridge: Cambridge University Press.

Sully, J. (1891). *Illusions*. New York, NY: Appleton and Co.

Thurston, L. (2012). *Literary Ghosts from the Victorians to Modernism: The Haunting Interval.* London: Routledge.

Van Ghent, D. (1950). The Dickens world: a view from Todgers's. *The Sewannee Review,* 58(3), 419–38.

About the Author

Peter Garratt is an Associate Professor in the Department of English Studies, Durham University. He has written and edited books about Victorian literature and culture and the cognitive humanities. He is currently editing a volume on British literature and philosophy, 1832–1872, for Routledge.

19

Voice-Hearing and Lived Space

Mary Coaten, South West Yorkshire Partnership NHS Foundation Trust

When people hear voices, they will often be asked whether it sounds like the voice is coming from inside or outside of their head, and whether it can be experienced as close or far away. But the spaces that voices occupy might be much stranger and harder to pin down. Might there be an embodied and spatially aware way in which to frame voice-hearing? This chapter will explore the lived body experience described by voice-hearers in the Voices in Psychosis (VIP) interviews, while also referring to the findings from my own research in dance movement psychotherapy (DMP), with a particular focus on trauma.

A striking feature of the VIP transcripts is the frequency with which voice-hearing is described in terms of being in communication with, or relating to, something that was moving or was described through a language of movement. This is of particular interest to me as a dance movement psychotherapist with considerable experience of working with people experiencing voice-hearing in the National Health Service (NHS). Drawing on the work of Heidegger and Merleau-Ponty, this chapter uses the theory and practice of DMP to consider the relationship between space, time, and what I describe as the 'mytho-poetic' experience of hearing voices.

Space has always been of interest in the psychiatric assessment of hearing voices. However, in DMP, there is interest not just in where voices are (as in the use of internal versus external location to guide psychiatric diagnosis), but also in something more dynamic, relational, and potentially disclosing of meaning. In the VIP transcripts, those hearing voices often describe the experience in terms of space, with the voice being located in or as coming from inside, outside, far away, upstairs, or through a wall. Consider the following examples from the transcripts (emphasis added):

> Sometimes. . . . It's something really close, like a presence *right here or behind, never in front*. (Grace)
>
>   [It] sounds as if he's just *sitting beside us or sitting on me shoulder* . . . it always feels like it's outside. (Iris)
>
>   I've heard them *on the left side* as well, but it's mainly *the right side that I'm hearing them*. (Xander)

Mary Coaten, *Voice-Hearing and Lived Space* In: *Voices in Psychosis*. Edited by: Angela Woods, Ben Alderson-Day, and Charles Fernyhough, Oxford University Press. © Mary Coaten 2022. DOI: 10.1093/oso/9780192898388.003.0019

> Yeah, sometimes it can sound like somebody's *right up next to your eardrum*. Saying the words into your ear . . . Or, if you, if you sort of *pick that up at the back end*, it can feel like it's happened inside of your head. (Bill)

Here voice proximity is registered in relation to the body, as well as in relation to how intrusive or uncomfortable that might feel to the hearer. For example, if you are sitting beside someone and they talk to you, right next to your eardrum, this might feel somewhat unnerving.

Additionally, the voice's location in one's personal space, whether near or far, might reflect something embedded in personal relations or affect. One could speculate that the voice-hearer's relationship to the voice might both reflect and be reflected in its spatial location. For example, are some voices more likely to be experienced as violations of privacy or personal space, as engendering a sense of suspicion or threat? In describing whether voices are, near, far, to the left, to the right, on the shoulder, next to the eardrum, and so on, voice-hearers are locating the voice less in an objective space than in one arising out of feelings and social relations. This next example further elucidates these points:

> Different angle, sometime here, sometimes there . . . And from that voice, from really far away, *it's like my uncle is staying in [place] and I'm in [place] so far, far away*. (Neil)

Neil's experience gives me a sense of movement (the voice appears here, there, and 'far far away') and of something changing in his personal space. What also strikes me is a connection to a disembodied voice which becomes carefully placed in specific locations, either very close or very far away. The reference to distance also seems important, not necessarily in the objective sense, but in a symbolic or metaphoric one. The metaphoric and relational sense of space expressed in these accounts can first be framed by looking into philosophical accounts of the phenomenology of space.

Phenomenological Approaches to Space

In the transcripts, the location of the disembodied voice is expressed in a variety of ways, often emphasizing qualities of nearness, remoteness, and orientation ('right next to my eardrum', 'far, far, away', 'on the right side, not the left side'). As we have already seen, these accounts emphasize location in embodied and subjective terms: what matters is the voice's place in relation to the voice-hearer, which is very different from what is traditionally understood as a more objective or measurable sense of space. Phenomenologically, according to Heidegger, it is our 'being-in-the-world' that makes the opening up of space possible. This 'being in'—defined as *Dasein* (Heidegger, 1953, p. 102)—is translated as presence, a sense of aliveness, existence, and 'being there'. In terms of spatiality, *Dasein* has its own 'being in space' and 'is possible only on the basis of being-in-the-world in general' (Heidegger, 1953, p. 56). This being-in-the-world is rooted in a familiarity of 'being-with-others' and concerns 'de-distancing and directionality' (Heidegger, 1953, p. 102). Here, 'de-distancing' is not to be understood as a specific measurable distance, but more existentially as space in which we are oriented. The existential constitution of 'being-in-the-world' also has a directedness—such as the right or the left, the forward or the back—and this emerges from one's innerworldly space and sense of being present in the world. This encounter with the 'other' through our 'being-in-the world' implies there is an existential and relational space that opens up between self and other, which is unique to the person, and reveals something about the relational in the process. When Neil describes the voice of his uncle as being 'far, far away', this seems as much an insight into Neil's sense of emotional proximity to his uncle as his physical proximity to the voice he hears.

Merleau-Ponty (2012, p. 298) agrees with Heidegger that space is related to existential existence but makes a unique contribution in relation to what he describes as a 'lived space'. In describing lived space, Merleau-Ponty refers to persons for whom 'spatiality exists through an inner necessity, [since] it opens to an "outside" such that one can speak of a mental space and of a world of significations and objects, and of thought' (Merleau-Ponty, 2014, p. 307). With regard to the VIP transcripts, I argue this inner necessity opens to the outside in the form of the disembodied voice: the voice creates a mental space in which something significant happens, and distance disappears in the objective sense.

Movement and Lived Space

The form of locating oneself in space that I have been discussing is not only experienced psychically, but also physically. Having explained that voices occupy a lived, relational space, it might seem strange to think about physical movement as being relevant or beneficial. But our own sense of space and the cues indicating where we are in space and time are inextricably linked. As a dance movement psychotherapist, I am interested in how individuals move and interact in space and time, both individually and as a group, and the impact this has on our feelings and emotions.

DMP provides an opportunity to explore people's sense of space and be able to help people reform/reshape their relationships in the light of it. As stated by the UK's Association for Dance Movement Psychotherapy:

> DMP recognises body movement as an implicit and expressive instrument of communication and expression. DMP is a relational process in which client/s and therapist engage in an empathic creative process using body movement and dance to assist integration of emotional, cognitive, physical, social and spiritual aspects of self.

DMP helps to increase awareness of self in space while also locating the relational other. In experiencing movement and dance as meaningful and emotionally significant, together with the bodily sensations that accompany them, a connection is forged between movement and emotional expression which helps the person to locate themselves spatially, in relation to the other and in relation to their own voices and their meaning. Techniques such as 'interactional synchrony', where the movement becomes finely attuned in response to the other, and 'non-directive improvised movement', where there is simply an invitation to move freely in the space in whichever way the individual chooses, help match the rhythmic components of the music being played to the movement qualities of the group or individual. A sense of agency can be developed through defining body boundaries, grounding, and 'mirroring' the movement of others. The feelings associated with this process and with the non-verbal group take place in conjunction with the symbolic and metaphoric aspects that arise (for example, DMP makes use of the movement metaphors 'jumping out of one's skin', 'going out on a limb', and 'jumping for joy'). Feelings become expressed in the space and one is able to forge more of a felt connection with the body.

The significance of space and time to the therapeutic mechanisms of DMP was highlighted by my recent study of DMP in an acute adult in-patient setting (Coaten, 2020). Analysing the qualitative dynamics of movement and the symbolic and metaphoric processes expressed during DMP sessions, I found that participants often expressed their distress through 'mytho-poetic' images such as cosmic egg, ancestors in trees, 'Smiley' acid image, aliens, spaceships, and ghosts. The group often then took these symbols up collectively by literally moving together with these visual images. Similarities to the experiences reported in the VIP transcripts—including the sense of the voice and the image moving around, and the changing spatial dynamics—were striking. Participants in the sessions, as in the transcripts, demonstrated an altered sense of space and time. Movement analysis, conducted using the Kestenberg Movement Profile (KMP) (Kestenberg-Amighi et al., 2018), indicated a specific imbalance in engaging with the future and the past. Interestingly, the study also revealed several gender differences in the use of space and sense of self. Both men's and women's movements in the space lacked structure, a lack compensated for through my movements as the practitioner–researcher. However, participants expressed their sense of self differently by gender, such that men engaged more with one another as a group and women focused more on the individual bodily self. Symbolic and metaphoric communications were strongly present, indicating a relationship with an altered sense of space and time.

One's relationship with time is expressed through advancing and retreating movements. In KMP terms, advancing with acceleration, rather than deceleration, creates a sense of rushing forward at speed. For example, one of the male participants Janek advanced towards me while accelerating. This movement indicated a lack of awareness of the other in space, giving me little opportunity to respond with consideration. Janek wanted to communicate with me. He wanted to let me know that he did not feel safe and that there was danger in the building from unidentified others. He communicated this by rushing forward towards me at speed and whispering in my ear. Here is an example of an altered sense of space and time in conjunction with a symbolic communication (i.e. an imbalance in the use of time through movement, combined with a sense of danger from others in the building and an urgency in conveying this).

My research with individuals in this acute in-patient setting found that movement dynamics act synchronistically with symbols and metaphors. For example, Alan used strong and descending movements in conjunction with the symbol of a dragon as he danced to the band *Imagine Dragons*. Hannah moved around the room in a light, indirect way, using a veil-like cloth over her head to symbolize the ghost of her father and calling to mind the metaphor 'light as a feather'. In DMP, we meet the person and move with them, paying particular attention to the imaginal realm, which is often where they find and express themselves. This, I argued, was at the heart of the therapeutic mechanisms at work in each session.

Notwithstanding the differences between a phenomenological interview and a group DMP session, the presence of mytho-poetic images in the VIP transcripts merits close attention. For instance, Orla, who does not describe herself as religious, tells us that her voice talks to her about heaven and hell:

> Sometimes talks about heaven and hell . . . nothing too bad, she's just . . . telling me where I'm going to go and all that, and telling me about hell, what it's like . . . She can like tell me what's going to happen the next day, what's going to happen next week, what someone's thinking, what someone's doing.

Why is it that mytho-poetic images populate the lived space of voices, as revealed in the analysis of temporality and spatiality in DMP and the VIP transcripts? In the final section of this chapter, I argue it is because trauma and dissociation, common correlates of the voice-hearing experience, open up the psyche to the archetypal mytho-poetic imagination, as described by Jung (1959), Schore (2012), and Wilkinson (2006). When people experience severe mental distress, this mytho-poetic imagination fills their lived world in order to communicate something of significance to them.

Trauma and the Mytho-Poetic

The prevalence of trauma in those experiencing psychosis has been highlighted by Read et al. (2014). Relational traumas—chronic childhood physical, emotional, and sexual abuse, neglect, mistreatment, and bullying—disrupt normal neurobiological and psychological development. Chronic childhood trauma is also linked to an increased incidence of post-traumatic stress symptoms, depression, dissociation, and affect dysregulation, and disruptions in self-perception, identity, and impulse control (Schore, 2012; Van der Kolk, 2006).

Drawing on the foundational work of John Read, Jim van Os, and others, Corstens et al. (2012, p. 1) view psychosis as a dissociative state related to trauma, noting that 'The fact that many people who hear voices have endured significant trauma is a much neglected aspect of the voice hearing (VH) experience'. Dissociation impairs the capacity for present-oriented and adaptive functioning. According to Levine and Frederick (1997, p. 137), dissociation presents itself as a kind of 'spaciness', and as a break in the continuity of a person's felt sense that often includes distortions of time and perception. Cassam (cited in Gallagher, 2011) talks about perception as being 'enactive' and something that we do involving action and a sense of knowing, partly through the proprioceptive system (whereby we locate ourselves in space). If perception being 'enactive' is altered through dissociation, it will be influenced, in turn, by movement, as perception also involves action. This is an important justification for the use of movement in dissociative states, and one which Maiese (2016) has explored in the context of DMP in the treatment of dissociative identity disorder (DID). In DID, she argues, 'Dance Movement Therapy offers a way for subjects to re-inhabit their bodies and remain present in a bodily way (rather than dissociating), which helps to reinstate a robust sense of bodily integration and ownership' (Maiese, 2016, p. 251).

Dissociative states are often expressed through the mytho-poetic. According to Schore (2012), Wilkinson (2006), Kalsched (2013), and others, affects-in-the-body are encoded as the implicit memories of early trauma and become more available through the mytho-poetic image-language of dreams, metaphor, and poetry than through the rational-interpretive language of insight. We see this in the VIP study as well, especially through mentions of ghosts, angels, archangels, Satan, and undercover operations. These mytho-poetic images could all be understood as taking place in a 'lived space' in the imaginal realm, potentially enabling the person, where necessary, to express their distress or trauma in a safe, creative, and contained way. The VIP transcript material presented here and my own research into DMP and psychosis bear testimony to this possibility.

When someone is hearing voices in the context of a DMP group, they are moving and dancing at the same time. As a dance movement psychotherapist, I attune to these movement communications as well as to the mytho-poetic images that arise. I take note of these changes in movement and the mytho-poetic images, all of which surface in the presence of the other.

The idea that trauma and dissociation lead to an opening up to the imagination is usually attributed to Jung. According to Donald Kalsched, a Jungian analyst who has written on the appearance of archetypes in response to trauma, Jung recognized 'a magical and mysterious world into which the person experiencing trauma falls when dissociation cracks open his/her psyche . . . an archetypal or mytho-poetic world, already there to catch them, so to speak' (Kalsched, 2013, p. 4). Referring to an imaginal matrix which lies between two worlds of ordinary and non-ordinary reality, Kalsched (2013, p. 5) goes on to say that 'survivors of trauma have a deep understanding of the sacred world that sustains them even in the most depriving and abusing of environments'. In addition, especially where there has been distress, trauma, or an erosion of trust, the lived space and mythical world function to 'provide a matrix and resource for the traumatized soul [core self] in "another world", before it can return to, or enter, "this one"' (Kalsched, 2013, p. 5).

Conclusion

In this chapter, I have explored the changes in the person's experience of space and time, especially in relation to the mytho-poetic, setting it in a phenomenological context. The VIP transcripts, perhaps unusually, give us powerful insights into the motion of voice-hearing, in that individuals seem to describe voices as if they are moving around in space and time. My own research in a related therapeutic context also highlights the importance of working in this complex imaginal realm through a mytho-poetic understanding, attending simultaneously to relational and movement-based dynamics, to the language of movement metaphor, and to the symbolic communications within the 'lived space' of music, movement, dance, and rhythm.

This chapter has also argued that the mytho-poetic expresses links between trauma and dissociation: that the lived space of psychosis can simultaneously express one's experience of being-in-the-world and being with the other. As a dance movement psychotherapist, I work within this unique space, meeting the person who may be hearing voices and expressing their own mytho-poetic imagery, where the specificity of location in time and space is of the utmost importance, as it seems to be in the transcripts. Going forward, 'knowing' the voices in this way opens up new and different avenues for exploration and dialogue, and signals the as yet insufficiently recognized importance of movement practices in this field. It highlights how we can be more holistic and more responsive as practitioners and therapists, and how studies in the creative arts and creative approaches help us pay much more attention to the value of the imaginal realm and lived space in particular. Therefore, a philosophical, existential, and indeed embodied approach in re-framing voice-hearing experiences contributes significantly to a better understanding of their meaning and significance.

References

Coaten, M. (2020). *Dance Movement Psychotherapy (DMP) in Acute Adult Psychiatry: A Mixed Methods study*. PhD thesis. Durham: Durham University.

Corstens, D., Longden, E., and May, R. (2012). Talking with voices: exploring what is expressed by the voices people hear. *Psychosis: Psychological, Social and Integrative Approaches*, 4(2), 95–104.

Gallagher, S. (2011). *The Oxford Handbook of the Self*. Oxford: Oxford Handbooks in Philosophy.

Heidegger, M. (1953). *Being and Time*. Translated from German by J. Stambaugh. Albany, NY: State University of New York Press.

Kalsched, D. (2013). *Trauma and the Soul: A Psycho-Spiritual Approach to Human Development and its Interruption*. London: Routledge.

Kestenberg-Amighi, J., Loman, S., and Sossin, K. M., eds. (2018). *The Meaning of Movement: Embodied Developmental, Clinical, and Cultural Perspectives of the Kestenberg Movement Profile*, 2nd edition. London: Routledge.

Levine, P., and Frederick, A. (1997). *Waking the Tiger: Healing Trauma: The Innate Capacity to Transform Overwhelming Experiences*. Berkeley, CA: North Atlantic Books.

Maiese, M. (2016). *Embodied Selves and Divided Minds*. Oxford: Oxford University Press.

Merleau-Ponty, M. (2012). *Phenomenology of Perception*. Translated from French by D. Landes. London: Routledge.

Read, J., Fosse, R., Moskowitz, A., and Perry, B. (2014). The traumagenic neurodevelopmental model of psychosis revisited. *Neuropsychiatry*, 4(1), 65–79.

Schore, A. (2012). *The Science of the Art of Psychotherapy*. London: W. W. Norton & Company.

Van der Kolk, B. (2006). Clinical implications of neuroscience research in PTSD. *Annals of the New York Academy of Sciences*, 1071(1), 277–93.

Wilkinson, M. (2006). *Coming into Mind: The Mind–Brain Relationship: A Jungian Clinical Perspective*. New York, NY: Routledge.

About the Author

Mary Coaten is a Dance Movement Psychotherapist in the South West Yorkshire Partnership NHS Foundation Trust. She completed her PhD 'Dance Movement Psychotherapy (DMP) in Acute Adult Psychiatry: A Mixed Methods Study' in 2020 as a member of Hearing the Voice at Durham University.

20

Vagabond Narratives

To Be Without a Home

Patricia Waugh, Department of English Studies, Durham University

On first reading the Voices in Psychosis (VIP) transcripts, I noticed a marked preponderance of references to lived space—neighbourhoods, rooms, walls—mostly in attempts to locate and situate voices, but often expressing concern with conditions of habitation, unsettled and unsettling domestic circumstances, eviction and evacuations, sofa surfing, the dreaded spectre of homelessness. I began to wonder what sorts of relations might be traced between descriptions of lived space, the location and auditory qualities of voices, and the construction of home as a powerful cultural imaginary, our first cosmos (or chaosmos): what Bachelard (1964, p. xxxvii) designates 'the *topos* of our most intimate being'. Exploring the resonances of the legalistic phrase 'of no fixed abode' might provide a way to fathom the coordinates of these perplexed and fretful descriptions of domestic space. The ordinary ambivalence associated with home—comfort and constraint—is here all too often devastatingly realized in the very real experience of struggling to live in many contradictory worlds and spaces at once. Home is safety, but 'I don't feel safe' (Hugh): nowhere is safe. Even as the interviewees describe their struggles to impose Manichean order— past and present, good and bad, in and out—the ground of 'I' and 'me', as addressor and addressee, becomes fissured, afloat, adrift, 'an inner voice but with an external point of view . . . my voice but it's not me' (Ryan). So too do the interviewees seem to experience their worlds as uncanny processes of creation, woven and unwoven, in their very struggles to narrate. Where is 'here' for Hugh when he says 'the more I'm in here, and the more I'm not going out, the more it seems as though the voices are . . . pushing us'. In what sense can voices 'push'? Walls figure strongly in locating voices: 'boundary voices', reported by a third of interviewees, are heard through, behind, and inside walls, or lurking in between, in corners or tantalizingly ever 'round the corner'. Atmospheres—a 'static-y feeling' (Emma)—congeal into riot shields 'closing in on me' (Dawn). Vibrations bring felt presences, touching from a distance, shrinking space so that 'there' becomes 'here'. Echoes and reverberations amplify and open space. Past voices invade the present, so that there is no 'now' and 'then' either; 'there is no here' (Page). Muffled whispers rise up from under beds as walls and floors move 'like they're kind of breathing' (Anthony). Space is plastic, often

Patricia Waugh, *Vagabond Narratives* In: *Voices in Psychosis*. Edited by: Angela Woods, Ben Alderson-Day, and Charles Fernyhough, Oxford University Press. © Patricia Waugh 2022. DOI: 10.1093/oso/9780192898388.003.0020 animistic, concretized inside and outside at once: 'I feel like if I'm in these four walls and she's talking to me all the time, constantly, I feel like they're closing in on me' (Dawn); something exists that 'I don't see behind the wall . . . something moving in my head' (Neil). Footsteps, barks, and cries come closer or move away; voices move across rooms, up from cellars and down from attics, through doors, windows, and out of neighbourhoods, 'shouted from down the street . . . [but] like thinking my voice' (Brad).

For all of us, home is a space never simply geometric, standing before us, bricks and mortar, at a distance from the eye; home is dispersed and inscribed within us as habit, living on in fragments. It is the lifelong hesitation on the staircase, anticipating the ghostly creak from fifty years ago, or the ambush of cold dread as the sound of footsteps presses up against the bedroom door. Home is an imaginary and a palimpsest, space as space-time. '[P]oetically endowed with . . . a quality with an imaginative or figurative value we can name and feel . . . space acquires emotion' (Said, 1978, p. 55). Home is a choreography of sound, words that first greeted you on arrival, delivered into the silo of 'boy' or 'girl', the official measurements of weight and mass, approval or disappointment ('he's a big one': already the shame of being *small*). The past occupies the present as disposition, habit, orientation. *Befindlichkeit,* how I find myself in the world, begins with an experience of 'home' grasped pre-reflectively, but also within culturally and politically specific imaginaries of belonging or exclusion, approval or disdain. As Rilke (1978) reflects in his *Tenth Elegy*, depression is 'landscape, settlement and fortress, / Our depth and Our home'. Wrought with feeling, home is unusually prone to shapeshift with mood and emotion—to expand, shrink, fissure, fuse, splinter, divide, and multiply—autopoetically playing back and consolidating basic affective orientations to the world. 'The nausea isn't inside me: I can feel it over there on the wall, on the branches, everywhere around me . . . it is I who am inside it' (Sartre, 2003, p. 35). In *In the Dark Room*, Brian Dillon, revisiting his earlier leave-taking of the childhood home, feels again the shock of sensation after his mother's death, how there was—and is now—'suddenly too much space': a rent or hole opening in the house as his mother departs it (Dillon, 2005, p. 35). Moods matter and change matter. For Dan, whose depressions are triggered by threats of homelessness, his voices too are driving him out, 'especially when it's inside the head, very, very loud and it's like it consumes all the space around you'. He observes that sometimes 'I can hear them inside in my brain', and 'my body feels . . . quite heavy'; in elation, though, the voices race outside, louder and faster, autoscopically heard from nowhere, bouncing off hard surfaces, opening out space, as his body is left behind.

Home is never merely the 'setting' for my lived experience. Spatiality mediates and is mediated through my intersubjectively constituted subjectivity, transforming things via internalized others into the meaningful objects of my world. The space of home is not occupied 'like a match in a box' (Merleau-Ponty 2014, p. 284) but is itself spatializing, living on in me shaping subsequent spaces. Romantically conceived as a disposition to return, home is more a place that was never left; *Heimlich* or *Unheimlich*, it lives on, a fastness, a prison, a hothouse, a place of dread. In the domestic worlds conjured up in these interviews, where the eye is relegated to the ear, where listening has become compelling, obsessional, and all-absorbing, the shape of space is traced through the dynamic event of sound—the disturbance of one body by another, of present by past, propagated in a medium, waves travelling through air—bouncing off hard surfaces, amplified as shouts, or muffled, whispers between walls. How and where voices are located and heard, whether moving or static, inside or outside (or both simultaneously), growing louder into proximity or fading into distance, shouting or whispering, is established through the medium of 'atmosphere' or *Stimmung* that is airy or dense, sonorous or muffled, hard or soft, conditioned through the intersections and blurrings of memory, perception, and imagination. Floors move beneath feet, walls breathe, atmospheric pressure bears down on body parts, 'as if the voices are . . . pushing us' (Hugh). Creating 'a buzz . . . I can't escape' (Gail), 'a big . . . whirring washer', 'Like a tornado' (Leah), tonal flows sink down as sadness, rise and radiate as elation, shrink into a minor key as fear. Voices begin as whispers, 'coming through' as laughter, commentary, building to crescendos, confiscating the space to breathe, so the self is felt to be shrinking and dying; voices diminish round corners, diverted to a horizon bristling with unlocatable significance, always just out of touch. They may arise in a symphony of clicks, knocks, animal shrieks, whispers, humming, murmurs, itinerant screams, often omnidirectional, drawing the ear out into distant space, then turning inward like a stethoscope fitted to the distant past. Inner speech, no longer primarily an aspect of an indivisible and weightless mental world attuning the listener's body to outer space, acquires ontological extension, corporeal substance, becoming too an acoustic event moving through space neither securely interior nor exterior, but experienced as divisible, bearing weight, mass, and volume. For Fred—who believes he can hear his partner having sex when he phones her—space has lost a dimension, its foreground disappearing: 'all I do is focus on what's going on in the background, instead of actually listening to the conversation'. Straining to hear, like the war veteran still focused on distant guns, his world is tuned to the arrival of the dreaded certainty of betrayal. Present space is buried under the weight of past and future, of shame and dread: a future that has already come to pass or is bearing down on the present, and a past that lurks in every corner. Reliving years of childhood abuse, Olivia's mind preys upon her vulnerabilities 'to vocate and make a kind of almost like a horror film' around her as the room shakes with a 'scratching' sound 'all over my walls', the writing on the wall heard synaesthesically, 'like a camera film like flickering . . . it's like a flicker . . . like a person's a flame', 'creepy echoing, like you can almost hear it echoing off the walls but it's like in your head'.

   In what Minkowski (1970, p. 429) calls the 'dark space' of psychosis, the feeling of an easy coincidence of the flow of consciousness with the embodied subject's sense of groundedness in space is lost. The subject's own spatiality is no longer organized and organizing through an *Umwelt* of embodied intentionality, just as home, as a space encircling and protecting the lived body, is never quite real—only ever a ghostly cultural imaginary, haunting in its absence. Home, constantly changing and disorderly, a place of violence and abuse, invested in as an imaginary of complete safety, is nowhere safe: atmospheres of foreboding prevail, always something coming ('you don't know what it is yet . . . you hear it but . . . you don't know where it's coming from' (Bill)). Is it safer to be inside or outside? The question perplexes many of the interviewees. Like a Mobius strip, one flips into the other, weirdly hylomorphic; as in the Aristotelian doctrine of the relation of soul to body, the mind is at once the form of the body that contains it and a space that has become its own spatially extended world. As the sedimented unsaid or unfelt is disrupted, ghosts are raised; there is no fixed abode. Not surprisingly, therefore, the interviews are marked throughout by struggles for prepositional exactitude, attempts to fix voices to sources and locations: under, above, below, up, down, and around. A 'pretty average four year old child' heard 'on the right hand side of me head, but like above me right eye' (Jane); voices that are 'in my head . . . but upstairs, in the flat above' (Sean); voices that come through 'from me gut . . . as if somebody's grabbed your location' (Leah); voices that 'consume all the space around you', or that can be 'inside the head, very, very loud' (Dan); voices that 'come out of the loft', or that hide 'in the garden . . . in the dark' (Emma). A grammar of equivocation likewise conveys the shifting, non-Euclidean, vertiginous experience of domestic space (one of the interviewees even wonders whether he is suffering from a vestibular disorder). Voices are at the same time inside and outside: 'like somebody's right up next to your eardrum' (Bill); 'like someone's whispering in your ear', but 'not necessarily at a whisperer's volume', and 'not necessarily pinpointed in one location' (Alex); 'out there, in sort of my brain . . . but inside as well' (Violet); 'either really close to me ear or like just round the corner . . . [or] in the back of me head' (Page). Ontological stability threatens to slip away entirely as desperate recovery measures are put into effect . Eric, describing a childhood home filled with the violence of his father, the rage of his sister, and the shame of his mother, where his escape from the hothouse on the hill was to step outside into the wind, feels its caress 'taking care' of him again in the steadying rhythm of music. But there is no long-lasting escape from the omnidirectional, unpredictably arriving voices, synaesthetically experienced as the maternal Blue and the abusive Yellow Ladies. '[M]aybe they were a mental replacement for a family', he reflects, a 'care model' for home carried, like a whispering gallery, in the moving soundscape surrounding his head: 'you don't just hear where it's coming from, it's . . . like you're inside . . . it's like having your head inside the bell rather than away from it'. As if an echo bounces his shame around the walls of a dome, the voice of the Yellow Lady reverberates 'from all directions, and she will keep going', resulting in 'a cacophony of like lots of bits of voices, but then the main voice will just come at you . . . there's no direction to it, so you can't hide, you don't know where it's coming from . . . [it] rings and rings and echoes and echoes'.

One might begin to draw up a topography of psychoses as materializing different kinds of dark space, different constitutions of 'home'. To my mind, six such houses declare themselves in these transcripts: I will call them bughouses, doll's houses, dreamhouses, glasshouses, ghost/houses, Unhoused. To focus on relations between affect, sound, and space in the context of the imaginary of home foregrounds what might be thought of as a pervasive mode of reverse Cartesianism, an attempt to stay the slipping-away of familiar space-time. For Descartes, as indeed for all of us in our operational mode of common-sense thinking, the primary attribute of corporeal substance or matter is that it takes up space; it has qualities such as divisibility, volume, mass, and weight, like the human body or tangible objects in the world. Descartes' corresponding assumption was that 'mind' or mental substance is indivisible, having no mass or volume, and therefore taking up no space. This is how we proceed at the level of common sense. But here, the reification of the mental, the concretization of thoughts into voices that brings a sense of the mental taking on the qualities of substance, builds a reverse Cartesian or mirror world of substance that slips disorientingly and devastatingly in and out of an ordinarily experienced extended space that is already filled with objects. Mind as the ghost in the machine, air, nothingness, suddenly thrusts out a hand as if it had acquired mass, volume, and extension. Descartes's *res cogitans* and *res extensa* change places.

In *bughouses* (circular paranoid worlds, bunker mentalities, bugged rooms), everything bristles with relevance, the ear strains perpetually to pick up confirmatory evidence of the source of the plot (another spatial metaphor), and fantasies arise of containment, defence against pollution, and the dangerous alien. Walls are fetishized. Fears accumulate concerning the never quite seen, the invisible flows that seem to penetrate matter; a spiralling obsession with barricades ensues. In *doll's houses,* space shrinks claustrophobically, threatening to suffocate the self, or it suddenly expands, amplifies, and threatens to swallow the self (as Dan experiences). In *dreamhouses* (kinetically non-Euclidean, their logic always either/and, slip-streaming, dynamic and always in movement), geometric points in the *res extensa* are endowed with mentality: organs speak, walls listen in. Space is extended and yet displays a dimensionless intentionality of its own, as in Hugh's perplexed sense of people from his past jostling into the present, 'as if a play was being played out . . . so many people there', all gathering in the studio flat below as he is 'trying to fish into me memories' to put them back in place. Or as space flattens, as background and foreground, depth, and perspective disappear, 'scenarios' from parallel universes intersect with, or penetrate, the domestic location, a quantum universe of action at a distance and of bodies occupying one space takes over the Newtonian world. In *glasshouses*, protective bubbles are sought, safe spaces that begin to implode or float free of anchorage, like Eric wrapping himself in music like the wind, or Will, 'trapped inside', finding there is 'another person inside me as well', his own voice 'there no more'. In *ghost/houses* (like Rachel Whiteread's 1993 Turner prize-winning 'House', a house modelled inside out), as outer space begins to slip, the minimal self is shored up as a homunculus (or several) in a container. Anthony has 'taken a seat . . . in the back of my mind', watching himself 'through my eyes' as the house heaves and moves around him. Orla describes how her head is 'split', like an apartment divided into rooms: 'one bit . . . mine', but with 'someone in me head . . . at the front' (at times, it feels like 'she's took over a little bit', until the pressure increases to the point of near implosion). But in *unhoused*, 'me soul' is 'raped' (Leah), body is occupied and mind is whirled and dispersed through a giant, whirring washing machine, describing a theodicy where agonistic fields of force vie for supremacy. The sacrificial limbs of a child, scapegoated, are being roasted and ego slips away, an excluded middle, as only supernatural forces or bodily organs retain intentionality. Lost children are rehoused in the body, their voices 'coming through' her ovaries, gut, and throat.

'Nomos can be descaled as a wall', writes Wendy Brown of the current political turn (Brown, 2010, p. 45); it might be descaled too as the 'four walls' of the house, the space, or 'Raum' (as in to make space), of home. The word 'home' itself foregrounds the relation between body, space, and emotion: *Heima* (ON) or *Haim* (OE) means to hold dear, where the heart is; but *Hein* also provides the root of *Nomos* or Law, from *Nemein*, a divide, a plot or a pasture. Etymologically, the imaginary of home points both ways, the roots of possessive individualism wrapped around the heart, the commons of care. King Lear's 'unhoused' wretches, that he 'has ta'en too little care of', live beyond the pale (the stake of the fence separating the homeland or homestead from the outlaw); like the bastard, Edgar, Poor Tom, they are the 'bare life' of Agamben's *homo sacer* (Agamben, 1998), persons beyond the sacral space of the law and its protection, who live as hunted creatures. 'I'm not worth being in this house', says Ryan, hearing its sounds as underwater acoustics, experiencing himself submerged, a near-extinct creature, literally drowned out by the others, the voices, in his head. The homeless and the uncomfortably and precariously housed, the psychotically unhoused, more powerfully than any other group, offer insights into, even as they become icons of, the current contradictions and limitations of liberal ideals of political and other kinds of sovereignty, enshrined in seventeenth-century law at the moment that 'vagabond' took on its current stigmatizing semantics. An estimated two-thirds of homeless people in the UK suffer from serious diagnosable mental illness at the same time that the imaginaries of home and homeland are being politically reinvested with possessive and nationalistic fervour. We need a new political phenomenology of home. Thinking home and homelessness through these interviews makes a small contribution to an exploration of the complex political relationship that holds between homelessness, the new 'vagabondage', and contemporary political fantasies of home and belonging that are inextricably bound to those of defence and exclusion—of keeping out the alien, the refugee, the foreign interloper, of purifying the tribe. We are reminded that driving people out of their homes drives them mad. Agamben (1998) suggests that sovereignty is achieved through subjection to the law or the normative, and its mode of operation determines how I appear before the other, how I take up space, feeling entitled to its possession or made to feel a shamefaced interloper unworthy of being homed. The neoliberal fantasy of global digital economies, of a world of money flowing unobstructed across borders (ontologically impossible as a mode of living), alongside the unsettling threats to the unity and autonomy of sovereignty of the new virtual worlds of terror and counter-intelligence, have revived an obsession with the powerful imaginary of 'home' as citadel, of sovereignty as theologically bestowed. Now it is paraded as theatrical spectacle, like the divine right of kings, in the physical erection of walls and borders, the modern tabernacles of the new neoliberal nationalisms. To lack a home, or even merely physical shelter, in this revived Social Darwinist climate is to be more than ever vulnerable to being radically 'unhoused' as a person. Like those early modern vagabonds, it is to suffer stigmatization beyond the pale.

References

Agamben, G. (1998). *Homo Sacer: Sovereign Power and Bare Life*. Translated from the Italian by D. Heller-Roazen. Stanford, CA: Stanford University Press.

Bachelard, G. (1964). *The Poetics of Space*. Translated from the French by M. Jolas. Boston, MA: Beacon.

Brown, W. (2010). *Walled States, Waning Sovereignty*. New York, NY: Zone Books.

Dillon, B. (2005). *In the Dark Room: A Journey in Memory*. Dublin: Penguin Ireland.

Merleau-Ponty, M. (2014). *The Phenomenology of Perception*. Translated from the French by D. A. Landes. London and New York, NY: Routledge.

Minkowski, E. (1970). *Lived Time: Phenomenological and Psychopathological Studies*. Translated from the French by N. Metzel. Evanston, IL: Northwestern University Press.

Rilke, R. M. (1978). *Duino Elegies*. Translated from the German by D Young. New York, NY: Norton.

Said, E. (1978). *Orientalism*. New York, NY: Pantheon Books.

Sartre, J.-P. (2003). *Being and Nothingness: An Essay on Phenomenological Ontology*. Translated from the French by H. E. Barnes. London: Routledge.

About the Author

Patricia Waugh is Professor in the Department of English Studies at Durham University and a Co-Investigator on the Hearing the Voice project. She is currently completing a monograph entitled *More than Ordinary Madness: The Novelist as Voice Hearer*.

21

Leah's Voices

Reflections on Auditory Verbal Hallucinations as Spiritual and Religious Experience

Christopher C. H. Cook, Emeritus Professor, Institute of Medical Humanities, Durham University

Introduction

Leah, a woman in her forties, is in contact with Early Intervention for Psychosis services provided by a local National Health Service (NHS) Mental Health Trust. At the time of her interview in the Voices in Psychosis study, she was under observation for a suspected mental disorder, having in the previous year suffered an episode of psychotic illness lasting a few months. We know very little about her personal history, but we know much about the voices that she hears and we gain some moving insights into some of the traumatic experiences that she has had, all of which have been at the hands of men who abused her or deserted her in her time of need. The lack of contextual history is frustrating both for the clinician and for anyone interested in understanding her spirituality and faith. We cannot be sure what the religious traditions of her family were, although references to Jesus, to church, and to aunts who were nuns with religious art in their homes would all strongly suggest a Christian affiliation within the family, probably as Roman Catholics. The structure of the interview, the ambiguity of some of Leah's responses, and the lack of clarity of the tape at some points together present an at times confusing and disjointed, if not self-contradictory, account. Despite this, a rich narrative can be pieced together, within which a picture of the phenomenology of Leah's voices emerges in some detail.

The congruence of the derogatory affective tone of the voices that Leah hears with the history of abuse that she has suffered is psychologically striking. No less striking are the senses of meaning and purpose that Leah finds within her experiences and her courage in coming to terms with them. As much as her psychotic episode might be seen as an understandable response—a 'breakdown'—in the face of severe trauma, it also presents (and re-presents) an ongoing experience of abuse by hostile voices that both remind her of the abuse that she suffered in the past and continue to provide ongoing verbal abuse in the present. Despite this, amidst the voices that she hears, Leah finds spiritual comfort, safety, reassurance, and protection. She also

Christopher C. H. Cook, *Leah's Voices* In: *Voices in Psychosis*. Edited by: Angela Woods, Ben Alderson-Day, and Charles Fernyhough, Oxford University Press. © Christopher C. H. Cook 2022. DOI: 10.1093/oso/9780192898388.003.0021 finds recourse to active spiritual and religious strategies for coping with the horror of what she is experiencing. Reflecting on what has happened, she is able to find meaning and purpose, and even to describe herself as 'blessed' and 'thankful'.

This chapter offers a narrative and phenomenological account of Leah's experiences of voices, with some reflections informed by research on religious coping.

The Voices that Leah Hears

Leah describes the voices (and non-verbal hallucinations) that she hears as localized in both internal (somatic) and external space. Thus, some of the voices come through her heart, as though through some kind of radio receiver and speaker that 'picks up other people's vibrations and other people's thoughts' and 'speakerises' them in a sound like a whisper, as though someone was speaking under their breath.[1] Similarly, she believes she picks up voices from TV and radio. However, she appears to find the radio receiver analogy only partially adequate because the voices get all mixed up with her own thoughts, and thus she also has recourse to images of a washing machine, or tornado, which mixes up her own inner voice with other voices. The whisper generally seems to distinguish the alien voices from Leah's own thoughts, and each voice has its own tone by which it can be recognized. Despite this, she sometimes finds it difficult to distinguish her inner voice from the other voices, a state of confusion which she finds upsetting.

Externally, Leah indicates that things she hears on the left she takes to be from Satan, whereas if she hears them on the right, then 'that's the good side'. Her voices are generally categorized as either good or bad. When they argue with each other, she finds herself taking sides. On the good side, the archangels protect and save her. One voice says, 'I'm not going to let them do this to you'. On one occasion, when she was planning to spend the night on a quayside, they moved her on, telling her that someone was raped there. The bad voices whisper 'nasty things', call her 'bitch' or 'slag', and tell her to kill herself. Although she does not explicitly say this, it is fairly clear that she sides with the good voices against the bad; however, the categorization is not always completely clear. Thus, with the voices from Satan 'you never know quite . . . whether he's doing bad, he's a bit mixed up'.

Leah says that she hears 'actual people's voices' and that they are 'very there'. However, she recognizes that other people do not hear them, and so she also qualifies this. They are there 'in spirit, not in physical'. At least some of the voices appear to be experienced in a mixture of sensory modalities—thus the angel voices are accompanied visually by shadows, like angels' wings, and by a sense of presence. When Michael is present, she experiences a somatic tingling sensation. The voices may be triggered by memories and places associated with past trauma, such as the

---

[1] The voices are also sometimes experienced as coming from her ovaries. These voices argue, 'as if I had one boy in each, talking to each'. One voice (Loki—see below) is experienced as coming from her gut.

place where she was raped and the house where she lived with her children (whom she is now not allowed to see). At the time of the interview, Leah reported hearing voices for about five hours each day, but this represents a considerable reduction in frequency. It would appear that the voices were virtually constant at the height of her 'break', ceasing only during sleep. Even then, she would dream vividly and the voices would make appearances in her dreams. Leah has tried talking back to the voices, but they either don't listen or tell her that she is wrong. They impact on her relationships with others, as she is ashamed and embarrassed by them. They 'could be nasty about me, and they can also be nasty about the people around'.

Through the course of the interview Leah struggles to identify exactly how many different voices she hears. Initially, she suggests that there were seven main voices, then five. At the end of the interview, she concludes that there are eight, but she actually describes ten different voices during the course of the interview. These are summarized in Box 21.1.

Only the two archangels, and perhaps her Grandma, are unambiguously positive voices. Only the voice of her uncle is unambiguously evil. The other voices are all ambiguous to a greater or lesser extent. Seven of the voices are male, and only three are female. Gabriel appears only as a sense of presence, and his voice is not actually heard.

Leah loves the angels and hopes that they will be with her forever. They are nice to her. The male voices 'are sometimes alright and sometimes not alright'. The male and female friends seem to be linked in some way to 'the bad stuff'; from them, 'it's general just piss take or nastiness'. They sometimes put a curse on her for being a grass. Despite all of this, Leah finds herself looking for them if they go silent: they 'keep us company'. Both the angels and the boys (the three male friends) bring messages, for example, 'they'll bring me that voice of me kids'.

Leah's Experience of Trauma

Leah's brief account of the voice of her uncle leads us to suspect that she was sexually abused by him as a child, although she now has no memories of this (a not uncommon experience in such circumstances).

Leah tells us of a number of significant life events that took place during the year before the interview. Her husband, who had been having an affair, left her when her mother was diagnosed as suffering from a life-threatening illness, thus leaving her to care alone for her mother and her children while also working and looking after the home. He also left her with a significant financial debt to repay. In this context, it is hardly surprising that she describes being depressed and anxious. Subsequently, the children were sent to live with their father. While this relieved her of some responsibilities, it also represented a significant additional loss.

On top of all of this, Leah says that she was raped. We are given few details of the assault, but it is clear that Leah knew the identity of her assailant. While she clearly

Box 21.1 The voices that Leah hears

Archangel Gabriel – experienced only as a sense of presence, a more recent addition to the 'voices' that Leah hears.

Archangel Michael – experienced as a sense of presence, visually as shadowy wings, and as a voice. When present, he is associated with experiences of a tingling sensation and a high-pitched noise. Leah feels very safe in Michael's presence; she experiences a 'protective sort of bubble, forcefield, when he's there'.

Three male friends – two of whom Leah has 'been intimate with'. Their arrival is associated with a clicking noise.

A female friend – a lesbian, with whom Leah was best friends for a long time. The voice (not the actual friend) calls Leah 'a prostitute', and 'in my voices', this voice is married to one of the three male friends (in real life, they have a close relationship but are not married). This voice 'bounces about the room' and is also associated with the clicking noise.

A gypsy – experienced as a positive voice, which 'comes in bubbles'. The gypsy has told Leah that she has 'got God in her heart' and is 'God's angel', and sends Leah on 'various tasks when I was begging and stuff like that, various tasks, like feed the ducks in the park'. The gypsy is also associated with the clicking noise.

Loki[a] – the 'black angel'. 'He does good things, he saves people but . . . he's, he's . . . he's vicious'. Although he is not nasty to Leah, he is nasty to the other voices. 'God brought him in'.[b] Loki protects Leah from the three male friends; 'He's a bad man, but certainly saved my backside'. 'I hope I haven't had to sell me soul to him like, because it's nay good that like, it's God's angel, she said, so I mustn't have sold me soul'. He tells Leah to pick up books and read things, and is also associated with the clicking noise.

Uncle – mentioned only at the very end of the interview and described as 'extremely evil', 'a bad, bad man. . . . I've asked for Jesus' help and everything with him. Absolute nightmare. Rapes me soul'. Leah's uncle was accused of abusing Leah when she was very young, although Leah does not have any of her own memories of this.

Grandma – at one point in the interview, Leah describes a vision of her grannie, although it is not clear that this occurred in a fully waking state. Little is said about this voice.

[a] Loki is a god of Norse mythology and also (more popularly in contemporary culture) a fictional character appearing in Marvel comics. The voice that Leah identifies as Loki bears a remarkable resemblance to the more ancient and ambivalent mythological character.

[b] Elsewhere, Leah says that the gypsy brought Loki.

acted responsibly in reporting this crime to the police, in her mind, she was being 'a grass' and 'where I come from grasses are not treat very kindly'. The act of reporting the crime to the police was thus a difficult one for Leah and associated with correspondingly mixed emotions. At this point, 'the voices started to get really, really bad', telling her that she would get stabbed and that she was a grass.

The Narrative

Following all of this, Leah became homeless for a period of some weeks, and then was placed in a hostel by a charity working with the homeless. The voices told her to jump under a train. At this point in the narrative, Leah tells us that the voices, and also her own thoughts, were 'crap', including racist content. In October of the year before the interview, Leah sought help from mental health services (the crisis team and the Early Intervention for Psychosis team).[2] It also seems to be at this point that she started attending church: 'I had to go to church and say, this is, you know, please forgive me, this is not me, you know what I mean?' She reports this as being a helpful coping strategy: 'I love church.'

Leah further describes writing down what the voices were saying and posting what she had written under the church door. On another occasion, the voices told her to turn to page 666 in the Bible and start reading.[3] They told her 'to spit in it and make a cross with it, and then take it back to the church'. Although the interviewer does not pursue the point, it appears that Leah had thoughts that she might be possessed or afflicted by demons in some way. She reports 'coughing up demons and stuff like that'. When Loki told her to read from a particular book, not long after she had been raped, the words 'lick it out' assumed considerable significance to her. 'I thought this guy was the devil, had got into me'. Her eyes went over the words again and again, and Loki said that he would 'lick it out of me heart'.[4]

Significantly, Leah believes that the voices are happening for a reason. On the negative side, the voices are associated with punishment. On the positive side, she is 'being told to change me life'. 'I think I've been on the wrong path, and I think I've been, I'm being placed on a different path.' There has been a significant spiritual and religious dimension to this change of path: 'I was spiritual, but I wasn't big into God or Jesus or anything like that, but I am now, like, definitely. . . . I certainly feel like I've been blessed now, somebody's put us back on the right path.'

Spirituality, Religion, and Psychosis

Religious content is not unusual in the psychopathology associated with the diagnosis of a psychotic illness (Cook, 2015). The nature of the relationship between religion and psychosis is complex, with religion neither protecting against psychosis nor predisposing to it. Stigma and lack of understanding of mental disorders within faith communities may be negative factors, contributing to the difficulties that people

---

[2] This leads to treatment with risperidone, promethazine, and antidepressants. She is also assigned to a Community Psychiatric Nurse.

[3] 666 is the 'mark of the beast' in the biblical book of Revelation (13:11–18).

[4] It's not entirely clear whether this is what Loki, as a voice, actually said or whether perhaps this is Leah's interpretation of the words that Loki had directed her to read.

with such a diagnosis face during the course of recovery. On the other hand, religiosity and spirituality provide important coping resources for many people and may come to the fore in times of illness (Heffernan et al., 2016; Huguelet and Mohr, 2009). Leah appears to be one such person, for whom renewal of appreciation of the faith tradition within which she was raised has helped in developing coping strategies and finding meaning and purpose in the midst of a distressing and disorientating illness.

The religious coping strategies that may be identified within the transcript include church attendance, prayer, and a practice of writing down the distressing things that the voices have said and posting what she has written under the door of the church. Perhaps more importantly, amidst overwhelming and enormously distressing experiences, Leah finds meaning in the context of her faith. Paradoxically, she understands her life as having been put back on track by what has happened to her. She is even able to see herself as blessed. Leah's faith gives her cause for optimism amidst circumstances that—at least initially—had been a cause only for depression and anxiety. Even though the voices tell her to kill herself, the word 'suicide' at no point appears in the transcript. It would not seem unreasonable to speculate that it is her faith that provides a significant defence against suicidal ideation (Cook, 2014).

Pargament et al. (1998) identify positive and negative types of religious coping, with the former generally being associated with better, and the latter with poorer, health outcomes. In psychosis, positive coping styles seem to be protective against depression, anxiety, and suicide (Rosmarin et al., 2013). Almost all of Leah's religious coping seems to be of the positive type, but there are two possible exceptions. She appears in places to engage in what Pargament would refer to as 'punishing God reappraisals' and 'demonic reappraisal'. However, the evidence that the transcript provides for these forms of negative coping is not strong. Although Leah refers to punishment in various places during the interview, and clearly understands the voices as punishing her, she nowhere states that God is punishing her. Indeed, in one place, she denies that she deserves punishment (for her uncle's death). Her understanding of punishment may therefore represent a more positive coping style than at first appears.

Leah only refers to demons once, and then in reference to coughing them up or expelling them from her body. She does understand some of the voices as having a satanic origin, but over and against this, others are protective, including angels who are (at least implicitly) sent by God. Her understanding of the interplay between demonic and divine powers in causing what is happening to her is actually quite theologically complex. Thus, although Loki is Satan's 'black angel' and is 'vicious', he also does good things and is nasty to the other voices who are nasty to Leah. She is even able to say at one point that 'God brought him in'. Leah always identifies herself with the good side in this struggle between good and evil, and the gypsy voice refers to her as 'God's angel'. Moreover, the most powerful figure in the panoply of voices is the protective Archangel Michael.

Overall, I would argue that Leah's religious coping style is thus firmly within Pargament's positive category, specifically including (among other strategies) benevolent religious reappraisal (redefining the stressor as positive), collaborative and spiritually connected coping (siding with the divine/good), and adoption of a religious focus. However, it contains elements of what might be interpreted as Pargament's negative category (reappraisals of the 'punishing God' and demonic kinds). Although Leah does not hear the voice of God directly, her voices are more than psychologically revealing. They reflect an attempt on Leah's part to find spiritual meaning and growth amidst adversity. Her voices are spiritually meaningful.[5]

Spiritual and religious voices occurring within the context of psychosis have traditionally not been understood as meaningful. Psychiatrists, generally less likely to be religious than their patients, have often not been sympathetic to finding any religious meaning within the phenomena that they view as 'psychopathology' (Cook, 2011, 2012). Others, subscribing to a discontinuity model of psychosis and spirituality, would distinguish between the meaningful (spiritual) and non-meaningful (psychotic), even if admitting that sometimes the distinction is blurred. Yet others would see a continuous spectrum of experiences in which the spiritually meaningful merges into the disintegration of meaning seen in severe psychosis (for a helpful collection of essays exploring these approaches, see Clarke, 2010).

Perhaps Leah may be located on this spectrum somewhere, maybe more towards the end of the meaningful? Perhaps she may, but the important thing is not the spectrum: it is the individual search for meaning within the experiences. The finding of meaning within Leah's voices is more than just a coping strategy; it is an affirmation of Leah's quest to find meaning amidst adversity.

Conclusion

Leah's voices represent a psychological and spiritual interplay of good and evil forces experienced as inhabiting both her own inner mental space and a threatening outer world. Arising in response to multiple traumas, they are both a further source of stress/trauma to Leah and also a way of making spiritual and psychological sense of what has happened and coping with it. This brief case study demonstrates that the voices of psychosis are not always (if ever) meaningless or chaotic and that there is potentially both spiritual and psychological benefit in paying attention to what they have to say.

References

Clarke, I., ed. (2010). *Psychosis and Spirituality: Consolidating the New Paradigm*. Oxford: Wiley-Blackwell.
Cook, C. C. H. (2011). The faith of the psychiatrist. *Mental Health, Religion and Culture*, 14(1), 9–17.

---

[5] For further discussion of voices as potentially theologically revelatory, see Cook, 2018.

Cook, C. C. H. (2012). Psychiatry in scripture: sacred texts and psychopathology. *The Psychiatrist*, 36(6), 225–9.

Cook, C. C. H. (2014). Suicide and religion. *British Journal of Psychiatry*, 204(4), 254–5.

Cook, C. C. H. (2015). Religious psychopathology: the prevalence of religious content of delusions and hallucinations in mental disorder. *International Journal of Social Psychiatry*, 61(4), 404–25.

Cook, C. C. H. (2018). *Hearing Voices, Demonic and Divine: Scientific and Theological Perspectives*. London: Routledge.

Heffernan, S., Neil, S., Thomas, Y., and Weatherhead, S. (2016). Religion in the recovery journey of individuals with experience of psychosis. *Psychosis*, 8(4), 346–56.

Huguelet, P., and Mohr, S. (2009). Religion/spirituality and psychosis. In: P. Huguelet and H. G. Koenig, eds. *Religion and Spirituality in Psychiatry*. Cambridge: Cambridge University Press, pp. 65–80.

Pargament, K. I., Smith, B. W., Koenig, H. G., and Perez, L. (1998). Patterns of positive and negative religious coping with major life stressors. *Journal for the Scientific Study of Religion*, 37(4), 710–24.

Rosmarin, D. H., Bigda-Peyton, J. S., Ongur, D., Pargament, K. I., and Bjorgvinsson, T. (2013). Religious coping among psychotic patients: relevance to suicidality and treatment outcomes. *Psychiatry Research*, 210(1), 182–7.

About the Author

Christopher C. H. Cook is an Emeritus Professor in the Institute of Medical Humanities at Durham University and was a Co-Investigator on Hearing the Voice. He has a special interest in spirituality, religion, and theology of voice-hearing.

22

'I Just Feel Like There's Just Lots of People in My Head!'

Reciprocal Roles and Voice-Hearing

Anna Luce, Crisis Skylight Newcastle

Nicola Barclay, Cumbria, Northumberland, Tyne and Wear NHS Foundation Trust

In this chapter, we explore how cognitive analytic therapy (CAT) may be helpful for voice-hearers, based on our experience of working within Early Intervention in Psychosis (EIP) services in the North East of England. CAT, largely developed by Anthony Ryle (e.g. Ryle and Kerr, 2002), encompasses both a structured, time-limited therapy and a theoretical model of human development in which the self is viewed as inherently dialogical, relational, and intersubjective. Humans' internal worlds can be viewed as a collection of voices in conversation, developed through real-life relationships and (social) experiences. Problems occur, however, when these voices become restricted or outdated, appear overly negative, powerful, or frightening, or become cut off from each other. Using two case examples from the Voices in Psychosis (VIP) study, we explore how the CAT concept of 'reciprocal roles' (RRs) might be helpful for understanding (and hopefully improving relationships with) voices.

Cognitive Analytic Therapy: An Overview

As it has evolved over several decades, CAT is highly theoretically integrative and continues to develop with contributions from new practitioners and in response to emerging research. CAT began as Ryle's attempt to bring together psychoanalytic and cognitive understandings (e.g. the works of Melanie Klein and Aaron T. Beck); it later embraced theories of learning, language, and child development (e.g. the works of Lev Vygotsky), and encompassed attachment, developmental trauma, and neurobiology (e.g. Jellema, 2005). CAT takes an essentially social view of human (personality) development and, by extension, the development of mental distress.

Anna Luce and Nicola Barclay, *'I Just Feel Like There's Just Lots of People in My Head!'* In: *Voices in Psychosis.*
Edited by: Angela Woods, Ben Alderson-Day, and Charles Fernyhough, Oxford University Press. © Anna Luce and Nicola Barclay 2022.
DOI: 10.1093/oso/9780192898388.003.0022

Our internal worlds are largely formed by our early interpersonal and wider social experiences, and we actively construct our 'reality' based on internalized models of relationships with others, ourselves, and the world. Difficulties and distress are caused by learnt 'procedures' (patterns of thinking, feeling, and responding) which were adaptive at the time, but which are no longer helpful or are restrictive, and now prevent us from satisfactorily achieving our aims in life.

Usually delivered over sixteen to twenty-four sessions, CAT is a relatively brief, time-limited therapy, which is goal- and change-focused, proactive, and structured. It takes an individualized, collaborative, and compassionate stance, with a focus on therapeutic alliance and on relational issues arising in therapy. The therapeutic task in CAT is to develop a joint understanding of how and why an individual has come to understand and respond to themselves, others, and the world as they do; to consider how these might relate to the difficulties they are experiencing (identifying unhelpful 'procedures'); and to explore alternative ways of being, relating, and acting ('exits') which allow for healthy personal growth and relationships. This jointly constructed understanding ('reformulation') is expressed in narrative (letters) and visual (diagrams) forms. CAT attempts to work alongside individuals at a level which is acceptable and yet effective for them in maximizing their learning and development (called the 'zone of proximal development' or, more snappily, the ZPD). Moreover, in CAT, issues around endings (e.g. complex feelings including disappointment and loss) are explicitly attended to.

Humans: Fundamentally Social and Dialogical

CAT views humans as fundamentally social animals in that we require interactions with others' minds ('intersubjectivity') for the development of our own minds. These interactions literally 'wire' our brains and form our internal world, personality, and sense of self. The requirement for social interactions, companionship, and community continues throughout our lives. Our interactions with others are mediated through signs, and as humans, this involves verbal language. Vygotsky argued that through a process of 'internalization' during childhood, our speech and language capacities cease to function solely for interpersonal communicative purposes, becoming also the medium of our thoughts ('verbal thinking'). Bakhtin's notions of dialogism have also informed CAT (Bakhtin, 1984, p. 287):

> I am conscious of myself and become myself only while revealing myself for another. The most important acts constituting self-consciousness are determined by a relationship toward another consciousness (toward a thou) . . . not that which takes place within, but that which takes place on the boundary between one's own and someone else's consciousness on the threshold . . . a person has no internal sovereign territory; he is wholly and always on the boundary; looking into himself, he looks into the eyes of another or with the eyes of another.

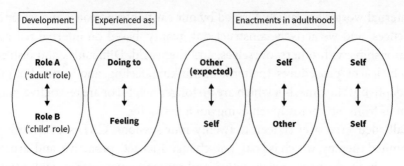

Figure 22.1 Development and enactments of reciprocal roles.

We are thus formed through our interpersonal, social, and cultural relational experiences. From this perspective, individual 'psychopathology' does not exist as such, only socio-psychopathology emerging from trauma and power inequalities. Therefore, CAT is not explicitly 'diagnostically driven' and assumes complexity.

Reciprocal Roles

Our experiences of relationships with caregivers in our early lives form the basis (templates) for future relationships—called 'reciprocal roles' (RRs) in CAT—with other people and, importantly, also with ourselves. These are complex, often unconscious, full body experiences, involving implicit relational memory, perception (including beliefs, values, and meanings), and affect (emotion), which can be associated with a dialogic voice. Importantly, both 'poles' of a relationship are internalized, so that we are able to assume or elicit both 'roles'. An example might be the criticized child who, in adulthood, continues to feel/fear criticism from others and is highly self-critical, but who is also (often without realizing it) experienced as critical by others. Enactment of a role always implies another, whose reciprocation is sought or expected. Diagrammatically, RRs can be expressed as shown in Figure 22.1 (adapted from Potter, 2019).

We predict and elicit expected roles from others using active (although often unconscious) strategies. These 'reciprocal role procedures' (RRPs) are thus stable patterns of behaviour which originated (and were highly adaptive) in early relationships, which have then been internalized and carried into the present. These form the templates (the 'dances') by which we continue to interact with other individuals, with wider systems (family, social, services), and with ourselves (including self-care).

Some RRs are supportive (e.g. caring ←→ cared for), while others can be less helpful (e.g. critical ←→ never good enough). However, we have multiple relational experiences during our lives, leading to a repertoire of RRs which forms all mental 'activity' and underpins the basis of our personality or 'self'. Sufficient or 'good enough' early care experiences enable us to develop a repertoire of generally helpful RRs which are integrated and flexible, and which equip us for healthy adult relationships, facilitate conscious self-reflection, and foster a coherent sense of self. However, for many of us, early caregiving experiences are characterized by abusive or neglectful RRs, where our attachment needs have not been consistently or adequately met. For some, this results in restricted or extreme RR repertoires, and frequently also in imagined or 'wished for' RRs (e.g. of being perfectly or ideally cared for, or of feeling special or unassailable).

Overwhelming experiences impair the ability to move smoothly and flexibly between roles, interfere with the development of a coherent sense of self and self-reflective capacities, and result in experiences of dissociation, disturbances in consciousness, and disowned or cut-off aspects of the self. The difficulties which bring many people into therapy or contact with services arise through extreme or restricted RR repertoires as a result of trauma or neglect, the intense feelings caused by unmet, unexpressed attachment needs, and difficulties with an integrated sense of a 'good enough' self. As Jellema (2005, p. 10) states:

> Much so-called 'psychopathology' has come about through the person's relationship with Magistral [that is, authoritative/dominating] voices of parents and abusers. The more abusive and neglectful the early experiences of the patients, the more damaged they are likely to be in later life. . . . suppressed, hidden voices in psychotherapy, can help make the power formulation clearer. These voices derive their power from embodied experience, from real-life experiences of not being allowed to speak.

CAT, Psychosis, and Voice-Hearing

Ian Kerr and colleagues have integrated CAT concepts within the bio-psycho-social 'stress-vulnerability model' frequently employed for understanding why a specific individual at a specific time may have developed psychotic experiences (Kerr et al., 2003). They propose that many who develop psychosis do, in fact, experience particularly harsh, deprived upbringings. People who have higher 'biological vulnerabilities' (e.g. neurocognitive impairment or difficulties processing social information) may be more likely to experience hostile or neglectful reactions from caregivers/society (e.g. lack of attunement, frustration, and stigma). The resulting 'maladaptive' RRs that we frequently encounter working in psychosis services (some common examples are shown in Figure 22.2) are then repeated within peoples' interpersonal relationships, within their self–self relationship (being abusive or neglectful of themselves), and with clinicians and the mental health system (resulting in poorer care).

Kerr et al. (2003, p. 517) propose that psychosis frequently involves disruption to the different aspects of personality structure: 'In more severe psychotic states, CAT would understand psychotic symptoms and phenomena to represent the muddled, amplified or distorted enactments of such RRs as well as their dissociated dialogic voices'. Voice-hearing experiences in psychosis are thought to have a basis in 'reality': the reality of relationships or our responses and attempts to cope with them

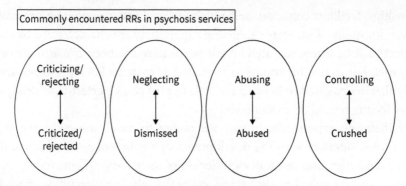

Figure 22.2 Commonly encountered reciprocal roles in psychosis services.

which have been misattributed or misinterpreted. Thus, 'psychosis represents an extreme version of being "out of dialogue" both internally and externally' (Kerr et al., 2003, p. 517). This resonates with our clinical experience of observing how unhelpful or unhealthy RRs are re-enacted around those with psychosis by families, mental health services, and society at large.

CAT has been applied to voice-hearing in psychosis explicitly by Perry (2012). In line with other researchers (e.g. Morrison et al., 2004), he highlights how individuals' relationships to their voice-hearing hugely influences their response to these experiences. Voices viewed as powerful and controlling are particularly distressing. Perry (2012) suggests that those parts of the self that are prevented from being expressed, from having a 'real' voice, are perhaps more likely to become 'voices'. These misconstrued, disowned parts are then experienced as coming from an external source. Understandably, people attempt to avoid or actively suppress 'negative' voices; however, as with all attempts at suppression, this only causes them to become more frequent, aggressive, or assertive. Since it is the embodied quality and emotional experience of certain roles that are internalized, 'voices' can evolve and develop beyond replays (or memories) of actual verbatim interactions, and frequently do not sound like people in our pasts. In addition, some 'voices' may represent the 'wished-for' or protective imagined/fantasy RRs described earlier. It is also important to note that positive and supportive voice-hearing is a common experience and most likely derived from 'healthy' RRs/caregiver experiences.

We turn now to offer a relational analysis of two participants ('Nina' and 'Grace') in the VIP study, starting with one such supportive voice.

Nina

Nina, a white woman in her late teens, reported hearing up to ten different voices, all with seemingly different roles and influences on her. We have hypothesized two RRs

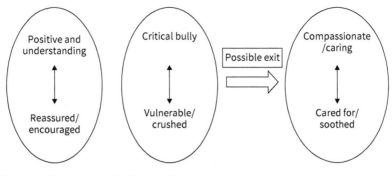

Figure 22.3 Possible reciprocal roles for Nina.

for certain of her voices in Figure 22.3. She notes that 'One of the positive ones reminds me of my granddad. . . . I lost him recently and ehm . . . I think he was there before like he passed, the voice, but he's kind of become a little bit stronger in my head'. This voice reflects how her grandfather treated her and made her feel when he was alive: 'he definitely acts like my granddad, like he's positive but in a very you know like stoic way'. As discussed earlier, humans are always in dialogue with an 'other', even if this is in our own mind. We internalize our relationships with others, and in Nina's case, this relationship template had been a helpful influence when trying to manage the more negative of her voice-hearing experiences: 'I can hear him like say "don't be stupid", "don't listen to them" . . . I mean the voice and everything's never insensitive about anything, he's always understanding'. However, 'grandad' can also take a more critical stance at times: 'he does call me like stupid for believing the negative voices', indicating another RR.

In contrast to her positive voices, Nina says, 'I think the negative voices, they definitely come from my past experiences with people my age'; 'It's always been hard at school. . . . I just seem to be bullied and everything.' These experiences continued to the point they seem to have become expected: 'To be honest. I've . . . ehm, a lot of people have been really horrible to me, ehm through my school life and I don't know, maybe just used to having people being mean to me.' Bullying RRs appear also to have continued into the present, informing Nina's way of relating to herself:

Sometimes when I'm, I feel upset, ehm . . . sometimes eh there's one, there's one voice that likes to, he likes to eh nag me and he likes to make me feel worse. . . . About myself. Usually it won't be for . . . normally I get upset about myself but sometimes I'm upset about something else, he'll start pointing out negative things about me and ehm . . . he'll make me feel bad . . .

Thus, Nina continues to be criticized and bullied (in her current, 'safe' adult life), which undermines any sense of achievement and her self-confidence, and increases anxiety and low mood.

Individuals internalize both 'ends' of RRs, which we can see in Nina's experience of a critical bullying voice which she fears may be voicing her own views:

> I know it's bad to say, I know it's really bad to say (!) but I don't really care about like … I do … (sighs) it's hard to say like … (sighs heavily) like the things that he says about some … the people in the streets, it makes me feel like bad that maybe I'm the one thinking it, but then on the other hand I'm like, it's like it's not me that he's talking about. [T]here's one that's horrible about other people and he'll like, he'll comment on what people are like, like oh he's got a big nose, he's fat or she's got cankles or something, and that can make me feel bad because … I feel like that's another part of me that wants to say those things out loud.

The 'Critical Bully' role becomes more prominent when Nina is feeling vulnerable, at risk, or distressed (e.g. when out of the house). This 'end' of the RR (and the associated thoughts/feelings) appears not to be fully 'owned' by Nina and is experienced as external voices, although she does wonder if they may be coming from her: 'the negative ones like to come out when I'm alone and I'm in public. . . . Because I'm not around anyone that I'm comfortable with. . . . I feel like they think that's where I'm most ehm . . . vulnerable, because I don't really have anyone that I can go to for comfort'.

If, as therapists, we were able to think about this together with Nina, we might offer a hypothesis that while these thoughts may be coming 'from her', they are based on templates of previous relationships and—rather than indicating that she is a 'horrible person'—are likely to be learnt responses for managing feelings of vulnerability (thus having a protective function). If we were seeing Nina in therapy, we might hope to develop and encourage more helpful and healthy RRs in Nina's repertoire to offer a more compassionate and caring perspective, particularly for when Nina is feeling vulnerable or uncomfortable. The RR of compassionate caring/cared for that we would attempt to establish in therapy would then enable Nina to foster caring RRs with herself and her voices in everyday life, as shown in a possible 'exit' in Figure 22.3. We could also seek to recruit the supportive granddad voice in this.

Grace

Grace, a white woman in her mid-twenties, tends to hear voices when she goes to certain places, particularly those that are associated with her mother or that remind her of traumatic incidents. She recognizes two of the voices, one as being that of her mother and the other, her aunty. She also experiences a male voice that she does not recognize. The voice that sounds like her mother and the male voice were described as angry and negative towards her.

When asked to describe her experiences of hearing voices, Grace responded:

[I]t's kinda like talking in me head that's not me. . . . Sometimes it's very quiet, it's always there, sometimes it gets really loud and aggressive. . . . I don't know [what makes me feel that it's not me], I just don't think I would say those things to myself.

It can be confusing when a voice says something that we feel we would not normally say, or certainly would not say to ourselves. From a CAT perspective, such experiences would be viewed as an expression of an RR that originates from a disowned 'role'/emotion. For some of us, experiences of aggression from others can make it difficult for us to 'own'/acknowledge our own rageful impulses or feelings for fear of becoming like the people who harmed us. However, because we learn and internalize both poles of the relationship (and also because life can be very annoying!), these feelings persist in our experience.

Grace states that her first experience of hearing a voice occurred when having a conversation with her manager at work:

I was at work, and I felt a little bit angry, there was something that my manager said that I didn't agree with, and then all of a sudden they were just there, and it was very intense, very loud. Ehm, and I just, I just . . . I just felt . . . I just fell to the floor, I just didn't know what to do. . . . [the voice said] multiple things, just . . . like . . . I'm a failure, I'm horrible, what are you doing, you're not doing anything right.

If we have experienced others as angry or abusive, it can feel intolerable when we experience similar emotions or reactions, and so they can become disowned/cut off from our consciousness and experienced as a voice. Grace first experienced a voice when she became angry towards someone more powerful than her. The voices were intense, loud, very critical, and, interestingly, directed inwards towards herself (see Figure 22.4).

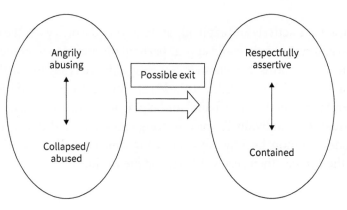

Figure 22.4 Possible reciprocal roles for Grace.

'Exits' for Grace may involve learning about the normality and function of difficult-to-experience emotions, finding ways of accepting and understanding them, and thinking about how they might be helpfully expressed. For example, anger warns us when our boundaries are being infringed upon in some way and can help us to assert or protect ourselves. Learning how to assert and respect her own needs, not only with others, but also with herself, could enable Grace to develop more re-spectful relationships with firmer, self-considerate boundaries (shown as a possible 'exit' RR in Figure 22.4).

Improving Relationship with Voices

In our clinical work, RRs help us to establish with our clients—in a simple, col-laborative fashion—an understanding of voice-hearing experiences as mirrors or echoes of, or responses to, previous life experiences and internalized relationships. Such sense-making work, even with those who are experiencing acute symptoms, supports the reflective capacity that we hope to develop within a course of therapy. While being mindful of an individual's ZPD, by considering the function of a voice and whether old, unhelpful, or abusive patterns may be playing out, we can then de-velop a more benign explanation of voice-hearing, suggest new relationships with, and approaches towards, voices, and hopefully reduce distress.

Compared with CBT, evidence for CAT with voice-hearing and psychosis is in its infancy (Taylor et al., 2019). However, while CBT has proven successful in helping clients gain a greater sense of power and control over their voices, Perry (2012, p. 20) suggests that:

> CAT provides some alternative ways to negotiate power from a person's voices in a way that maintains a dialogue and relationship. This approach also means that (even when a person is entirely convinced that a voice is not part of them), power and freedom from un-helpful procedures are negotiated between the person and the voice, as they would be in any other relationship.

In addition, as CAT actively and explicitly attends to, and works with, the therapeutic relationship and ruptures, it would appear particularly suited to working with those who experience psychosis, for whom therapeutic alliance is key to whether therapy is beneficial or harmful (Goldsmith et al., 2015). The CAT concept of RRs therefore offers a useful therapeutic 'short-hand' for helping to make sense of, de-stigmatize, and contextualize an individual's voice-hearing experiences. They can also provide explicit models for more healthy ways of relating which people can work towards in relation to their voices, themselves, others, and the world.

References

Bakhtin, M. M. (1984). *Problems of Dostoevsky's Poetics*. Translated from the Russian by C. Emerson. Minneapolis, MN: University of Minnesota Press.

Goldsmith, L. P., Lewis, S. W., Dunn, G., and Bentall, R. P. (2015). Psychological treatments for early psychosis can be beneficial or harmful, depending on the therapeutic alliance: an instrumental variable analysis. *Psychological Medicine*, 45(11), 2365–73.

Jellema, A. (2005). An animal living in a world of symbols. *Reformulation*, 25, 6–12.

Kerr, I. B., Birkett, P. B. L., and Chanen, A. (2003). Clinical and service implications of a cognitive analytic therapy model of psychosis. *The Australian and New Zealand Journal of Psychiatry*, 37(5), 515–23.

Morrison, A. P., Nothard, S., Bowe, S. E., and Wells, A. (2004). Interpretations of voices in patients with hallucinations and non-patient controls: a comparison and predictors of distress in patients. *Behaviour Research and Therapy*, 42(11), 1315–23.

Perry, A. (2012). CAT with people who hear distressing voices. *Reformulation*, 38, 16–22.

Potter, S. (2019). From map and talk to relational awareness. In: *Shared Thinking Space: Innovations in Reflective Practice in Forensic Settings* [conference]. Middlesbrough: Tees, Esk & Wear Valley NHS Foundation Trust.

Ryle, A., and Kerr, I. B. (2002). *Introducing Cognitive Analytic Therapy: Principles and Practice*. Chichester: John Wiley & Sons.

Taylor, P. J., Perry, A., Hutton, P. M., Tan, R., Fishers, N., Focone, C., Griffiths, D., and Seddon, C. (2019). Cognitive analytic therapy for psychosis: a case series. *Psychology and Psychotherapy: Theory, Research and Practice*, 92(3), 359–78.

About the Authors

Anna Luce currently works at Crisis UK and was previously a Clinical Psychologist and CAT Practitioner in Early Intervention in Psychosis at the Cumbria, Northumberland, Tyne and Wear NHS Foundation Trust. She is particularly interested in therapeutic approaches which seek to improve relationships with distressing voices, experiences, or emotions through an understanding of their origin and possible functions, with a view to developing more rewarding and compassionate lives and relationships.

Nicola Barclay is a Clinical Psychologist in Early Intervention in Psychosis and At-Risk Mental State (ARMS) services at the Cumbria, Northumberland, Tyne and Wear NHS Foundation Trust. She is interested in how unusual sensory perceptions develop and, for those who find these experiences problematic, working to reduce distress, develop understanding of these sensory experiences, and improve quality of life.

23

Learning to Navigate Hallucinations

Comparing Voice Control Ability During Psychosis and in Ritual Use of Psychedelics

David Dupuis, Quai Branly Museum, Research Department

Far from being reducible to the biological and psychological dimensions to which they have been confined in the West since the nineteenth century, hallucinations are also deeply shaped by culture. As the meaning attributed to them originates outside individuals, in collective ways of doing and thinking, the social environment is able to affect frequency, meaning, and even phenomenological features of hallucinations (Larøi et al., 2014). In opposition to contemporary Euro-American societies, many cultures value hallucinations and place them at the heart of their social life. For example, historical and ethnographic studies have documented the importance of hallucinations in Native American societies and the wide variety of techniques that can be used to induce them, such as fasting, isolation, sensory deprivation, and the use of psychotropic substances. Hallucinogenic plants, such as ayahuasca, occupy a central place in the life of Amazonian societies, as do peyote and psilocybin mushrooms in the Mesoamerican region, or the San Pedro cactus in the Andean world (Furst, 1972).

If the pathological model is indisputably dominant in Euro-American societies since the end of the nineteenth century, diverse perspectives on hallucination have recently been opening up. Indeed, techniques for the voluntary production of (arguably hallucination-like) visual mental imagery have been developed for sports and professional performance as part of coaching practices (visualization techniques), while new Western religious movements, whether New Age or evangelical, also give a central place to hallucinations (Luhrmann, 2012). More recently, psychiatric service users have claimed a new social identity as 'voice-hearers' through the emergence of progressive self-help groups.

The institutionalized use of hallucinogens, long mostly confined to Native American societies, has benefited since the second half of the twentieth century from a growing interest from Euro-American societies. In the context of the emergence of the counter-cultural and psychedelic movement, these practices have benefited from significant transnational diffusion, which has placed these indigenous practices in an intercultural dimension frequently referred to as 'neoshamanic'. As a result,

David Dupuis, *Learning to Navigate Hallucinations* In: *Voices in Psychosis*. Edited by: Angela Woods, Ben Alderson-Day, and Charles Fernyhough, Oxford University Press. © David Dupuis 2022. DOI: 10.1093/oso/9780192898388.003.0023 hallucinations perceived in these contexts began to be used in Euro-American societies as vectors of political emancipation, psychotherapy, personal development, or new forms of syncretic religiosity (such as new age religiosity).

Inspired by the craze for the psychotropic ayahuasca drink and the mythicized image of the 'primary' forest, an influx of travellers headed towards the Peruvian Amazon from the 1990s onwards, giving rise to what some have called 'shamanic tourism'. In order to meet this new demand, many reception centres have developed over the past twenty years on the borders of the metropolitan areas of the Peruvian Amazon (Iquitos, Pucallpa, Tarapoto). These institutions, which anthropologists have called 'shamanic centres', are often founded on the partnership between Westerners and mestizo or indigenous locals. They offer participation in ritual activities presented as part of 'traditional Amazonian medicine'. Combining discursive and pragmatic elements from very diverse cultural backgrounds, the mechanisms implemented by these institutions are more or less freely inspired by certain practices specific to Peruvian Metis shamanism, most notably the ritualized use of hallucinogens such as ayahuasca.

I conducted eighteen months of ethnographic fieldwork at one of the region's leading institutions, studying the use of these substances by approximately one hundred Westerners in this context by sharing their daily lives and rituals. Conducting interviews and longitudinal follow-up with around forty individuals, I observed that in these contexts, hallucinations were highly valued and most often invested with an educational and therapeutic dimension.

The interviews collected with psychiatric service users during the Voices in Psychosis (VIP) study offer an opportunity to compare hallucinatory experience as perceived by two Western groups experiencing hallucinations in very different contexts.

Looking at the data collected in the VIP study, it is striking to see that, while in shamanic centres, voices are voluntarily sought out and frequently valued as therapeutic, in the psychotic experience, voices are perceived spontaneously, involuntarily, and most often as disruptive and negative. How are the voices perceived by users of psychiatric services similar to, and different from, those perceived by shamanic tourism clients? What can this comparison tell us about the attribution of a pathological dimension to voice-hearing phenomena? How do the institutionalized practices of hallucinations, in the indigenous cultures of the Americas and more recently in the West, invite us to take a fresh look at voices in psychosis?

It is to these questions that I will propose some answers. Comparing the data collected in the Peruvian Amazon with the VIP interviews, I will show that the ability to control voices is the main distinguishing criterion between these two groups, and will explore the implications of this difference for a better understanding and treatment of 'voices' in psychosis.

Hearing and Controlling Voices in a Shamanic Centre in the Peruvian Amazon

Takiwasi: A Shamanic Centre in the Peruvian Amazon

Founded in 1992 by the French doctor Jacques Mabit and Peruvian and Spanish collaborators, the therapeutic community of Takiwasi is both an addiction treatment clinic and one of the main places welcoming Western travellers to the region to 'meet ayahuasca'. These travellers—men and women, aged between twenty and sixty—come mainly from the middle and upper classes of the urban areas of Western countries. Their biographies are often marked by the accumulation and repetition of different registers of misfortune (death, chronic pain or pathology, accidents, academic or professional difficulties, 'loss of meaning'), the resolution of which is presented as the main reason for their coming. The resistance of these difficulties to the treatments offered by Western medicine and the dominant forms of psychotherapy (psychiatry, psychoanalysis, behaviourism, etc.) has most often initiated a journey of experimentation with alternative therapies that leads them to the Amazon. Coming to Amazonia is also rooted in a form of religiosity characteristic of Western modernity, built on the accumulation of 'spiritual experiences' from various cultural horizons and a modular, individual, and irregular set of practices.

In Takiwasi, these travellers join 'seminars' which bring together about fifteen participants for a period of two weeks. Alongside introductory lectures, discussion groups, and individual interviews, the courses include ayahuasca rituals and days of retreat in the jungle involving the consumption of other plant preparations. Participation in these activities requires compliance with various food, relational, and sexual prohibitions. The use of ayahuasca is combined with complex ritual devices. During these rituals—which take place at night in a collective room (*maloca*) and extend from six to nine hours—the healers (*curanderos*) use ritual songs (*icaros*), perfumes, and other techniques characteristic of Peruvian mestizo shamanism, such as the practice of *soplada* (which consists of blowing tobacco smoke or perfumes on the patient's body) or the use of *chakapa* (a rattle constructed of bundled leaves which is shaken while singing by the *curandero* around the patient), in order to comfort, protect, or purify participants. The next day, the participants' experiences are shared in speech groups that aim to help the participants interpret their experiences.

Hearing Voices in Takiwasi

The ingestion of ayahuasca most often involves the perception of visual, tactile (sensations of brushing and touching), olfactory, gustatory, and auditory (sounds, melodies, voices) hallucinations. Participants testify in particular to the production of rich mental imagery—a property that has given the plant preparation its reputation as 'hallucinogenic'. These mental images are generally composed of bright and colourful geometric shapes, but can also take on more figurative forms. Many participants report the perception of animals, anthropomorphic beings, or beings mixing human, plant, and animal elements that emerge and evolve within rich, visionary landscapes.

In this context, visual and auditory verbal hallucinations—here called 'voices' and 'visions'—are most often not interpreted as hallucinations (as defined by psychiatry as perceptions without objects), but as acts of communication from usually invisible entities, allowing the development of a lasting relationship with them. The so-called 'hallucinogenic' substances are consequently, from an emic point of view, invested as a relational tool. If hallucinations are perceived by the participants as a sign of the presence of agents with initially undetermined identities, these identities gradually tend towards a correspondence with the supernatural entities postulated by the local cosmology: demons, nature spirits, entities of the Christian pantheon, or ancestors. These entities are distributed according to a configuration described by ritual specialists as a spiritual struggle between malicious and protective entities. In the Takiwasi context, strongly influenced by Christianity, participants have to learn to distinguish in a dual way between the voices and visions they perceive. Voices are, for instance, distributed according to the emotional properties of their content. Those containing insults, depreciation, and invitation to guilt, fear, or discouragement are attributed to malicious entities of an evil nature, while those consisting of encouragement or advice, inducing joy and appeasement, are attributed to protective entities such as protective ancestors, nature spirits, the ayahuasca spirit, or entities of the Christian pantheon:

> At one point I had a vision with the archangel Saint Michael who was piercing a demon with his sword, as in the religious images. Later I felt the presence of Jesus Christ, who looked behind my back, where chains were hung attached to a cage. I saw demons laughing because I had to drag my cage to move forward in life. They jerked me around all the time, like they were raping me. When Jesus Christ saw the chains and the cage, he said it had nothing to do here and kicked to kick it all out. (Philip)
>
> There were all these demons parasitizing me inside, but I saw the ayahuasca that was chasing them, like a lot of little bright snakes inside my body that were circulating and cleaning all that up. . . . Later I saw the ayahuasca spirit. She was a kind of woman with a snake-like lower body, showing me how the demons got in, what I had done, and therefore what I had to do to stop them from entering. (Mary)

Learning to Control Voices

While beings manifested through voices and visions are often initially perceived both as persecutors (demons, witches, etc.) and as allies (ancestors, entities of the Catholic pantheon, spirits of nature, etc.), it seems that over time they are increasingly perceived as protective, educational, and therapeutic. This seems to be one consequence of the techniques transmitted to participants during their visit. During speech groups or individual interviews in which the experiences are discussed, ritual specialists encourage the participants to view voices as coming from intentional agents whose behaviour is likely to be affected by the way the participant relates to them. Participants are consequently encouraged to adopt control techniques designed to affect—by reducing or stimulating—their occurrence, intensity, and frequency. These cognitive, affective, or behavioural control strategies, transmitted both vertically from ritual specialists to participants and horizontally between participants, generally aim to modify the relationship with voices. Here are some examples, as described to me by participants in the hallucinogenic rite in Takiwasi:

> When I feel it's difficult, when I lose control or have bad visions, I do as the healers told me, I focus on the songs. It's like a rope you hold on to, and it allows you to get through difficulties. (Eric)

> I think about the people I love, and it helps me. I feel their presence encouraging me, comforting me in the struggle, and it eventually passes. (Juliet)

These strategies consist, as we can see, of active efforts to stand up to the voices of evil entities and attempts to control them in order to no longer perceive them. They may include strategies of confrontation or opposition, achieved through dialoguing with the voices (ordering a compelling voice to remain silent) or attempting to diminish or transform the emotional tone created by the perception of certain voices through the use of a vigilance strategy (directing attention to the disturbing voice in order to prevent and control it). They may also include avoidance strategies involving alternative activities (directing attention to other perceptions such as ritual songs or positive voices), or compensatory behaviours like fleeing the ritual space, sleeping, praying, or using an artefact. After a period of learning, the majority of participants seem to be able, during ritual practices, to cultivate hallucinations inducing joy and appeasement and to reduce or even eliminate those perceived as disruptive. For most of them, the presence and influence of voices perceived as abusive and controlling ('demon voices') decreases, while the presence of voices suggesting ways in which they could improve their life, complimenting them on their achievements, and praising their good qualities (mainly identified as the 'ayahuasca spirit voice') increases. These techniques of hallucination control, first implemented during rituals, are then frequently used by participants in their daily lives in order to achieve more control over their mental states (emotions, compulsive behaviours, etc.), and consequently increase their self-esteem and confidence.

Hearing and Controlling Voices in Psychosis

If we compare these observations with the first-person reports in the VIP interviews, it is striking to note that here too, voices are very frequently perceived as acts of communicative felt presences, rather than as simple perceptual signals:

> It's like voices are telling us to do stuff that I never usually would do. . . . These voices are, telling us to do the opposite of what I would normally do. . . . Like somebody else is telling us that basically there's either an arsehole or something like this or that. (Matt)

This point has been noted in recent work on voices in a psychosis context (Bell et al., 2017; Deamer and Wilkinson, 2015). While in the VIP interviews, the degree of voice personification is most often minimal and few participants experience a supernatural narrative, voices are frequently perceived as a sign of an externally individualized agency. These acts of communication, which sometimes take the form of real conversations, are most often expressed in the form of commands.

The second striking point emerging from the comparison is that voices are predominantly described in a negative way—as unpleasant or even horrific. While just over one-third of participants reported positive emotions in relation to their voices, every single participant in the study associated their voices with negative emotions, including anxiety, depression, fear, paranoia, sleep disruption, and suicidality. Voices are predominantly experienced by participants as abusive or violent and as having a negative impact on their relationships, and this feature does not appear to change over time.

Finally, the majority of participants reported little ability to influence or control voices and their disruptive effects. Those coping strategies reported by participants were mainly techniques for redirecting the participant's attention. Faced with the voices, Ulrich 'does things' to entertain himself, Dawn goes for a walk, and Violet talks to her friends and family or decides to go to the museum. Many of them, like Violet, Will, and Anthony, use music to divert their attention from voices, while others, like Chris, play games or use a more radical solution, like Xander, who prefers to sleep. Most participants described these coping strategies as distraction techniques, but the diversity and effectiveness of these techniques seem limited.

Conclusion: Towards an Inventory of Techniques for the Control of Hallucinations

This brief comparison first serves as a reminder of the property that has sometimes been attributed to hallucinogens (previously referred to as 'psychotomimetic' substances): that of mimicking certain features usually associated with psychosis, such as auditory verbal hallucinations and their attribution to external agents. The observation of the use of hallucinogens as carried out in Takiwasi suggests also that the relationship with hallucinations and their content is highly influenced by the social environment. In previous work, I have proposed to model this process, which I have called 'socialization of hallucinations' (Dupuis, 2021a), exploring the underpinnings by which social interactions shape the individual's relationships to their hallucinations and their very content through education of attention, structuration of expectations, and categorization of perceptions.

A question still arises from this comparison. Could the coping strategies observed in Takiwasi, which are leading users of shamanic practices to discriminate and control the frequency and content of their voices, benefit voice-hearers in the context of psychosis where voices are also perceived as acts of communication by agents?

This is what new therapeutic techniques such as AVATAR therapy (Leff et al., 2014), Relating Therapy for Voices (Hayward et al., 2009), and hearing voices peer support groups (May and Svanholmer, 2019) seem to suggest. These different techniques have a common approach in that they treat hallucinations not as perceptual phenomena, but as acts of communication (Deamer and Wilkinson, 2015) which are experienced as a social and relational phenomenon (Bell et al., 2017). In this relational approach, voices are perceived primarily as communication hallucinations, rather than as auditory ones. As the VIP study shows, the voices are indeed frequently experienced as personified, having identities and agency, and are consequently perceived as being coherent communicative speech acts:

> I've had bad voices and good voices, like nice ones and bad. One was called Mark, and one was called Martha. Mark was the bad one, he used to tell us to kill myself and self-harm, like tell us that I don't, like no one wants us here and stuff like that. And then on the other hand, I've got Martha telling us that, that I'm a good lass, like a nice lass and stuff. (Violet)
>
> It's like every single day I hear three different voices, ehm, there's a female voice, she's called Roxy, she actually introduced herself to me. Ehm, and then there's an angry male voice, who's like there all the time, I don't know his name, but he's there like constantly unless I'm asleep, he like, he's like . . . a boy in a way but like he just, he's a bully to everyone. Ehm, and then the third one is very quiet and . . . just he doesn't, like I don't hear him like every day, it might be like once a week that I hear him. (Xander)

As the experience of hearing voices is increasingly understood within this relational framework, new methods such as AVATAR therapy, which consists of encouraging the voice-hearer to construct a visual 'avatar' using a computer program, invite the voice-hearer to relate to the voice in order to modify the hearer–voice relationship. Even if this relationship can involve a variety of relational possibilities (conflict, alliance, etc.), the voice-hearing phenomenon in psychosis is, as observed in the VIP study, frequently characterized by domination and intrusion, with the voice-hearer feeling as if they are in a passive and submissive position, persecuted by the voice. The goal of these relational therapies is to transform this relationship by enhancing awareness of the reciprocal nature of this relationship, and inviting the voice-hearer to engage voluntarily with voices through dialogue. The seminal studies on relational therapies (Hayward et al., 2009) show that these practices increase the controllability of, and decrease the distress linked to, the voice-hearing phenomenon. In a nutshell, these studies show that the more the patient is engaging assertively with voices, the more they are able to control them: the higher the control of voices, the lower the distress and frequency of negative voices reported by the participants. It is striking to observe that these emerging therapies propose using some of the coping strategies that can be observed in so-called neoshamanic practices, such as directly instructing the voice to be silent. I also learnt during conversations with members of the Hearing Voices Network in Paris (France), with whom I have been collaborating since 2017, that during peer support groups, voice-hearers are sharing these kinds of strategies of interaction with their voices, which often has the consequence of reducing distress (May and Svanholmer, 2019; Ruddle et al., 2011).

These observations highlight the importance of documenting cultural practices surrounding the perception of hallucinations, as they offer promising areas for investigation towards the creation of an inventory of the techniques used to control hallucinations. This seems particularly true for social contexts that value and seek hallucinations. Among evangelical prayer practices (Luhrmann, 2012), techniques related to the creation of imaginary companions ('tulpas') in Euro-American societies (Veissière, 2016), and ritual practices surrounding the use of hallucinogens in Amerindian indigenous and mestizo shamanism (Dupuis, 2021b) or Vajrayana Buddhism meditation practices, a common feature emerges: if hallucinations are frequently valued and sought after, they are indeed only tolerated if they are the subjects of a process of social learning, allowing individuals to control the occurrence, nature, intensity, and frequency of their hallucinations.

The techniques developed within these social settings, to the extent to which they give a central place to the perception of hallucinations, seem to have a potential clinical application. As they are likely to be learnt, they appear as potentially efficient alternative therapeutic tools in regulating the distress linked to voice-hearing for so-called psychotic patients. Documenting these control techniques and the coping strategies they involve through ethnographic surveys therefore appears likely to enrich the repertoire of techniques within emerging relating therapies for people who hear persecutory auditory hallucinations, especially when they do not respond, or respond minimally, to antipsychotic medication.

References

Bell, V., Mills, K. L., Modinos, G., and Wilkinson, S. (2017). Rethinking social cognition in light of psychosis: reciprocal implications for cognition and psychopathology. *Clinical Psychological Science*, 5(3), pp.537–550.

Deamer, F., and Wilkinson S. (2015). The speaker behind the voice: therapeutic practice from the perspective of pragmatic theory. *Frontiers in Psychology*, 6, 817.

Dupuis, D. (2021a). The socialization of hallucinations Cultural priors, social interactions and contextual factors in the use of psychedelics. *Transcult. Psychiatry* [Epub ahead of print]. doi: 10.1177/13634615211036388

Dupuis, D. (2021b). Psychedelics as Tools for Belief Transmission. Set, Setting, Suggestibility, and Persuasion in the Ritual Use of Hallucinogens. *Front. Psychol.* 12, 730031. doi:10.3389/fpsyg.2021.730031

Furst, P. T. (1972). *Flesh of the Gods: The Ritual Use of Hallucinogens*. New York, NY: Praeger Publishers.

Hayward, M., Overton, J., Dorey, T., and Denney, J. (2009). Relating therapy for people who hear Voices: a case series. *Clinical Psychology and Psychotherapy*, 16(3), 216–27.

Larøi, F., Luhrmann, T. M., Bell, V., Christian, W. A. Jr, Deshpande, S., Fernyhough, C., Jenkins, J., and Woods, A. (2014). Culture and hallucinations: overview and future directions. *Schizophrenia Bulletin*, 40(Suppl. 4), S213–20.

Leff, J., Williams, G., Huckvale, M., Arbuthnot, M., and Leff, A. (2014). Avatar therapy for persecutory auditory hallucinations: what is it and how does it work? *Psychosis*, 6(2), 166–76.

Luhrmann, T. (2012). *When God Talks Back: Understanding the American Evangelical Relationship with God*. New York, NY: Alfred Knopf.

May, R., and Svanholmer, E. (2019). *Self-Help Guide to Talking with Voices. Ideas for People Who Hear Voices and Want to Try Engaging in Dialogue with Them* (2nd version), 1st edition. https://openmindedonline.files.wordpress.com/2019/09/self-help-guide-to-talking-with-voices-r.-may-and-e.-svanholmer-sep-2019.pdf (accessed 26 April 2021).

Ruddle, A., Mason, O., and Wykes, T. (2011). A review of hearing voices groups: evidence and mechanisms of change. *Clinical Psychological Review*, 31(5),757–66.

Veissière, S. (2016). Varieties of tulpa experiences: the hypnotic nature of human sociality, personhood, and interphenomenality. In: A. Raz and M. Lifshitz, eds. *Hypnosis and Meditation: Towards an Integrative Science of Conscious Planes*. Oxford: Oxford University Press, pp. 55–74.

About the Author

David Dupuis holds a PhD in Social Anthropology and an MA in Clinical Psychology. He is currently working in the Research Department of the Quai Branly Museum (Paris). He has been a Research Fellow in the Laboratory of Social Anthropology (Collège de France, Paris) and a member of the Hearing the Voice project at the University of Durham. Based on fieldwork conducted in Latin America and Europe over the past decade, his work focuses on contemporary recharacterizations of psychedelic substance use and the relationship between hallucinations and culture.

24

'Then I Open the Door and Walk into Their World'

Crossing the Threshold and Hearing the Voice

Akiko Hart, National Survivor User Network

'When It's Dark, I Think Someone Is Standing There.' (Violet)

She is watching me now, as I write this, the smell of the words drawing her in. The words, a spell, conjuring her into being, and yet her presence also fading as the paragraphs take shape on my screen. Why doesn't she want me to write about her? I'm not sure. As I write, she seems less real. She becomes the thing I write about.

As I read the Voices in Psychosis (VIP) transcripts, I can't help but respond with my own stories. A small act of disclosure—atonement, perhaps, for the many disclosures I've read. The transcripts are alive with intimacy, but they are also data. I find myself wanting to bear witness to the testimonies by letting them breathe, and yet they also compel me to reply, to be inspired by them, to use them. Can one bear witness when one does research? Perhaps. But there is also a disconnect between researchers and the objects of their research. There is an us and a them: a separation between those who write and those who are written about. So here, I choose to play both roles. I sit outside and alongside Hearing the Voice, as neither a researcher nor a voice-hearer, but as someone who, through my work developing Hearing Voices peer support groups, is deeply engaged and enmeshed with the many worlds circling this area. Here, I share my experiences of presences, wrapping them loosely around three themes—interiority, panopticism, and possibility—in order to unshackle them from my urge to understand them.

There is no agreed name for some experiences which rest on the hinterlands of perception. Sometimes referred to as 'threshold phenomena' (Blackman, 2013), sensed presences, or felt presences, these 'silent companions' (Alderson-Day, 2016) are persons or agents felt, but not directly seen or heard.

> [Y]ou know that feeling you get when you've, when like there's another person there? . . . Do you know what I mean? If you go in an empty house and there's someone in

Akiko Hart, *'Then I Open the Door and Walk into Their World'* In: *Voices in Psychosis.* Edited by: Angela Woods, Ben Alderson-Day, and Charles Fernyhough, Oxford University Press. © Akiko Hart 2022. DOI: 10.1093/oso/9780192898388.003.0024 there that . . . I don't know, it's hard to . . . like that . . . static-y feeling, you know that, as if someone is there. (Emma)

Presences can occur in a number of contexts, from hypnagogic or hypnopompic hallucinations in the borderlands of sleep and wakefulness, to sleep paralysis, bereavement, and extreme survival situations, to neurological or psychiatric conditions such as Parkinson's disease or Lewy body dementia (Alderson-Day, 2016). Or they can simply be a part of daily life. There are a striking number of direct and indirect references to presences in the transcripts, as the participants mobilize the inadequate words at our disposal to describe what is happening.

While conceptualizations of the self as bounded and autonomous have been challenged and shattered, interiority is often indexed to a singular 'I' and buffered by a protective layer of skin. Our movements may be tracked by CCTV and our conversations intercepted by Alexa, but inside our heads, inside ourselves, we might still be able to guard a private realm inaccessible to others. For the VIP participants, however, this is not always the case. For Liam, the presence is always there, by his side: 'I just feel the presence of someone with me all the time, watching me'. Gail's voices follow her: 'it makes me feel quite trapped and . . . because no matter where I go, they're still there'. Jane shares space in her head with 'Onin' and is clear about the demarcation between them:

Because like do you know when you think, like have thoughts in me head, as in like your voice and it's your personality and things, well with Onin, it's completely like separate, like . . . emotions, feelings, that sort of thing, completely separate.

Cultural theorist Lisa Blackman re-situates these 'threshold phenomena' in a liminal space, 'between the self and other, inside and outside, and material and immaterial' (Blackman, 2012, p. xii). It is perhaps no coincidence that Orla sees 'Kay' around doorframes, neither in nor out. These 'boundary voices', hovering or proliferating at the edge of known and immediate space, hold the uncanny. Their rendering into being, their stepping into the room, is yet to come.

This invites us to consider whether blunt spatial distinctions adequately render the permeability and fluidity of these experiences, when we extend in the world, and are of the world—and yet are asked to remodel them as interiority (Blackman, 2012, p. 151). Grace refers to a 'bubble' surrounding her when the presences become more aggressive, her personal space expanding: 'So I feel like nothing can get in, nothing can get out, and it's just, that's just, and it's pressure building on . . .' But if one's inner life is thronged with observers and interlocutors, if we share our space with multiple voices, parts, or persons within us, if there is no silence, then this opens up the possibility that interiority might be neither singular nor private.

'I Feel Like There's Constantly Someone Watching Me.' (Gail)

And it was the word that made her flesh, as she eased herself out of the pages of the book I was reading and into my home, like Sadako crawling out of the TV towards us in *Ring* (1998). She was alive while I read about her. When I closed the book, she stayed alive, her presence no longer confined to its pages. She lived somewhere in the house. I was never sure where. At night, she would come and visit me. She would stand in doorways, hide behind closed doors, and watch me while I slept. I never saw her, I never heard her voice: I am not a voice-hearer, after all. But I know when she is here. As it is for Emma, it is that 'static-y' feeling.

Being watched can be imbued with love or desire, but is more often associated with 'an active and malevolent observer' (Harper, 2002). The 'red one' in Eric's life doesn't communicate through words, but through watching: 'I used to just sort of feel so much guilt and shame because he would be staring at me from a corner.' Gail identifies being able to hear what the voices are saying and the feeling of being constantly watched as the most distressing parts of her experience. Being watched is paradoxically both an intensely personal experience, bound as the gaze is to the individual, and also one that is shared and discursive (Harper, 2002).

Bentham's panopticon, as reimagined by Foucault, proves itself a malleable conceptual tool in this regard. Originally a prison designed in such a way that inmates are always visible to the guards in the central watchtower, but do not know exactly when they are being observed, it becomes a psychic internalization of modernity in Sass's reading, and then a post-modern panoptic regime which mobilizes surveillance in order to create better consumers (Woods, 2011, p. 214). Recovery in the Bin, an activist collective, repurposes this imagery in the context of punitive welfare reforms in the UK. Here, the panopticon is embodied by, and activated through, the Department of Work and Pensions (DWP), which is responsible for welfare policy and administration. The Welfare State, that post-war triumph in the public imaginary designed to protect those in most need from cradle to grave, now becomes scourge and jailor: 'I live inside an invisible cage built by the DWP' (RITB, 2019).

The asylum, long since closed, is no longer the prison. There is seemingly no way to escape the tendrils of the many-headed Hydra of the State (see Image 24.1) (Rowan Olive, 2018), scrutinizing with its peripheral vision the activities of claimants in order to track, trap, shame, and sanction them. The DWP panopticon becomes the locus of pain and trauma, sustaining and feeding the distress and disability it is appointed to monitor. Its pervasive suspicion is internalized by claimants (Dylan, 2018), as it attempts to peer into their souls and expose them through assessments:

I am more than the sum total of my mental health, but this 40 page bible of me demands to know all the worst aspects of who I am and how I am. The stuff I am really ashamed of, the

(a)   (b)

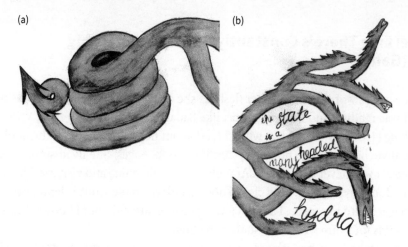

Image 24.1 Hydra of the State.
Credit: Rachel Rowan Olive, 2018.

stuff I hate about myself. Here is a list of all the things I can't do because I am broken. Here are the bones of my despair.

In her poetic exploration of paranoia, coloniality, and surveillance, the critical psychologist Rachel Liebert introduces the concept of psycurity, an 'abstract machine' channelling paranoia to animate a neo-colonial security state in order to police and dehumanize marginalized bodies (Liebert, 2018, p. 85). The coils of psycurity wind themselves around public spaces, but also the private sphere, where they wage a war on imagination. Being watched is pathologized as paranoia, a deliberate misdirection drawing our attention away from the political reality of surveillance, but also foreclosing it as an experience which might hold meaning or possibility for the individual. And yet, before I start to think about what these possibilities might entail, I want to stay with the experience of being watched. We are sometimes too quick to want to find meaning. For me, being watched was paralysis. It was my world getting smaller until it atrophied to a single dot which felt safe. There was no meaning, beyond surviving the moment.

'She's in the House, It's not in My Head.' (Emma)

They call her Bertha. That isn't what I call her. She is alive because she hates. She is real, but she is not a person. She is me, and she is not. She is what I fear and what I might become.

In my dreams, I see her, a flash of skirt, a figure running. I have touched her: she is real, you see. She is usually far away, these days. She is preoccupied with herself. She doesn't want to harm me anymore. I don't think she watches me, most of the time.

I have tried to find her, through words, again. I read *Wide Sargasso Sea*, Jean Rhys's retelling of *Jane Eyre*, so that I could see the woman before she becomes monster, the character before she is representation. But there, I also found Rhys and our shared haunting.

In Teale's play *After Mrs Rochester*, Bertha/Antoinette steps out of the book and onto the stage, as an older Jean Rhys sits beside her in a room in the Devon countryside. Her story is locked with Bertha/Antoinette's, both white Creole women trapped and alone in England, both desiring and rejecting whiteness and respectability. Rhys retells Charlotte Brontë's story because Brontë 'had never tasted a mango or seen one rot in the midday heat. She didn't know that fabric rots. That furniture falls apart. That everything decays as quickly as it grows. That the road they built returned to forest. (*Beat.*). She had never seen the Wide Sargasso Sea' (Teale, 2003, p. 72). What kind of risks did Rhys take as she let the porosity between worlds slip away and disintegrate, until she found herself using 'I'?

I tried to find her in psychology and was told, with great certainty, that she was in fact my mother, my terror materialized. (*The child voice must be the baby she lost. The male presence the father she fears.*) This interpretative act was violence, not least because it was impossible to deny. But it was also impoverished. Anchoring my experience to a familial psychodrama tethers her to my world, as an object which needs to be studied, understood, and resolved. But she is also not of the world: she is also possibility.

A topography of the borderlands of perception invites us to welcome shade and silence as a decolonizing praxis (Liebert, 2018, p. 110). Moving beyond the false hermeneutic binary of voices as symptoms of illness *or* voices as psychodrama made manifest requires us to 'plung(e) vertically through the border between imagination and reality' (Liebert, 2018, p. 112). In this endeavour, we are perhaps hampered by our need to make meaning, to understand, to know. Any reading risks colonizing experiences, indexing them to the logics to which we ourselves are bound. I find myself looking at the transcripts and holding myself back, unsuccessfully, from analysis and interpretation. I struggle to give the participants space, to let them breathe, to follow them where they go. How then, to proceed?

Freeing ourselves from the urge to know might compel us to be open to the transgression of reality, and to different ways of listening and attending to voices, presences, and related experiences. It asks us to pause, lightly, to move beyond framing voices as an experience to be understood, towards finding a way to let the voices speak. To imagine, and to open ourselves up to different forms of knowing and not-knowing. Grace Cho speaks of transgenerational and diasporic haunting as 'a secret that takes the form of a ghost', who speaks the unspeakable and comes into being because of silence (Cho, 2008, p. 164). She gives space to the *yanggongju*, the Korean ghost who speaks of trauma, sexual violence, and shame, through performance art, auto-ethnography, and psychoanalysis. Liebert attempts to reclaim paranoia as possibility by staging an encounter between the prodrome (the early signs or symptoms thought to be a forerunner to, and therefore predictive of, psychosis) and

Coatlicue, a Mesoamerican goddess of the serpent who inhabits borderland spaces. Both Cho and Liebert speak to their own experiences, unsettled, unbound, and offer a hand to the reader: first, they invite us to look inside. Here, I have also drawn inwards—whether as a prelude to connection or a move to introspection, I don't yet know.

'She lives here', says Jean Rhys to her younger self Ella in Teale's reconstruction (Teale, 2003, pp. 31–2), as Ella reads *Jane Eyre* and stares at Bertha in front of her on stage:

ELLA: I don't want her here. I travelled 5000 miles to get away from her . . . How did she . . .

JEAN: You brought her here.

ELLA: Tell her to go away.

JEAN: She can't.

She is with me, she is beside me, and she is also far away. She is part of me, and she is not. I found her through words, and that is where I will lose her. Can I, perhaps, find a way of hearing her voice, this other I have never heard? To step aside, for a moment, let her speak, and see my world through her eyes (Rhys, 1966, p. 148):

[W]hen night comes, and she has had several drinks and sleeps, it is easy to take the keys. I know now where she keeps them. Then I open the door and walk into their world. It is, as I always knew, made of cardboard.

References

Alderson-Day, B. (2016). The silent companions. *The Psychologist*, 29, 272–5.

Blackman, L. (2013). *Immaterial Bodies*. Los Angeles, CA: Sage.

Cho, G. (2008). *Haunting the Korean Diaspora: Shame, Secrecy, Silence, and the Forgotten War*. Minneapolis, MN: University of Minnesota Press.

Dylan, R. (2018). The life and times of a modern day mental. *Asylum Magazine*, 25(3), 10–11.

Harper, D. (2002). The politics of paranoia: paranoid positioning and conspiratorial narratives in the surveillance society. *Surveillance and Society*, 5(1), 1–32.

Liebert, R. (2018). *Psycurity: Colonialism, Paranoia, and the War on Imagination*. London: Routledge.

Recoveryinthebin.org (2019). The invisible prison—panopticon of the DWP. https://recoveryinthebin. org/2019/07/27/the-invisible-prison/ (accessed 20 April 2019).

Rhys, J. (1966). *Wide Sargasso Sea*. London: Penguin.

Rowan Olive, R. (2018). The state is a many headed hydra. [artwork]. *Asylum Magazine*, 25(3), cover.

Teale, P. (2003). *After Mrs Rochester*. London: Nick Hern Books.

Woods, A. (2011). *The Sublime Object of Psychiatry: Schizophrenia in Clinical and Cultural Theory*. Oxford: Oxford University Press.

About the Author

Akiko Hart is the CEO of the National Survivor User Network (NSUN). She is the Chair of the International Society for Psychological and Social Approaches to Psychosis (ISPS UK), which advocates for social and psychological approaches to psychosis, and is a trustee of Hearing Voices Network England and National Voices.

PART SIX
VOICE-HEARING AND MENTAL PROCESSES

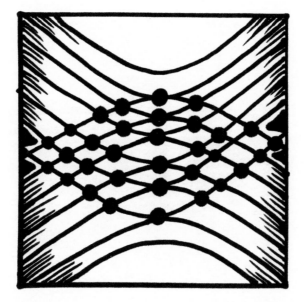

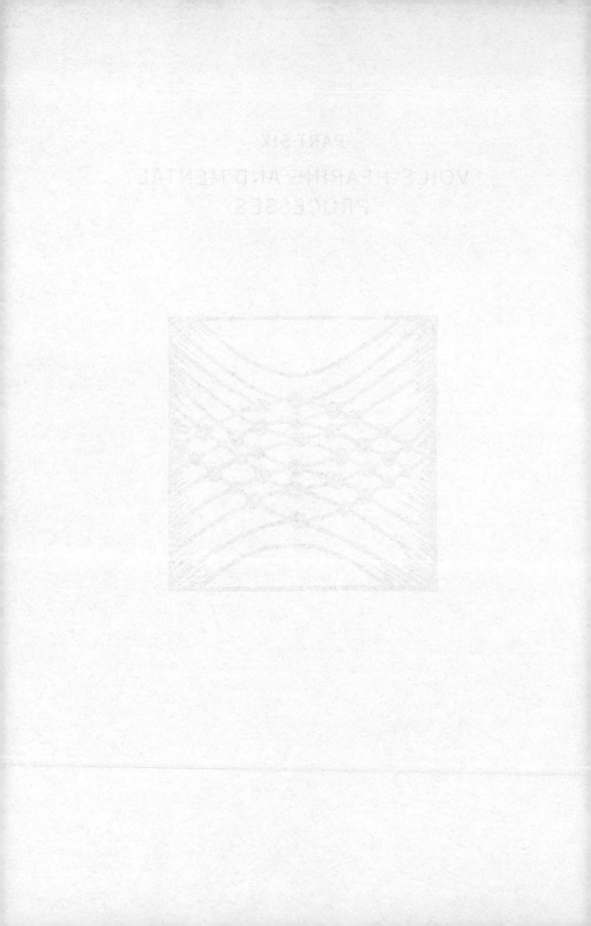

25

Remembering Voices

Charles Fernyhough, Department of Psychology, Durham University

Early in the Hearing the Voice Phenomenological Interview, participants are asked about their memories of the time when their voices started. For Dan, it was connected to a vision of his recently deceased grandfather: 'I was in school, and I was sat in just a science lab, and I heard my granddad, who had just died, talking to me, eh, and I saw his body on the table . . . [T]hat was the first time I ever had a sort of experience like that, ehm, and it was about two weeks after he'd died.'

What are the challenges in giving an account of the beginning of an unusual and frequently distressing experience like voice-hearing? How do they exceed the difficulty of answering *any* question about an experience that—by definition—no one else can share? In this chapter, I want to propose that thinking about memory in relation to voices gives us a unique perspective on some troublesome characteristics of human memory, and that the Voices in Psychosis (VIP) interviews can help us untangle some of the issues they raise.

In a sense, *all* reports on subjective experience are memories. Giving detail on any moment of experience must happen after the moment in question, unless it is happening at the instant in which the experience unfolds—in which case the telling of the experience is presumably part of the experience. Even the most sophisticated methods for describing inner experience (such as the Descriptive Experience Sampling method developed by the psychologist Russell Hurlburt (Hurlburt, 2011)) minimally depend on some kind of retrospective account of the experience in question. Whether it happened an hour or ten years ago, talking about a voice-hearing experience means talking about something that happened in the past. For that reason alone, it is inevitably going to be shaped by the vagaries of memory.

We are in the realm of what psychologists call *autobiographical memory*: our memory for the events of our own lives. Although the roots of the contemporary consensus can be traced back to the 1930s and earlier, a profound change in our understanding of autobiographical memory has occurred in the last four decades, with the recognition that it is a creative, recombinative process. Rather than *reproducing* events like the playing back of a video recording, autobiographical memory involves *reconstructing* events in the present moment, integrating different sources of information, and, in doing so, drawing on a variety of cognitive and neural resources (Fernyhough, 2012).

Charles Fernyhough, *Remembering Voices* In: *Voices in Psychosis*. Edited by: Angela Woods, Ben Alderson-Day, and Charles Fernyhough, Oxford University Press. © Charles Fernyhough 2022. DOI: 10.1093/oso/9780192898388.003.0025

The various colourful errors that people make in remembering events have proved highly instructive to scientists attempting to understand memory's mechanisms, while their personal implications have been explored with great insight by artists and writers throughout the centuries. As someone who doesn't hear voices, I assume that it's hard enough to talk about the experience under any circumstances. But it may be particularly challenging to talk about the origins of an experience that no one else has shared, which is widely met with stigma and misunderstanding, and which—for those very reasons—was likely not disclosed to others at the time.

One striking thing about recent research in autobiographical memory is the extent to which it has been shown to be a social process. Many of the things we remember we actually *co*-remember; we live through many of the same events as others, and we negotiate shared representations of them, correcting each other's biases and adopting our confederates' mistakes. For example, research has focused recently on the phenomenon of *memory conformity*, whereby individuals incorporate information provided by other people into their own memory reports. When an experience cannot, by definition, be shared (because it has happened to one person only), and when it is then not talked about (because of shame, stigma, or anxiety about how it will be received), the task of remembering is presumably made that much more difficult.

That is not to suggest that memories of voice onset are unreliable—or at least that they are more unreliable than any of our memories. But it might help to account for the occasional vagueness in voice onset reports. Will, for example, struggled to pin down the beginning of his voices: 'I don't know, it just felt like when I got to like eight or six year old, I just felt like something changed, like I didn't feel right or . . . like . . . I just felt like . . . ah, it's hard to . . .'.

The slipperiness of some voice onset reports is likely counterbalanced by one obvious fact. Starting to hear a voice is inevitably a highly emotional experience. Bill, for example, describes it in one word: 'Frightening'. In Olivia's words:

> I remember feeling, like when I was a teenager, they were really, they were like telling me to hurt other people and things like that, and I remember that used to really scare me, because I thought I'm an evil person, because I didn't understand that these weren't my own thoughts, but I was like there's some part of my brain that's horrible and I didn't know why I was like that.

We know from a substantial body of research that intensely emotional events are more likely to stick in memory. One example is what have become known as 'flashbulb memories': memories of highly emotional world events (such as the terrorist attacks of 9/11) that are extremely vivid and accompanied by details about the context in which the individual first heard of the event. Such memories are no more likely to be reliable than ordinary, less emotional memories. Research into flashbulb memories, such as a study following up the trauma memories of those in the

Manhattan area who were eyewitnesses to the 9/11 atrocities, shows that they are just as susceptible to distortion as any other memories (Hirst et al., 2009).

Memories of voices should therefore be persistent, but also prone to distortion. In considering the emotional valence of the remembered experience, it is important to distinguish between the upsetting nature of particular voices and the distress that might be caused merely by the hearing of a voice that no one else can hear, no matter what its emotional weight. For some VIP participants, the first appearance of voices was not distressing because they were initially benevolent or neutral, and only later became distressing. For example, Eric's first voice (the Blue Lady) was a source of comfort and reassurance to him at a time of emotional turmoil. Chris's first voice-hearing experience was benign: 'I just thought it was somebody taking the mick out of us to be honest.'

A key event might therefore not be the first time the voice was heard, but the moment of first recognition of its possible significance—such as the fact that no one else was able to hear it or that it might be a sign of mental illness. Will, for example, wasn't sure that he could pin down a time when the voices started, but he remembered becoming more aware of them in his first year at school, when the bullying started. 'Once you hear the voices', the author Mark Vonnegut wrote of his experiences of mental illness, 'you realise they've always been there. It's just a matter of being tuned to them' (Vonnegut, 1975, p. 137). Xander told a similar story: 'I don't know if it's been there forever or it's just that I can't remember a time without them.' One moment of increased awareness coincided with Xander's recognition that this experience wasn't 'everyone's normal'. Anthony, in contrast, remembers only becoming aware of the unusual nature of his experience relatively late: '[W]hen I first started hearing it, and for a long time after, I just thought it was normal, I didn't really find anything too alarming about it then, but again, I was a young teenager I suppose, I was quite naïve I suppose.' Memory of the first moment of awareness of the experience's significance (as 'normal' or otherwise) might therefore be as important in some of these accounts as memory for the onset of the actual experience.

So far I have focused on a person's memory for these unusual experiences: what it is like to remember a voice speaking to you when no one else can hear it. In balance with the growing awareness that memory involves processes of reconstruction, there has been an equally significant shift in our understanding of voice-hearing, with the recognition (always clinically appreciated, but now also thoroughly substantiated empirically) of a strong link between trauma and at least some cases of voice-hearing (Bentall et al., 2012). A significant proportion of the VIP participants relate their voice-hearing to experiences of trauma. For example, Fran clearly linked her initial voice-hearing experience to being bullied for the first time in high school. Leah's voices were more likely to occur in places associated with 'bad memories'. For others, the link is not so clear. Zara's abuse by two men at the age of fourteen was not clearly linked with the onset of her experiences: 'I can't remember hearing voices. I remember talking to meself a lot but I can't remember hearing voices.'

Could some voices even *be* memories? Many mental health professionals, including those aligned with the worldwide Hearing Voices Movement, understand voices as stemming from traumatic events that have led to unresolved emotional problems. It has become accepted that many voices are messages from the past, bearing information about previous hurt (Romme and Escher, 1989). Could at least some of them actually *be* memories of those buried events?

Although the idea has a long history in clinical psychiatry, this is a question that has only fairly recently been addressed in empirical research. One way to tackle it is to ask whether voices have any of the qualities of ordinary memories. A recent study analysed in-depth interviews with nearly 200 voice-hearers, most of whom were diagnosed with schizophrenia. More than a third said that the voices they heard were in some way akin to previous conversations with other people. But relatively few of these conversations seemed like verbatim replays of what was said; most of the reports claimed that the voices were 'similar' to what had been said in the past (McCarthy-Jones et al., 2014).

This is actually just what you would expect if voices had their roots in memories of actual events. Memory does not reproduce; it reconstructs. Memory for verbatim information is known to be particularly prone to distortion. We rarely recall the exact words that someone has said; it is much more useful to us to recall the gist or meaning of a person's words, with the result that the specifics of word choice and syntactic structure are often lost.

This points to a way of understanding voices as reconstructions of past, highly emotional events, rather than undistorted memories of them. As a result of the extreme emotion at the time when the details of the event were encoded, memory for traumatic events can often involve a failure to integrate the various aspects of the memory, leading to decontextualized elements of the memory persisting in a 'freefloating' state. Certain forms of trauma-based therapy for voice-hearing make use of the fragmentary, decontextualized nature of some voices, with promising results (Hardy, 2017).

The VIP transcripts show plenty of evidence of the reconstructive nature of voices. Jane attributed the cause of her voices to memories of past events that were not actually her own memories, but which had nevertheless affected her emotionally. Nina described her negative voices as coming 'from my past experiences with people my age'. The voices did not stay fixed in time, however, but aged with her, pointing to the kind of dynamic reconstruction which is a feature of autobiographical memory. This might explain why Nina was not entirely confident in the cause of her voices, and was even able to put a number on her uncertainty: '60% def . . . that it's from past experiences, 40% that's just from my head.'

The age at which the trauma occurred is likely to be relevant here. Most people cannot recall events from earlier than three or four years of age, a phenomenon known as childhood amnesia. Although the causes of this phenomenon are not well understood, they likely relate to the fact that autobiographical memory is a process with many moving parts which requires several different cognitive and neural systems to be up and running. In early childhood, before this suite of capacities is fully developed, the individual does not have the ability to construct memory representations that can later be recalled. If the trauma in question occurred in early childhood, one would expect that the related memories would be focused on emotions and physical sensations, rather than on narratively organized, language-based accounts (Fernyhough, 2016). This might be one source of the predominately somatic, non-auditory experiences that VIP participants describe. Memories of a trauma that happened later in life would be more likely to be associated with verbatim linguistic information, such as the remembered voice of an abuser.

It is also important to consider what voices are *for*. An important tenet of the Hearing Voices Movement is that voices fulfil certain functions in a social relational context, such as acting as emotional defences (Romme and Escher, 1989). Jade, for example, felt that her voices were defending her from malevolent forces: 'So they were keeping an eye on me too. . . . [T]hey were there as a protection.' If voices can be understood as aspects of the self that exist in a dynamic and fluctuating equilibrium, they might be expected, on occasion, to be protective of the self, as well as challenging its integrity. Such voices would not be expected to be literal replays of traumatic events, but they may well be emotionally related to them.

We have seen plenty of evidence of how the vagaries of memory can shape accounts of hearing voices. The VIP transcripts also show influence in the opposite direction: voices sparking memories. Bill described his voices as triggering flashbacks, described as 'unwanted memories that you can't escape, no matter what you do there's nothing to distract it because as you're trying to forget these thoughts, get them out of your head and distract yourself with something else, you know, there's other things going on in your head'. Chris's voice-hearing experiences reminded him of an instance when he was violent to another person, and also brought back memories that he had suppressed: 'I'll think of something that I would never think about or . . . I think of memories that I've locked away that I don't want to think about, so I don't feel like I've thought of them on me own.' For some participants, like Dan, the voices prompt instant forgetting: 'I know that sounds really odd, but I sort of, whenever I hear this one, I black out and I only remember the start of it, and so I can't be fully sure if it's this person or not.'

As we have seen, memory for voice onset can be as much about the nascent awareness of something that is already ongoing as it can be about the beginnings of a new experience. (Whether those two scenarios can actually be distinguished is a tricky philosophical question which we can't go into here.) The same can apply to the disappearance of voices. It is fairly common to hear people whose voices have gone away describe it as a gradual appreciation that something that was present is not present any more. Alex's account, at the follow-up interview, of the disappearances of his voices is full of the language of doubt:

I mean . . . nearer the end, you, I . . . I sometimes think it could have been exactly the same, it's just I've managed them better. . . . So you think they're easing off, or you think they're not as bad, but like I say, after a while you're just sorta . . . trying to get on with, with it as you're hearing them, you know?

There is also a note of regret about their passing: 'And you think, oh, I cannot wait for them to stop and then when you do, you think things are too quiet now almost, you know!'

Memory for voices and other unusual experiences warrants a great deal more careful investigation. How voice-hearers reconstruct their experience through memory can have significant implications that are only beginning to be explored in research. In turn, those implications might be difficult to separate out from the interpretations that individuals are encouraged to place upon their voices by clinical professionals as part of the process of therapy. A deeper understanding of how voices relate to memories of trauma is already paying dividends in clinical practice, with the development of new trauma-based approaches (Steel, 2016). There are also implications for stigma, including both self-stigma (negative thoughts about one's own worth) and the scathing judgements of the community. Any vagueness of voice onset reports needs to be understood as a natural corollary of the workings of human memory, rather than as a reason to suspect the authenticity of a voice-hearer's testimony. Remembering is the work of a complex, fragile machine; remembering an experience that is ultimately ineffable tests those workings to their limits.

Acknowledgements

I am grateful to Luke Collins for his helpful input to this chapter.

References

Bentall, R. P., Wickham, S., Shevlin, M., and Varese, F. (2012). Do specific early-life adversities lead to specific symptoms of psychosis? A study from the 2007 The Adult Psychiatric Morbidity Survey. *Schizophrenia Bulletin*, 38(4), 734–40.

Fernyhough, C. (2012). *Pieces of Light: The New Science of Memory*. London: Profile Books.

Fernyhough, C. (2016). *The Voices Within: The History and Science of How We Talk to Ourselves*. London: Profile Books.

Hardy, A. (2017). Pathways from trauma to psychotic experiences: a theoretically informed model of posttraumatic stress in psychosis. *Frontiers in Psychology*, 8(697).

Hirst, W., Phelps, E. A., Buckner, R. L., Budson, A. E., Cuc, A., Gabrieli, J. D. E., Johnson, M. K., Lustig, C., Lyle, K. B., Mather, M., Meksin, R., Mitchell, K. J., Ochsner, K. N., Schacter, D. L., Simons, J. S., and Vaidya, C. J. (2009). Long-term memory for the terrorist attack of September 11: flashbulb memories, event memories, and the factors that influence their retention. *Journal of Experimental Psychology: General*, 138(2), 161–76.

Hurlburt, R. T. (2011). *Investigating Pristine Inner Experience: Moments of Truth*. Cambridge: Cambridge University Press.

McCarthy-Jones, S., Trauer, T., Mackinnon, A., Sims, E., Thomas, N., and Copolov, D. L. (2014). A new phenomenological survey of auditory hallucinations: evidence for subtypes and implications for theory and practice. *Schizophrenia Bulletin*, 40(1), 231–5.

Romme, M. A. J., and Escher, S. D. M. A. C. (1989). Hearing voices. *Schizophrenia Bulletin*, 15(2), 209–16.

Steel, C. (2016). Psychological interventions for working with trauma and distressing voices: the future is in the past. *Frontiers in Psychology*, 7, 2035.

Vonnegut, M. (1975). *The Eden Express: A Memoir of Insanity*. New York, NY: Praeger.

About the Author

Charles Fernyhough is a psychologist and writer. The focus of his recent scientific work has been in applying ideas from mainstream developmental psychology to the study of psychosis, particularly the phenomenon of voice-hearing. He is the Principal Investigator and Director of the interdisciplinary Hearing the Voice project, supported by the Wellcome Trust.

26

Voices and Reality Monitoring

How Do We Know What Is Real?

Colleen Rollins, Department of Psychiatry, University of Cambridge

Jane Garrison, Department of Psychology, University of Cambridge

The Subjective Reality of Hearing Voices: Knowing What's Real and What's Not

> [It's] difficult to differentiate between what is real and what isn't and . . . what are my thoughts and . . . then . . . I don't know how much I have control over these kind of things which come into my head . . . it makes me question myself and . . . I can't quite differentiate from whether it's real or not . . . it makes me doubt my reality. (Gail)

How do we determine which aspects of our internal mental experiences correspond to information presented in the external world? That is, how do we know what is real? This question, which has excited philosophers for millennia, bears particular relevance to the experience of hearing voices, auditory percepts arising in the absence of the appropriate sensory stimulus. To the voice-hearer, voices can carry a compelling sense of reality. Indeed, as these reports from the Voices in Psychosis (VIP) study attest, voice-hearers may perceive voices with the same acoustic properties as external speech and therefore react as they would to an external speaker, turning around to see who called their name or responding verbally:

> [I]t just feels real, as if it was anybody else. Just things like that, name being called, sometimes laughter, that other people can't hear. (Bill)

> [N]umerous of times I've asked me little sister and I've asked me mam, can you hear that? And they're like no, Toby, we can't hear it. That's when I know something serious is happening. (Toby)

> Like you know when they're shouting and you say stop, stop, because it's so . . . And it does feel really real, like I still sometimes struggle to believe that it's not! (Dan)

Colleen Rollins and Jane Garrison, *Voices and Reality Monitoring* In: *Voices in Psychosis*. Edited by: Angela Woods, Ben Alderson-Day, and Charles Fernyhough, Oxford University Press. © Colleen Rollins and Jane Garrison 2022. DOI: 10.1093/oso/9780192898388.003.0026

The strong subjective reality of hearing voices similarly holds true of experiences in other sensory modalities: seeing, feeling, tasting, or smelling things that are not there.

> [S]ometimes I can see a person just walking down a street, or walking behind us, thinking that someone's following us, and I'll look and I'll keep seeing that they're there, and then I'll realise that they're not actually there. (Grace)

> You can feel . . . people slapping you or like . . . touching your back. . . . And they're not there. (Brad)

Even voices with properties different from external speech, such as those experienced within the head or having thought-like qualities, can carry the same sense of reality. While personal accounts of voice-hearing reveal considerable variability in the types and qualities of voices, a common denominator may be the subjective reality of the experience and the inability to discriminate internal from external sources of information. Or, as Brad puts it: 'often I'll struggle to know what's real and what's not'.

In this chapter, we review the cognitive mechanisms for distinguishing internally generated events from information present in external reality, a process termed 're-ality monitoring'. We then review the brain mechanisms that support people's ability to discriminate reality, and their role in the experience of hearing voices for people with and those without a psychiatric diagnosis. Understanding the neural and cognitive substrates responsible for hearing voices is important for informing treatment strategies and providing insights into how the brain constructs our reality.

Reality Monitoring and Hallucinations

Imagine walking home in the dark, late at night. You hear the wind whistling, leaves rustling behind you—or was that the sound of footsteps, of someone following you? Reality monitoring processes help us to distinguish whether such experiences are internally generated (as for thoughts, imagery, or reasoning) or derived via our senses from the outside world (Simons et al., 2017). Under the theoretical Source Monitoring Framework (SMF) (Johnson and Raye, 1981), individuals may make judgements about the source of information, such as whether it was perceived or im-agined, by comparing its content with characteristic internal or external memories of similar sensory events. Information which is high in sensory detail would thus be assessed as externally derived, while information high in internal cognitive con-tent would be assessed as self-generated. As such, it is suggested that voice-hearing arises from a failure in reality monitoring processes when an individual's internal monologue (or 'inner speech') is judged, for whatever reason, as being high in sen-sory content and is thus misattributed to an external source (Jones and Fernyhough,

2007). Voice-hearing may also include non-speech sounds or voices without speech. Indeed, the material for the reality monitoring judgement does not need to be speech; the focus of the SMF is on the reality testing of the current holistic perceptual experience.

> I'm not joking . . . it literally feels like just having a conversation with somebody, it sounds like . . . it's so weird, ehm . . . And I always thought, you know, oh they must be able to tell you know . . . he must know that it's like fake, and he must be able to think, oh you know I'm hearing it and it's there but it's not, you know, it's not real. But it's, it's really convincing, and you do like genuinely believe that it is happening and someone is speaking to you. And it's, it's really hard to convince yourself that it's not. (Dan)

Experimentally, reality monitoring can be measured with psychological tasks in which participants are asked to make judgements about their memory of the sources of different percepts, like words or pictures. An example is a word pair task, in which participants are shown a series of two commonly associated words (e.g. 'Bacon and eggs'), with the second word in the pair sometimes left blank ('Bacon and _____'). In both cases, the participant is asked to speak aloud the complete word pair, but in the second case, they have had to imagine the missing word ('eggs') in their head. Participants are then shown the first words ('Bacon') and asked to recall whether the second word in the pair had been seen or imagined. Research studies have reported that people with a diagnosis of schizophrenia are more likely to make errors in reality monitoring tasks, compared to people with no psychiatric diagnoses and, more specifically, that patients who hear voices show an increased bias towards misidentifying imagined stimuli as being real, compared to patients who do not hear voices. Some studies have found that this bias exists even while recognition memory is preserved, suggesting a possible specific role for reality monitoring processes in the manifestation of voices in schizophrenia (Simons et al., 2017).

Although 60–80% of people with a diagnosis of schizophrenia report hearing voices, this is also a trans-diagnostic human experience occurring in people with other clinical diagnoses such as Parkinson's disease, as well as in people with no psychiatric history whatsoever (Rollins et al., 2019). This has led researchers to understand voice-hearing as a dimensional phenomenon, occurring on a continuum from health to illness, which raises the question of whether there are common or distinct mechanisms in patient populations compared to people without a clinical diagnosis. A predisposition or proneness to experiencing unusual sensory experiences can be measured in the general population using questionnaires asking about the vividness and nature of people's perceptions. Several studies have reported that healthy individuals who hear voices or are prone to similar visual or other sensory experiences show the same externalization bias in reality monitoring tasks as individuals with a schizophrenia diagnosis, suggesting that reality monitoring may be a key component of both clinical and non-clinical experience. However, other studies have found no evidence of source monitoring deficits in non-clinical samples, nuancing the

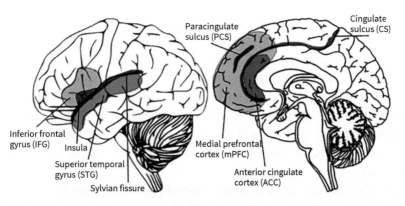

Image 26.1 Brain regions implicated in voice-hearing and reality monitoring.
Credit: The authors, 2021.

question of whether hallucination-like events experienced by the general population are continuous with clinical voice-hearing.

The Brain Basis for Hallucinations and for Monitoring What Is Real

The way in which we perceive the world and understand or model our reality is underpinned by the structure and function of the brain, which can be assessed using neuroimaging methods such as structural (sMRI) and functional magnetic resonance imaging (fMRI). Using sMRI, researchers can quantify different morphological indices of neuronal health, such as the amount of grey matter, cortical thickness, and gyrification (the degree of folding in the cortical surface), whereas fMRI can be used to measure brain activity by detecting changes in blood flow, either during a specific psychological task or when the participant is resting. Using these techniques, neuroimaging studies have identified a number of brain regions involved in hearing voices and reality monitoring (see Image 26.1). These include: the medial prefrontal cortex (mPFC), implicated in processing and attributing self-referential information and attending to the mental states of oneself and others; the superior temporal gyrus (STG), involved in speech processing and language perception; the inferior frontal gyrus (IFG), involved in semantic processing and the activity of which during voice-hearing in individuals with schizophrenia correlates with the reported subjective reality of the voices; and the insula, involved in a range of subjective feelings, including self-awareness, which, together with the anterior cingulate cortex (ACC) region, constitutes a node in the brain's salience network that is associated with directing attention to important stimuli (Raij et al., 2009; Rollins et al., 2019, 2020; Zmigrod et al., 2016).

Recent research using sMRI has shown that the length of a specific structural feature on the medial surface of the brain, a fold called the paracingulate sulcus

(PCS), is associated with reality monitoring ability in the general population and with lifetime history of voice-hearing and general hallucination status in schizophrenia patients (Buda et al., 2011; Garrison et al., 2015; Rollins et al., 2020). Thus, common brain regions appear to support both reality monitoring and voice-hearing, adding weight to the argument that the two processes are linked. Broadly, this list of brain regions outlined above unsurprisingly shows that it is the neural substrates underlying self-referential processing, reality monitoring, speech and language, and subjective awareness that are implicated in the manifestation of hearing voices.

Much of the research undertaken to investigate the brain basis for hearing voices has focused on people with a diagnosis of schizophrenia. A recent meta-analysis and review of the brain structural correlates of the broader category of hallucinations across different sensory modalities and diagnoses has shown that psychiatric and neurological patients have distinct neuro-anatomical signatures (Rollins et al., 2019). This suggests there may be a plurality of neurobiological mechanisms responsible for the genesis of these perceptual experiences. Clearly, understanding whether overlapping or distinct neural mechanisms underpin voice-hearing in clinical and non-clinical voice-hearers would nuance the question of a continuum for these experiences. In characterizing how aspects of voice-hearing are supported by the structure and function of the brain, neuroimaging research can help us understand how differences in processes like reality monitoring contribute to the voice-hearing experiences that deeply affect people's lives.

From Brain Folding to Phenomenology

The folding of the cerebral cortex is thought to be crucial for higher-order cognitive functions, but the mechanisms underlying the developmental process of folding (gyrification) remain unclear. The human brain begins early in gestation as a smooth (lissencephalic) surface, but begins to fold at around 10–15 weeks of fetal life, with dramatic folding and surface expansion occurring during the third trimester of pregnancy to result in the complex and familiar pattern of troughs and crests known as sulci and gyri. Folding patterns are largely similar across individuals and stable across the lifespan; however, they influence surrounding brain morphology—grey matter density, cortical thickness, the degree of opening, and depth of folds—features that can change with ageing, learning, and experience. Despite similarity in the primary sulci of the brain, there is huge inter-individual variability in smaller brain folds which is associated with differences in functional connectivity (the communication between different brain regions), cognitive abilities, and risk of psychiatric illness. Recent research has also highlighted the role of folding patterns in the experience of hearing voices for people with a diagnosis of schizophrenia. Notably, the PCS on the medial surface of the prefrontal cortex of the brain (described above; see Figure 26.1) is one of the last to form before birth and shows considerable variability in size in the general population. Absence of the PCS in both hemispheres is associated with reduced accuracy in the reality monitoring abilities of healthy adults (Buda et al., 2011). Other features of voice-hearing have also been associated with the folding of the brain (Cachia et al., 2015; see Rollins et al., 2019 for a review).

The sulcal pattern of the posterior Sylvian fissure (see Figure 26.1) is linked to whether voices are attributed to being internally generated or originating from external agents:

[T]he worst ones [voice-like experiences] are when it's my own voice . . . they've got their own personalities, but it's my voice in me head. . . . But I don't believe it's me. (Brad)

I hear three different voices, ehm, there's a female voice, she's called Roxy, she actually introduced herself to me. Ehm, and then there's an angry male voice, who's like there all the time, I don't know his name, but he's there like constantly unless I'm asleep, he like, he's like . . . a boy in a way but like he just, he's a bully to everyone. Ehm, and then the third one is very quiet and . . . just he doesn't, like I don't hear him like every day, it might be like once a week that I hear him. (Xander)

A local displacement in the position of the right superior temporal sulcus is associated with whether voices are heard inside or outside of the head:

[S]ometimes it sounds like it's somebody maybe within the same room as me, or sat next to me, but then when I look around it's like they're not there, but I swear like I can hear it. And sometimes it's like within my head and it's like someone's put it in my head, or like it's just come out of me somehow, and it's like been, it's like you can hear it inside your brain, but sometimes it's out. So it really depends. (Dan)

Finally, reduced sulcation in the right parietal cortex and left Sylvian fissure has been observed in schizophrenia patients who experience both voice-hearing and visual hallucinations, compared to individuals with the experience of voice-hearing alone:

Yeah, sometimes along with the whispering, I will hear . . . see like little shadows out of the corner of me eye, or like someone will be like waving at us like that, and I'll look and there'll be nothing there. Just like that, they tend to go together, them two. (Page)

Together, this research suggests that specific phenomenological facets of voice-hearing may also have a neurodevelopmental component, in addition to the prominent role of life experiences (and trauma in particular). As such, an understanding of both nature and nurture, and the complex interaction between the two, is needed to help us understand the brain basis of hearing voices.

Importance of Understanding Cognitive and Neural Bases for Hearing Voices

Understanding the cognitive and neural basis for how people perceive, generate, and interpret models of their reality, and why they sometimes struggle to know what is real and what is not in particular, offers advantages for helping voice-hearers and others make sense of this often confusing experience. As the VIP participants make clear, although voices can be benign or contribute to meaningful personal experiences, they can also be abusive, distressing, and frightening:

> [I]t was absolutely, it was really terrifying, because I didn't understand what was happening to us. (Leah)

> They can be physically, emotionally draining, in every way. (Bill)

> It just repeats hurt, hurt meself. . . . Hurt yourself all the time. (Ian)

> I've had bad voices and good voices, like nice ones and bad. One was called Mark, and one was called Martha. Mark was the bad one, he used to tell us to kill myself and self-harm, like tell us . . . no one wants us here and stuff like that. And then on the other hand, I've got Martha telling us that, that I'm a good lass, like a nice lass and stuff. (Violet)

Clinical treatments for distressing voices range from medication to peer support to cognitive behavioural therapy, and there is active research assessing the efficacy of new treatment options, including AVATAR therapy and non-invasive brain stimulation. However, little is known to help guide the choice of which treatment will be effective for a given individual, and efforts to develop more personalized treatment will likely require an understanding of the underlying brain and cognitive mechanisms.

Investigating the brain basis of voice-hearing also sheds light on some of the puzzling questions raised by people's personal accounts of their experience, such as why voices are experienced with such a compelling reality, why they can sound as though they are coming from inside or outside the head, and why people can hear different numbers of voices with different identities. The variability in subjective experiences may be related to different anatomical instantiations. Moreover, the relationship between phenomenological reports and brain science is reciprocally informing: knowledge of the brain mechanisms can help explain differences in experiences, and knowledge of people's experiences can direct attention to which aspects of voice-hearing are important to study. As such, individuals' lived experience is an indicator of the specific brain mechanisms involved, which, in turn, may move us closer towards more targeted treatments. Furthermore, appreciation of voice-hearing in people without psychiatric diagnoses has highlighted the question of whether voice-hearing exists on a continuum of experience, with gentle abnormalities in perception at one end and distressing hallucinatory experiences at the other. Understanding the neuroanatomy and cognitive underpinnings for hearing voices speaks to this debate by elucidating the extent to which voice-hearing occurs by a common mechanism in clinical and non-clinical groups. Finally, as perception is thought to be an active process (meaning that we think percepts are constructed through the ability of our brains to make their best guess of the external world from incoming sensory signals), studying voice-hearing can provide valuable insight into the cognitive processes of perception.

Hearing voices can carry stigma and impact interpersonal relationships, leading to a loss of social support, preventing access to care, and increasing distress:

> It seems to just be like a . . . just a big black shadow and it just follows you everywhere. You always feel like you're keeping this secret from people and you know it's hiding it and trying to act normal. (Bill)

By understanding the neural and psychological processes that occur when a person hears voices, we hope to make these experiences more understandable and reduce associated fear and stigma.

References

Buda, M., Fornito, A., Bergstrom, Z. M., and Simons, J. S. (2011). A specific brain structural basis for individual differences in reality monitoring. *Journal of Neuroscience*, 31(40), 14308–13.

Cachia, A., Amad, A., Brunelin, J., Krebs, M.-O., Plaze, M., Thomas, P., and Jardri, R. (2015). Deviations in cortex sulcation associated with visual hallucinations in schizophrenia. *Molecular Psychiatry*, 20(9), 1101–7.

Garrison, J. R., Fernyhough, C., McCarthy-Jones, S., Haggard, M., The Australian Schizophrenia Research Bank, and Simons, J. S. (2015). Paracingulate sulcus morphology is associated with hallucinations in the human brain. *Nature Communications*, 6, 8956.

Johnson, M. K., and Raye, C. L. (1981). Reality monitoring. *Psychological Review*, 88(1), 67–85.

Jones, S. R., and Fernyhough, C. (2007). Neural correlates of inner speech and auditory verbal hallucinations: a critical review and theoretical integration. *Clinical Psychology Review*, 27(2), 140–54.

Raij, T. T., Valkonen-Korhonen, M., Holi, M., Therman, S., Lehtonen, J., and Hari, R. (2009). Reality of auditory verbal hallucinations. *Brain*, 132(11), 2994–3001.

Rollins, C. P. E., Garrison J. R., Arribas, M., Seyedsalehi, A., Li, Z., Chan, R. C. K., Yang, J., Wang, D., Lio, P., Yan, C., Yi, Z.-H., Cachia, A., Upthegrove, R., Deakin, B., Simons, J. S., Murray, G. K., and Suckling, J. (2020). Evidence in cortical folding patterns for prenatal predispositions to hallucinations in schizophrenia. *Translational Psychiatry*, 10(1), 1–14.

Rollins, C. P. E., Garrison, J. R., Simons, J. S., Rowe, J. B., O'Callaghan, C., Murray, G. K., and Suckling, J. (2019). Meta-analytic evidence for the plurality of mechanisms in transdiagnostic structural MRI studies of hallucination status. *EClinicalMedicine*, 8, 57–71.

Simons, J. S., Garrison, J. R., and Johnson, M. K. (2017). Brain mechanisms of reality monitoring. *Trends in Cognitive Sciences*, 21(6), 462–73.

Zmigrod, L., Garrison, J. R., Carr, J., and Simons, J. S. (2016). The neural correlates of hallucinations: a quantitative meta-analysis of neuroimaging studies. *Neuroscience and Biobehavioural Reviews*, 69, 113–23.

About the Authors

Colleen Rollins is a Gates Cambridge Scholar and a PhD student in the Department of Psychiatry at the University of Cambridge. Her research explores how the structure and function of the brain supports the experience of hallucinations, primarily in the context of people with a psychiatric diagnosis.

Jane Garrison is a University Lecturer in the Department of Psychology at the University of Cambridge. Her work as a cognitive neuroscientist explores the brain basis of reality monitoring, the process by which we distinguish internally generated information from information presented in the external world. Jane's current research focus is on developing understanding of the relationship between the brain's structural morphology and hallucinations by investigating the determinants and implications of paracingulate morphological variation.

27

Supernatural Presences

Medieval and Modern Narratives of Voice-Hearing

Corinne Saunders, Department of English Studies and Institute for Medical Humanities, Durham University

What can a medieval perspective offer to our understanding of voice-hearing in the present? Do medieval and modern phenomenologies speak to each other? How do their explanatory frameworks compare? And what value might that have for voice-hearers now? The medieval period is of special interest because its Christian thought world—including God, the devil, and a spirit world between—allowed for the possibility of visionary, voice-hearing, or more generally supernatural experiences. Medieval psychological models posited a faculty of inner, 'common sense', which put together sense perceptions; these, in turn, were understood to pass through the imaginative and cognitive cells of the brain, to be stored in the memory as multisensory *phantasmata* or thought-images. Such *phantasmata*, it was believed, might be influenced by divine or demonic forces, or emerge unbidden in situations of extreme emotion, creating the effect of voice-hearing or visions. While theologians were most concerned with the possibilities of divine vision and demonic influence, medical theorists recognized the effects of mental illness, which they connected with imbalances in the bodily humours. If, for example, the melancholy humour was overly dominant, the cognitive processes were affected, potentially resulting in depressive illness; if the choleric humour predominated, then the imagination was affected, bodying forth too many images, potentially resulting in mania, which might include hallucinations. Voice-hearing, however, was not explicitly pathologized or identified as a symptom of psychosis; rather, medieval discourses focus on the experience. The phenomenological approach taken in the Voices in Psychosis (VIP) study, with its comparable emphasis on experience, reveals some surprising continuities, despite the radically different contexts of medieval and contemporary accounts.

Medieval records do not provide us with case histories or qualitative interviews, and we must look to other sources to probe the experience of medieval voice-hearers. This chapter reads the modern narratives collected in the forty VIP interviews alongside two English visionary works: Julian of Norwich's *Revelations of Divine Love* (ed. Windeatt, 2016; trans. Windeatt, 2015), and *The Book of Margery*

Corinne Saunders, *Supernatural Presences* In: *Voices in Psychosis*. Edited by: Angela Woods, Ben Alderson-Day, and Charles Fernyhough, Oxford University Press. © Corinne Saunders 2022. DOI: 10.1093/oso/9780192898388.003.0027

Kempe (ed. Windeatt, 2004; trans. Windeatt, 2019). Little is known about Julian of Norwich (*c*.1342–*c*.1416) other than that she was an anchoress or recluse living in a cell adjoining St Julian's Church in Norwich. Her book, the first known work by a woman in English, exists in two forms: a short version, probably written soon after the revelations it describes, which were experienced during extreme illness in 1373, and a longer version written some twenty years later. Though not an autobiography, its narratorial voice is unique and immediate. The revelations stem from vivid personal experience: Julian of Norwich (2016, Long Text, ch. 2, p. 30) recounts how she prays to be brought near to death, so that she may 'lyven more to the worshippe of God'. Her visions occur when this prayer is fulfilled.

Although her name is frequently linked with that of Julian, the life of Margery Kempe (*c*.1373–*c*.1440) could scarcely have been more different: she was married, bore fourteen children, ran a brewing business, and travelled on pilgrimage as far as Rome and Jerusalem. She was also, however, a visionary who adopted a strongly ascetic life, and whose spiritual experience was marked by unusual physical behaviours, in particular, compulsive cryings. Her *Book* (*c*.1436–1438) is mediated by two amanuenses, or copyists, and, like Julian's, was written some twenty years after the earliest experiences she describes. While Margery's second amanuensis clearly played a role in shaping the book, it is distinguished throughout by her lively and idiosyncratic voice.

Contemporary parallels to visionary experiences such as those of Julian and Margery may seem most likely to be found in present-day accounts of Christians hearing the voice of God, such as those recounted by T. M. Luhrmann (Luhrmann, 2012) and Christopher C. H. Cook (Cook, 2019), rather than in the voices of those experiencing psychosis. There is also, however, an ancient connection between the extremes of mental and visionary experience (see McCarthy-Jones, 2012). As with St Paul, blinded on the road to Damascus, conversion experiences may be deeply distressing, debilitating in both body and mind. Such experiences are by their nature life-changing. Julian's (2016, ch. 1, p. 27) sixteen 'sheweings or revelations' occur during life-threatening illness, and with them begins a sustained pattern of hearing the Lord's voice, which offers interpretation of the visions. Kempe's first visionary experience too is extreme, an invasive encounter with the supernatural in the madness following the birth of her first child (probably post-partum psychosis). As demons paw and shout threats at her, she is restored by a vision of the Lord, in the likeness of a 'most bewtyvows, and most amyable' man, seated by her bedside and speaking directly to her: '"Dowtyr, why hast thow forsakyn me, and I forsoke nevyr the?"' (Kempe, 2004, ll. 228–32). Again, the pattern is of conversations with Christ alongside multisensory experiences of revelation. For both Julian and Margery, as for so many contemporary voice-hearers, traumatic experience is a catalyst; trauma and voice-hearing are intimately connected.

There are also differences. In the secular world of the twenty-first century, there is less ready resort to a thought world in which voices and visions are possible, supernatural forces are assumed, and spiritual explanations are credible. Those interviewed in the VIP study very rarely identify their voices as spiritual. Yet religious or spiritual references are more common than this implies, occurring in fifteen of the forty accounts, and perhaps indicating deeply ingrained familiarity, even in a secular age, with the concepts of God and Satan, angels and demons, ghosts and spirits. It seems almost inevitable that these age-old conceptions would figure, often unconsciously, both in how mental experience plays out and in understandings of it.

The experiences of Leah provide the richest and most conscious example: her voices include those of the angels, in particular the archangel Michael, whom she also sees, and Gabriel, who is present but does not speak. Leah's narrative to some extent mirrors the quality of strange specialness conveyed by Julian and Margery. Leah's experience is also rooted in Norse mythology (possibly via Marvel comics): one of her voices is that of Loki, in Norse myth the duplicitous trickster god, whom she equates with Satan and characterizes as a 'black angel'. Leah's world is one in which she is actively engaged in religious practice: she identifies her aunts as 'nuns' (perhaps meaning virgins and extremely religious), has grown up immersed in a household where angels were often referenced, regularly attends church, and has had profound experiences related to church and the Bible. The angels, including Loki, play an actively protective role in her life, rendered visible in the shadows of wings she sees. It would be false only to see her experience as positive: she also reports 'coughing up demons', feels she has been punished, feels panic and anxiety, and appears to suffer from post-traumatic stress disorder (PTSD). Yet while the voices might seem symptomatic of mental illness, for Leah, they are protective, and she defines herself as 'blessed' in the ability to hear them. Like the voices and revelations of Julian and Margery, Leah's voices offer counsel and protection within a life marked by traumatic experience, including episodes of homelessness. They are an integral part of the imaginative spirit world in which she is immersed.

Other participants too participate in a spirit world. Most comparable to Leah's experience, perhaps, is that of Jane, who hears the voice of a four-year-old child Onin who has been dead for 149 years and lives in the 'good part' of hell: she is a 'demon, but not a bad demon', fair-haired and green-eyed, with wings. Her presence is beneficent, an antidote, it seems, to the trauma Jane has suffered. Kath, meanwhile, believes in God but does not identify her experience as spiritual: one of her two voices, however, is that of an 'angel', a good, young voice, while the other is that of an old man, much more negative and admonitory—but also a figure with whom she can discuss religion. Liam feels that God is talking to him, and that he is becoming religious; his voices are conflicted, some evil, some protective or saying he is 'chosen'. Opening onto a spirit world and bringing its messages, they seem to come from beyond the planet, which he feels he may have a role in protecting. While Will does not himself seem to be religious, his voices seem to be of people from the past, 'old-talking', 'very religious', speaking in a 'traditional' fashion, prophetic and threatening, some of them 'demonic'. Page states she is not religious but believes in magical possibilities such as crystals; she feels the voices may be supernatural, ghosts, or worse. The idea of a malevolent supernatural resonates with medieval accounts of demons. Anthony, though also not religious, tries to think of his voices as 'spiritual'; he believes in something higher and wonders if voice-hearing is a gift. While his voices are negative, 'almost demonic'—in particular, one loud, barking, abusive voice that urges harm—he has also experienced what he thought was a guardian angel, which seemed at the time a 'saving grace'. Olivia practises wicca and believes her voice-hearing is a special skill: she can hear thoughts and pass on messages from people's loved ones, speak to nature, communicate with animals, and hear birds speaking. Perhaps her experience is most reminiscent of Margery's, for whom a series of sounds heard with the bodily ear signal the presence of the Holy Ghost: the sound of bellows evoking the wind typically associated with Spirit, the breath of God, the voice of a dove, and the song of a robin, all followed by 'gret grace' (Kempe, 2004, ll. 2965–74).

Even for those interviewed who do not identify their voices as spiritual, spiritual contexts can inform understanding. Zara does not understand her voices, some calm and some angry, as coming from a 'spirit world'—they are 'too clear'—but thinks regularly about church and has attended spiritualist readings, where she has experienced people 'coming through' after death. She believes in the afterlife and accepts the possibility of seeing the dead, a partial context for the shadow figures she sees. Alex has grown up religious, though he does not understand his voices as supernatural. Fred finds a sense of well-being in church and believes in God, though he has not turned to his faith in relation to the paranoia and trauma that have been caused or exacerbated by his time in the Armed Forces. Kate, by contrast, though she so vividly experiences what seems to be a haunted house, does not believe in spirits.

Positive responses like Leah's, Jane's, and Olivia's are rare in the interviews; for most, voices are unwanted, hated, distressing, a curse. Religion, now as in the past, can be connected with, and can seem to explain, punitive, abusive, and negative experience. Toby believes in Satan, though he does not elaborate. Ryan attended a Church of England school, has held strong beliefs, and at one point had faith in God, yet lost that faith because when he prayed for death God did not kill him. His voices are described as being like an angel and a demon. The two forces, like Leah's, recall Margery's references to both demonic and angelic voices. For Margery, as in the VIP interviews, self-harm is a recurrent theme. The first chapter of the *Book* describes how, in response to the voices of devils, she bites her hand so hard she bears the scar for life and would have killed herself 'many a tym'; physically restrained, she tears at her own body with her nails (Kempe, 2004, ll. 214–17). Later, the devil 'bad hir in hir mende' (Kempe, 2004, ll. 4869–70) to choose which man she will prostitute herself with, a description that suggests the experience of intrusive thoughts. Margery's prayer provokes the return of 'hir good awngel' (Kempe, 2004, l. 4887) and of the Lord's voice. For Ryan, however, both voices want the same: his suicide.

Dan too has a religious background, members of his family have seen ghosts, and his mother sees herself as perfect, analogous to Jesus. While she explains Dan's voices in terms of religious experience, for him, they are much more conflicted and disturbing, both friendly and nasty, ranging from the sometimes abusive voices of relatives to manipulative, instructive, and whispering voices that urge self-harm or warn him of bombs. He has been 'obsessed' by religion in the past:

> I'd spend every day . . . copying out ehm . . . Bible verses about a hundred times a day, things like that. And I was in a chapel, and I was copying out my Bible verses, and I didn't see anything this time, but I heard a voice screaming in my head that I was going to be stoned, that I was going to hell, that I was a terrible person, I needed to kill myself, that I needed to cut myself until it stopped, and . . . just really nasty things like . . . 'go jump off a bridge' . . . 'everyone's going to hate you, nobody likes you'.

This kind of experience seems a long way from the divine revelations that counter demonic voices in Margery's narrative. Yet, as Barry Windeatt has recently argued (in Powell and Saunders, 2020), from another perspective, Margery's God seems a 'manipulative bully'; his voice can be oppressive and controlling, urging suffering without sympathy and revelling in it. Reading Margery's *Book* against the VIP interviews suggests that her voices may not have been so different from the fearful and distressing voices experienced by those in psychosis, though the meanings attributed to them could scarcely be more so.

Medieval writing does not prioritize voice-hearing, although there is a strong tradition of revelation extending back to classical oracles and to the Bible. Hearing voices is often only one aspect of visionary experience. The revelations of both Julian and Margery involve seeing, hearing, felt presence, and sometimes smell, and are often three-dimensional. Julian's 'sheweings', from her vision of the blood trickling down from Christ's crown of thorns (Julian of Norwich, 2016, ch. 4) to that of His body withering on the Cross (Julian of Norwich, 2016, chs. 16–17) and the crucifix before her eyes bleeding (Julian of Norwich, 2016, ch. 66), are graphic and frequently multisensory. Her experience of the Lord is similarly multisensory: 'hym verily seand and fulsumly feland, hym gostly heryng, and hym delectably smellyng, and hym swetely swelowyng' (Julian of Norwich, 2016, chs. 43, 98). Margery experiences and enters into three-dimensional scenes of Christ's life; she sees the Passion 'as yf Crist had hangyn befor hir bodily eye' (Kempe, 2004, ll. 2265–6), and the Sacrament fluttering like a dove (Julian of Norwich, 2016, ch. 20). Her 'gret comfortys' are both 'gostly' and 'bodily': sweet smells, sounds and melodies, delicate and comforting white specks explained by the Lord as tokening angels (Julian of Norwich, 2016, ll. 2863–89), as well as the flame of love burning in her breast. We might expect this to be a major difference from voice-hearing experience now. Yet while voice-hearing is the focus of the project and of the interviews, a repeated theme is that of multisensory experience. Certain kinds of visual experience are especially prominent, such as seeing shadows 'out of the corner of me eye' (Brad), 'shadows and things flying around' (Carl—perhaps akin to Margery's angels), and 'shadow-y figures, they don't really have a face' (Grace). Kate sees things scuttling, Dan sees figures in mirrors, Xander sees black figures at night, and Hugh sees the dead. Olivia sees people, shadows, animals, and bleeding things, and feels her ex-partner's touch on her arm. Eric, whose voices are synaesthetic, sees a red face staring, Anthony sees flashes of colour before his eyes, and Yan sees figures that seem to be made of flat, transparent colours, 'like stained glass'. Emma sees writing everywhere, and sometimes people. Jade experiences unpleasant smells, Hugh senses his grandparents through their smell, Orla smells burning, and Kate smells a sweet, sickly odour and also sees and smells smoke. Will senses his voices' presence and has touched the hair of one; he refers to an old, fusty smell 'when they come in the room'. Brad senses his former girlfriend breathing next to him and feels the bed move. Kath sees things and smells violets, and feels things creeping under her skin when she hears voices.

Dan's 'voice-hearing' is strikingly multisensory: he sees the body of his grandfather, sees people bleeding, smells smoke, and, as well as voices, hears screams, crashes, and explosions. Julian's vision of Christ's bleeding body, horrific yet wondrous, is similarly physical: 'I saw the bodyly sight lesting of the plentious bledeing of the hede' (Julian of Norwich, 2016, ch. 7, p. 39). Margery recounts a comparably graphic vision 'in a maner of slep', of someone mutilating Christ's dead body by cutting along the breast-bone with a dagger (Kempe, 2004, ll. 7005–10). Medieval accounts of the incubus, the nightmare demon that attacks the body, are recalled by Kate's remarkably multisensory experience: she feels the dead weight of something sitting on her chest and senses things creeping near her in the dark. Ryan too experiences sleep paralysis and sees black crawling figures. A number of those interviewed experience nightmares and vivid dreams, and one of Xander's voices introduces itself in dream, a feature of both Margery's and Julian's accounts. Perhaps most analogous to these fearful multisensory experiences is that of Julian in the sixteenth and last revelation: she experiences in sleep the terrifying presence of the devil, grinning, red and black-spotted, taking her by the throat; waking, she sees the smoke and smells the stench of fire and brimstone (Julian of Norwich, 2016, ch. 66, p. 137). For Julian, the fire is 'bodily', but those with her do not perceive it: it is experienced through the inward senses, on which God works.

Both medieval and modern experiences are strikingly embodied. For Julian and Margery, illness is a catalyst. Margery's experience across the *Book* is shaped by her physical responses, most strikingly her compulsive weeping, which metamorphoses when she travels to Jerusalem into something stranger, 'krying and roryng' (Kempe, 2004, l. 2216). Her cryings are the cause of suspicion and annoyance: 'summe seyd it was a wikkyd spiryt vexid hir; sum seyd it was a sekenes; sum seyd sche had dronkyn to mech wyn'—although they persuade others of her holiness (Kempe, 2004, ll. 2245–50). Her crying is sometimes accompanied by falling on the ground and turning blue. Margery's behaviours have attracted a variety of medical diagnoses, from hysteria to psychosis to temporal lobe epilepsy and migraine (Lawes, 1999, pp. 147–67; more generally on the psychology of mysticism, see Kroll and Bachrach, 2005). For Margery, however, as for voice-hearers now, physical symptoms are not causes of, but responses to, their experience. Hugh experiences dizziness, Chris has pins and needles at the back of his head, and Jane has muscle weakness and spasms. Headaches or migraines are also prominent in the VIP accounts; for instance, Iris has daily migraines which she knows will not go until her voice does. For many, voice-hearing causes panic, fear, and anxiety symptoms, and sometimes, paranoia; several also experience PTSD, insomnia, and flashbacks. Harry has had a breakdown: he is 'dead behind me eyes', his head aches through stress, and he also experiences mania. Dawn's body shudders with anxiety and fear, and hearing her voice like a ghost next to her makes her feel ghostly. Mike has a strange sense of déjà vu. Grace sometimes feels ill when hearing her voices and, on first experiencing them, fell to the floor, screaming. Liam frequently feels he may lose consciousness and says that his voices are 'doing me head in'. Fran has blackouts and feels paralysed by the voices; Dan blacks out and feels he is floating out of his body, as does Nina; Xander feels he is floating, looking in at life; Anthony's experience is dream-like and ethereal, and at times it seems that the walls are breathing. Olivia seems to fall and feels her balance has been lost. Leah experiences the voices in her body and especially her ovaries. Matt's experiences begin with a fit. These accounts echo the embodied, powerfully affective quality of medieval spiritual experience and the long-standing connections of revelation with illness and extreme physical response, seen in both Julian's and Margery's narratives.

The interviews repeatedly describe voices as coming from different places, both in and outside the head. This range of experience is also signalled by Julian and Margery, and they too attempt to characterize the qualities of voice-hearing. Julian asks in her first vision, of a tiny thing like a hazelnut, ' "What may this be?" ', and hears the spoken answer, ' "It is all that is made" ' (Julian of Norwich, 2016, ch. 5, p. 35). She repeatedly conveys the impression of a voice speaking directly to her (e.g. 'our good lord seid' (Julian of Norwich, 2016, ch. 14, p. 52)), sometimes within her mind (e.g. 'And I was answered in my reason' (Julian of Norwich, 2016, ch. 10, p. 45); 'Than had I a profir in my reason, as it had be frendly seyd to me' (Julian of Norwich, 2016, ch. 19, p. 60)). Seeing may be like hearing instructive words: 'And al this shewid he ful blisfully, meneing thus: "Se, I am God" ' (Julian of Norwich, 2016, ch. 11, p. 48). Voices may also be heard in the soul, the effect of the soundless voice sometimes described by contemporary voice-hearers: 'Than he, without voice and openyng of lippis, formys in my soule these words' (Julian of Norwich, 2016, ch. 13, p. 50). Margery too distinguishes between interior and exterior voices: lying in bed, she hears 'wyth hir bodily erys a lowde voys clepyng: "Margery" '; on waking, God speaks directly to her, ' "Dowtyr" ' (Kempe, 2004, ll. 4381, 4386). She describes 'how owyr Lord dalyed to hir sowle in a maner of spekyng' (Kempe, 2004, ll. 2577–8)— perhaps also the effect of a soundless voice. The interviews show a comparable range of kinds of voice-hearing—both interior and exterior— thought insertions, aspects of felt presence. Whispering is a prominent feature: Olivia hears 'evil whispering', Orla hears whispers and screams, Emma hears people whispering and laughing, and for Hugh the voices are 'whispering demons'. The fearful intrusiveness of whispering is vividly captured in Julian's late vision of the devil, which is accompanied by a vision of two people chattering earnestly yet inaudibly, intended, Julian writes, 'to stirre me to dispeir' (Julian of Norwich, 2016, ch. 69, p. 142). For Julian, God's power is also evident in the terrifying obscurity of the mind and the failure to understand. The description of the experience and the despair that it evokes are echoed by those interviewed in their accounts of the distressing effects of whispering voices.

Talking to their voices helps Alex and is possible for many others; such conversations resonate with those which Julian and Margery have with the Lord. Margery's primary emphasis is on the 'wonderful spechys and dalyawns [conversations] whech owr Lord spak and dalyid to hyr sowle' (Kempe, 2004, ll. 52–3), perhaps most similar to Leah's experience. Margery also converses with the Virgin, and with other saints (Peter, Paul, Mary Magdalene, Katherine, and Margaret (Kempe, 2004, ll. 7245–8)). But as well, the Lord's voice fulfils a much more mundane role, particularly later in Margery's narrative, offering a dialogic commentary on her life: assurances of well-being, interpretative frames for events, and practical advice of all kinds, from where she should go and what she should say to ascetic practices and attire. The descriptions evoke the repeatedly instructive, commenting quality that can intrude on everyday experience in contemporary accounts of voice-hearing.

Julian's and Margery's narratives also signal the trauma of voice-hearing. Doubt and uncertainty colour their experiences, even within a world where a supernatural explanation comes readily to hand and where visionary experience is valued and authorized. A crucial aspect of Julian's journey of faith is the process of believing that the 'sheweings' are not madness. Paradoxically, her doubts are answered when bodily seeing is complemented with spiritual vision: 'he shewid it al agen within, in my soule, with more fulhede [detail]'; she hears the Lord 'seyand these wordes full mytyly and full mekely, "Witt it now wele, it was no raving that thou saw this day"' (Julian of Norwich, 2016, ch. 70, p. 144). Margery's feeling is so extreme that she is as 'a woman wythowtyn reson' (Kempe, 2004, l. 6523), while others repeatedly place her as mad. She seeks Julian's counsel about her strange experiences in November 1413. Is there 'any deceyte,' she asks, in the 'ful many holy spechys and dalyawns [conversation] that owyr Lord spak to hir sowle' and her 'many wondirful revelacyons' (Kempe, 2004, ll. 1339–41)? Such revelations are dangerous, Julian responds: they may reflect 'nowt the mevyng of a good spyryte, but rathar of an evyl spyrit' (Kempe, 2004, ll. 1349–50), and must be judged by whether they move the soul to love, chastity, and compassion. If the *Revelations* and the *Book* emphasize the positive, they also convey a strong sense of more troubling possibilities. Julian contends with fears of insanity and despair, and a terrifying sense of the devil; Margery's revelations are countered by demonic and grotesque sexual visions, and she herself grapples with the radical quality of her experience. For both, visionary experience is extreme and opaque, only ever comprehensible in part, for it engages with the ineffable.

As the VIP interviews show so acutely, voice-hearers continue to seek explanations. They repeatedly see themselves as being in some sense controlled, even when this is not in a spiritual sense (occasionally technology provides a twenty-first-century explanatory model instead). Neil believes his voices may be a form of telepathy, Mike a kind of government surveillance. For Yan, microwaves as if from the radio seem to 'tap straight into his head', and he wonders 'how you could do it'. For Bill, voice-hearing is demonic, a curse, a secret like a black shadow cast over his life. Chris thinks his voices may be memories locked away coming out: the past is trying to 'push back'. The difficulty of comprehension, even for writers whose work has come to be influential and authoritative, and who had a clear framework for placing their experience, should not be underestimated.

Reading comparatively across time and genre, putting two such different thought worlds together, illuminates both past and present. The experience of modern voice-hearers draws attention to the traumatic and complex experiences of visionary writers, reminding readers that revelation is intimately connected with difficulty and uncertainty, and is often rooted in life-changing trauma. While vision is highlighted, such experience is typically multisensory and revelation is deeply embodied. Putting the interviews into conversation with visionary writing also means reading the accounts of voice-hearers today not in clinical, but in literary terms. The phenomenological approach of the study captures texture, affect, and ethos. Reading attentively alongside the voices of the past reveals the complexity of voice-hearing as an experience, its intersections with belief, context, and culture, its profoundly multisensory and embodied aspects, and the deep impulses of those speaking towards not diagnosis, but understanding. The urgent wish of voice-hearers now to place and explain their experiences, and to illuminate the experiences of others, finds an echo in the questions, doubts, and incomprehension of individuals nearly 600 years ago. The authority of the voices of the past, the power of their words to reanimate their experience, and the enduring quality of their writings may also offer inspiration in the present.

References

Cook, C. C. H. (2019). *Hearing Voices, Demonic and Divine: Scientific and Theological Perspectives.* London: Routledge.

Julian of Norwich (2015). *Revelations of Divine Love.* Translated from the Middle English by B. Windeatt. Oxford: Oxford University Press.

Julian of Norwich (2016). *Revelations of Divine Love,* ed. B. Windeatt. Oxford: Oxford University Press.

Kempe, M. (2004). *The Book of Margery Kempe,* ed. B. Windeatt. Cambridge: D. S. Brewer.

Kempe, M. (2019). *The Book of Margery Kempe.* Translated from the Middle English by B. A. Windeatt. London: Penguin.

Kroll, J., and Bachrach, B. (2005). *The Mystic Mind: The Psychology of Medieval Mystics and Ascetics.* New York, NY: Routledge.

Lawes, R. (1999). The madness of Margery Kempe. In: M. Glasscoe, ed. *The Medieval Mystical Tradition: England, Ireland, and Wales. Exeter Symposium VI: Papers Read at Charney Manor, July 1999.* Cambridge: D. S. Brewer, pp. 147–67.

Luhrmann, T. M. (2012). *When God Talks Back: Understanding the American Evangelical Relationship with God.* New York, NY: Alfred A. Knopf.

McCarthy-Jones, S. (2012). *Hearing Voices: The Histories, Causes and Meanings of Auditory Verbal Hallucinations.* Cambridge: Cambridge University Press.

Powell, H., and Saunders, C., eds. (2020). *Visions and Voice-hearing in Medieval and Early Modern Contexts.* London: Palgrave Macmillan.

About the Author

Corinne Saunders is Professor of English Studies at Durham University. She specialises in medieval literature and the history of ideas, and is interested in how medieval texts and frameworks can illuminate contemporary understandings of voice-hearing. She is Co-Director of the Institute for Medical Humanities at Durham University.

28

Maelstrom

David Napthine, Writer

Where do the voices come from? Where do the voices go when we can no longer hear them? These two questions hovered as I read the Voices in Psychosis interviews.

I'm neither a clinician nor an academic, so let me tell a story in response to these questions, one that draws upon the transcripts and steals from my colleagues.

I once met someone I've never seen since who told me something I'd not heard before: that beneath the waves at Corryvreckan[1] 'voices' congregate in a deep cave within the seabed. Not always the same voices, for they congregate at similar places throughout the world. They are universal and eternal voices without hearth or home; sometimes Echo, sometimes the Banshee and her friends, Lorelei and her sisters, and countless others. Insistent, insidious voices that command, seduce, and undermine. Voices of the dead, spirit voices, saintly and demonic. Voices from ancient worlds and our every day. Some hear some voices, and others hear others. Some hear no voices no matter how hard these voices persist; all these voices, out of sight and unheard until disturbed.

When the clash of tides and conflicting currents swirl the deep waters of Corryvreckan, the voices are roused from their cave and whirlpool to the surface where they churn on the waves before soaring and swooping to the skies above. They move like the summer swallows flying south for the winter, searching for the familiar where they can rest and reside. Look up and you may see these voices. Then again, you may not.

This is what I was told by someone I've not seen since.

One Friday evening, the whirlpool forms at Corryvreckan. The noise can be heard at Ardfern, a village on the Craignish Peninsula, some miles away. Those drinking in The Galley of Lorne take little notice. They've heard it all before. Robert hears them. He knows that for some, it is the sound of fear and that soon he will be needed. In the morning, he'll head to Ardfern Yacht Centre and amble his way between the boats that squat on wooden supports on the hard-standing, awaiting the paintbrush, the scraping of barnacles, the caulking and burning to make them ready for Scottish

---

[1] Corryvreckan, also called the Gulf of Corryvreckan and the Strait of Corryvreckan, lies between the islands of Jura and Scarba off the west coast of mainland Scotland. The name derives from Gaelic *Coire Bhreacain* (the 'cauldron of the speckled seas' and the 'cauldron of the plaid'). It is a whirlpool (the third largest in the world) created by strong Atlantic currents and an unusual underwater topography. The roar from the resulting maelstrom can be heard many miles away.

David Napthine, *Maelstrom* In: *Voices in Psychosis*. Edited by: Angela Woods, Ben Alderson-Day, and Charles Fernyhough, Oxford University Press.
© David Napthine 2022. DOI: 10.1093/oso/9780192898388.003.0028

waters. He will chat with one and laugh with another, and at the chandlers he'll buy what's needed for those who might or might not arrive while shooting the breeze with whoever is there.

Saturday morning, in a semi-detached suburban house in Birmingham, handy for the buses and handy for the schools, Christie, eating toast and marmalade, looks out on her garden as spring sunshine envelops her five-year-old Ella. She's playing with the morning and with Tina, her imaginary friend, who will have to play elsewhere when Katy arrives. For Katy and Ella will scooter to the park with juice and biscuits. Ella and Katy—friends forever.

Once the girls are park-bound and laughing, Christie flicks through last night's paper for the Sudoku not completed. Her husband Steve, knackered from the night-shift, snores in his bed and dreams of Villa winning later that day. Not that he'll be there. For while the crowds roar at Villa Park, he'll be on a husband-and-wife garden centre visit. It's that time of year.

Loading the dishwasher she doesn't think of the voices. Why should she? She can't hear them. There's no chitter-chatter, no threats or urging. She's taken her tablets—her husband reminded her before he grumbled to sleep. Wiping down the surfaces, she tries not to think of that question he asked before climbing the stairs. It came out of the blue and now whines just out of reach like small-fly buzzing on a summer's day.

Robert is at his boat. A shabby specimen, the boat that is, yet bobbing contented between the pristine craft of the weekend sailor. On board, he fastens and secures, checks the coiling of ropes and tidies below, all shipshape and Bristol fashion as you'd never hear him say. He rolls a cigarette and looks out at waters patterned by sunlight. The breeze is light and gentle from the south west, rattling the cables that await the sails. The forecast is good. He'll be ready should someone arrive. At some point, someone will. Because of that Ceilidh of the waters, the joyous roar of dancing voices laughing with release. It can get unruly at Corryvreckan.

The question Christie's husband had asked was simple:

'Where are the voices when you can't hear them?'

She didn't know.

'So where do they come from?'

She didn't know.

'When they've finished in your head where do they go?'

She didn't know.

'So how are you now?'

'Fine.'

'No voices?'

Christie shook her head.

'Even when the voices aren't there, are you still unwell?'

Pause for reflection.

Then her husband said, 'I live with you and you're as fit as a fiddle and twice as bonny', and he shook his head while looking at the carpet as Christie looked perplexed and wished that they could go to the garden centre now.

'Do you really want to know?' Christie asked.

'Yes. Don't you?'

She doesn't wonder where the voices are when they aren't there. Let clinicians and academics explore cause and correlation. All she wants is for the voices to stay away.

But they won't.

Just after lunch

Steve still sleeping

Ella at Katy's

The air moves

Tingling sensations

Heart rate faster

Here they come.

To taunt, tease, accuse, and threaten, tumbling through her skull in all directions, along her skin, riding her thoughts like a merry-go-round.

'What did I do to bring them to me?'

But her story lies hidden deep inside a labyrinth that, thread-less and alone, she daren't explore.

Now separate from herself, now homeless in her home, she sits staring at everything and nothing in particular.

Steve enters. He looks at her. She's hearing voices. He makes two mugs of tea, then sits, quiet and watchful, as she sits silenced by voices that cyclone inside her, then snipe around her, moving in and out and around and about. Steve takes her hand until the voices fall quiet enough for Steve to be heard.

'What can I do?'

'Take the voices away.'

'How?'

Her counsellor (the lady who helps pick apart submerged events that, seemingly forgotten, continually summon the voices to settle within her) said, 'visualize placing the voices into a bag, a box, anything that will hold them. Then seal it tight and throw it away.'

She tells Steve this.

'What she on about?' asked Steve.

Christie stays silent.

'These voices, you know, well aren't they just thoughts that won't do what their told? I have that all the time.'

'No.'

'Well they're not things, are they? I mean you can't touch them, can you, cos they're not there.'

'But they are there, Steve.'

'They are there, I know, love, of course they are, but it's not like, you know, in that way that I can see this mug of tea and pick it up and put it over here. Is it?'

Christie stays silent.

'Bollocks', says Steve.

Christie looks up.

'I've spilt tea on the new carpet.'

He cleans his spill as they struggle for the words to find a way to understanding.

'I must do something, Steve. I must.'

So he searches for something to hold the voices and returns with an Asda Bag for Life.

'Do you need any help to pack the voices?' he asks.

She says nothing for only she can herd these voices, these scattered fragments of her being, bring them together, and then into the bag. Once done, she holds it tight and closed. Steve secures it with Sellotape, masking tape, and gaffer tape. He has no idea what he's doing, but he loves his wife and that's enough to be going on with.

'Now what, Christie?'

'I take them away.'

'Where to?'

'I don't know.'

'I'll come with you.'

'No.'

'How will you know where to go?'

'I don't know but I will.'

'It scares me, Christie.'

'It scares me.'

She packs an overnight bag. Just in case. She waits. Then all of a sudden, she drives away, leaving Steve not knowing if he's coming or going. She is scared and worried about her husband who is scared and worried about her.

When Ella bounds in from the park asking for mum, Steve tells her that she's gone out. Will she be long? He doesn't know. When will she be back? He doesn't know. Where has she gone? He doesn't know. Over a bowl of soup, Ella asks if it's to do with her voices; is that why she's gone away?

'You know about mum's voices?'

'Yes.'

'Has she told you about them?'

'No.'

'So how do you know about the voices?'

'Tina said.'

Tina? Steve doesn't know any Tina. He switches on the radio to see if Villa had won. They hadn't.

Rain lashes the motorway as the winds on Shap try to shove her car into hurtling wagons. On her own and far away, the dark watches her white-knuckled grip and coat-hanger shoulders keep her tight in the inside lane. She wants to turn back, but she knows if she does, she'll betray the moment and sabotage tomorrow.

On she drives into Scotland, there to sit overnight in her Travelodge room, watching the voices as they push and pull in her Bag for Life, waiting for darkness to fade to light.

Robert waited all Saturday, but nobody came. Well sometimes he's busy and sometimes he isn't. He sleeps soundly, refreshed by the company in The Galley of Lorne. When he wakes with a Sunday morning head, he'll go to the ship's chandlers, to chat with one and laugh with another.

Tired, tired in her car, driving on nerves through Glasgow traffic that's out to get her, skirting Loch Lomond, leaving all cities behind, seeing nothing but the road ahead, and indifferent to Ben Lomond that looms above, she heads into a land of fewer people or no one at all.

The road bending into the unknown, a convoy forms behind her of flashing lights and blaring horns that scream at her 'Get out! You're in the way'. Forced to a lay-by, she hears the silent threat of an empty landscape.

Sunday morning and two people wait for Robert, one with a bag and one with a box. He nods a greeting and gestures them on board. They hesitate. He waits. It's up to them.

The clouds, massed together in mourning black, beckon Christie to drive further and further. She wishes she couldn't, but follows an instinct that might be false.

At the head of Loch Craignish, she turns for Ardfern and stops by the entrance to the Yacht Centre, where she shakes and shivers to stillness.

Is this the place?

She can go no further.

This is the end of the journey.

It is the beginning of the journey.

She looks at the yachts tied up along the boardwalks. Which way now? What if she's wrong? Clutching her Asda Bag for Life, she takes careful steps looking at each yacht.

Robert can see her. He can see the voices moving in the bag, but he can't hear them. If he could hear them, he couldn't do what he does.

He watches and waits. She reaches his boat. She looks at this man. He walks towards her and holds out his hand.

Uncertainty engulfs her and the contents of her bag become restless.

'Come aboard', says Robert, 'before it's too late.'

'I'm terrified of the sea.'

'And the voices?'

'I'm terrified of them.'

'The choice is yours.'

She turns away.

But she doesn't leave.

One of the passengers speaks. 'You've come this far.'

She turns, surprised to see two other people.

'It's not just you.'

'I didn't think it was.'

'Yes you did. It's what the voices want you to think. That it's just you.'

Christie steps aboard.

Robert casts off and motors to the deeper channels. Not the best of weather. Christie clutches her bag and closes her eyes.

Sails hoisted, Robert tacks with the wind, dipping and rolling with wind and wave. Three passengers, pale and anxious, eyes shut tight.

'Have you sailed before?'

'No.'

'Focus on the horizon.'

'Why?'

'It's the one still point we have.'

Christie looks at the horizon.

'But you need to open your eyes.'

Christie does so.

Her physical world settles.

'Do you know where we're going?'

'No.'

'Do you know why you're going?'

'Yes.'

'That's all that matters.'

As they sail for the north tip of Jura, Ella and Steve visit grandma as they always do for Sunday tea.

'Christie not with you?'

'No.'

'Has something happened?'

'Nothing out of the ordinary.'

'Mum's gone away with her voices.' says Ella.

Grandma looks at Ella and wonders if Christie has found religion.

Corryvreckan

Is quiet

When they arrive.

Robert asks, 'Are you sure you want to empty your voices into the waters?'

They look confused. That's why they're here.

'Aren't the voices part of you? If you tip them into the waves, aren't you throwing away something of yourself?'

They cannot answer.

'You are brave enough to come here, but are you brave enough to become a different person?'

One by one.

They open their packages and tip their voices into the waters, sending them home to the cave below.

Some voices are angry and some are sad.

But all tumble into the waters.

To wait until the tide comes again.

'Will the voices come back?' Christie asks Robert once they're moored and secure. He just smiles and makes his way to The Galley of Lorne.

Christie gets in her car and heads out of Ardfern.

How does she feel?

She doesn't know.

Will the voices come back?

She doesn't know.

And if they do?

She'll face them again.

Then settle them back.

Where they belong.

Author's Note

Storytelling is regarded as a powerful therapeutic mechanism. In twenty-first century Britain, tales of lived experience and survival often appear as recovery narratives, living witness accounts, and personal testimonies. In writing *Maelstrom*, I wanted to place the experience of voice-hearing within a different form of storytelling: the myth and the epic.

To do this, I have drawn upon the work of Joseph Campbell, notably his identifying of the Hero and the Heroic Journey in stories found in many cultures both extant and extinct.[2] In its simplest form, this story structure has the Hero summoned to undertake a perilous journey to achieve a specific aim, deal with fear and danger, and then return home with greater self-knowledge and understanding of the world. It is a familiar format much favoured by Hollywood.[3] I believe this story structure—and the way it is told—allows us to deal with the difficult, the frightening and disturbing, that which threatens our physical and psychological well-being.

The hero is an archetype and belongs to us all. With this in mind, I have cast those who have disclosed their personal conditions in the role of the hero, so that we (voice-hearers or not) can hopefully identify and empathize with their experience. Essential for the hero and the heroic journey is that we see something of ourselves in both the heroic character and what and who they encounter.

The key distinction between this epic/mythic story structure (e.g. *The Odyssey, Beowulf, Gawain and the Green Knight*) and the more personal forms of storytelling is that the storyteller is neutral. The story told is of an individual, but it is not the story of the person telling. It is told in the third person, a device that admits the audience to the story world and enables them to become active in that world. It elevates the individual story to the universal and allows the audience to

---

[2] Joseph Campbell, *The Hero with a Thousand Faces.*

[3] The highly acclaimed video game *Hellblade: Senua's Sacrifice*, created by Ninja Theory with significant input from Hearing the Voice, draws upon the heroic structure (in this case, Norse and Celtic mythology) to enhance our understanding of hearing voices.

empathize with the character and the situation and relate what they hear to their personal circumstances. The use of metaphor, imagery, and symbol—all common to myth and epic—along with storytelling tropes (such as allegory) is familiar to audiences and facilitates our understanding of particular worlds. Further, it can engender fellow-feeling when the story is told to an audience, rather than read by the individual.

I would like to suggest that in the world of psychosis and other adverse states, stories told within the universal and ancient 'epic' and mythic structures may offer a more open and inclusive way to talk about, understand, and find ways of dealing with those conditions than the accepted therapeutic storytelling structures.

Have I answered the two questions? Maybe. Maybe not.

Conversations

Maelstrom has asked me to say how much it has enjoyed, and is still enjoying, the conversations with the other chapters in this book. It has not met them all (it intends to at the earliest opportunity), but those it has met are proving, not surprisingly, to be both stimulating and engaging company. The chapters it has met so far are:

Chapter 5: The Sound of Fear (*Ben Alderson-Day and Thomas Ward*)
Chapter 7: Bodily Sensations During Voice-Hearing Experiences: A Role for Interoception? (*Jamie Moffat*)
Chapter 9: Lost Agency and the Sense of Control (*John Foxwell*)
Chapter 14: Relating to Leah's Voices (*Angela Woods*)
Chapter 17: Silences in First-Person Accounts of Voice-Hearing: A Linguistic Approach (*Elena Semino, Luke Collins, and Zsófia Demjén*)
Chapter 18: Household Ghosts and Personified Presences (*Peter Garratt*)
Chapter 20: Vagabond Narratives: To Be Without a Home (*Patricia Waugh*)
Chapter 21: Leah's Voices: Reflections on Auditory Verbal Hallucinations as Spiritual and Religious Experience (*Christopher C. H. Cook*)
Chapter 25: Remembering Voices (*Charles Fernyhough*)

Maelstrom is looking forward to further conversations and is not adverse to a walk by the sea followed by a bag of chips and a pint or two.

About the Author

David Napthine is a scriptwriter who works for radio, theatre, and film. He was Writer in Residence at the world's first major exhibition on voice-hearing *Hearing Voices: Suffering, Inspiration and the Everyday*, and has continued collaborating with Hearing the Voice through the Writers' Inner Voices project. He has recently been writer/researcher for *Northern Heartlands*, exploring the impact of landscape on people's lives and aspirations in North Pennines. He is currently creating a new work *Singin' Jerusalem* (funded by the Arts Council), an exploration of Jerusalem as symbol, image, and metaphor.

Index

For the benefit of digital users, indexed terms that span two pages (e.g., 52–53) may, on occasion, appear on only one of those pages.

Boxes are indicated by *b* following the page number

affect 50–58
  cause–effect relationship 54–56
  history 51–53
  phenomenology 53–57
affordances 79–80
Agamben, G. 174–75
agency 74–81
  actions and 77–78
  agents and 121
  control 75–76, 78–79
  core-optionality 78–79
  fear 47–49
  four forms 120–21
  movement 163–64
  multimodal hallucinations 71
  multiple facets 77
  phenomenology 76–77, 78–79
  post hoc attribution 76–77
  pre-reflective aspects 77, 78–80
  reflective aspects 77, 79–80
  thin (phenomenologically recessive) 76
agents
  multimodal hallucinations 68–69, 71, 72
  relationship with agency 121
  social agents 6–7
  speaker behind the voice 130–31
Alber, J. 111–12
alien control 76
anterior cingulate cortex 223
antipsychotics 25–26
anxiety 50, 53, 54
appraisal 62–63, 83–84
approximations 138–40
arcuate fasciculus 6–7
artistic voice hearers 4
asceticism 95
assertive engagement 25
assessment 20–21
at-risk mental state (ARMS) 21–22, 27–28
atypical antipsychotics 25–26
auditory quality of voices 128–30, 131–32, *see also* speech-like voices

autobiographical memory 213, 214, 216–17
automatic action 76, 77–78
AVATAR therapy 45–47, 200–1
Avdi, E. 148
ayahuasca 195, 196–98

Bartholomew of Farne 94
behavioural family therapy 27
being-in-the-world 162–63
being watched 205–6
Bell, V. 120–21
Benjamin, L. 118–19
bodily sensations 33, 59–65, 234–35
  dissociative experiences 63
  emotional processing 61–63
  interoception 59, 60–61, 62, 63, 64
  touch 34, 64
body, as culture 84–85, 89
Boldt, M. 88
boundary voices 43, 169–70, 204
brain mechanisms 6–7, 71, 223–25
bughouses 173–74
bullying 33, 36, 50

CAARMS (Comprehensive Assessment of At Risk Mental States) 20–21
care coordination work 23–25
Cassian, J. 97
Charteris-Black, J. 135
childhood amnesia 216–17
Cho, G. 207–8
Clouston, T. 52
cognitive analytic therapy 26–27, 184–93
  humans as social and dialogical 185–86
  overview 184–85
  reciprocal roles 184, 186–87, 188–90, 192
  relationship with voices 192
cognitive behavioural therapy 26–27
cognitive mechanisms 6–7, 44–45
cognitive neuroscience 71–72
Cohn, D. 113
common ground 137, 139

communication
  grounding 137–38
  hearing voices as 127–28, 197, 199, 200
  negation 143
  silence 142–43
Comprehensive Assessment of At Risk Mental
    States (CAARMS) 20–21
Conrad, J. 113–14
conspirations 101–7
  looking for absences 105–6
  narratives 103–5
  therapeutic 102–3
continuum of experiences 63, 115, 222–23, 226–27
control
  affordances 79–80
  agency 75–76, 78–79
  being controlled by voices 236–37
  fear 48
  learning to control voices 197–99
  silence 142–43
conversational grounding 137–38
coping strategies 148, 180–82, 199
core-optionality 78–79
Corryvreckan, story of tipping voices
    into 239–47
Culler, J. 111
cultural practice 6–7, 194, 201
Cuthbert 97–98

dance movement psychotherapy 161, 163–66
Deamer, F. 130
de-distancing 162–63
Deleuze, G. 122–23
delusions 51–53
Demjen, Z. 136
demons 33, 41–42, 93–100, 177, 180, 181,
    197, 231–32
Department of Work and Pensions
    panopticon 205
depression 50, 53, 54, 135, 140
devil (Satan) 93–95, 97, 177, 180, 181, 231,
    232, 234
diagnosis
  early intervention in psychosis 23
  subjectification 112–13
Diagnostic and Statistical Manual of Mental
    Disorders (DSM) 50–51, 53
dialogues 46–47
Dickens, C. 153–59
  Christmas Carol 153–54
  Drunkard's Death 154
  Great Expectations 156–57
  Household Words 153–54, 157–58
  Martin Chuzzlewit 155–56
  Master Humphrey's Clock 156–57

Signal Man 158–59
  Sketches by Boz 154, 155–57
Dillon, B. 170
disappearance of voices 217–18
dissociation 63, 165–66
doll's houses 173–74
double-awareness 104
Douglas, M. 83, 84–85, 86, 87, 89
dreamhouses 173–74
drug therapy 25–26
Dunstan 94

early intervention in psychosis (EIP) 3, 8, 17–31
  Access and Waiting Time Standard 18–20
  assertive engagement 25
  assessment 20–21
  at-risk mental state (ARMS) 21–22, 27–28
  care coordination work 23–25
  care coordinators 20–21
  conceptualization of voice-hearing 20–22
  cost issues 18–19
  course of care 27–28
  development 17–19
  diagnosis 23
  ending care 27–28
  evidence base 18
  first-episode psychosis (FEP) 22, 27–28
  hard to engage users 25
  inter- and intra-team variance 23
  local context 19
  medications 25–26
  non-distressing voice-hearing 21
  physical health care 25–26
  psychosocial interventions 26–27
  referral routes 19–20
  services offered to voice-hearers 23–27
  treatment delays 19–20
emotionally unstable personality disorder 23
emotions
  bodily sensations and interoception 61–63
  cognitive approach to psychosis 45
  first appearance of voices 214
  memory and 214–15, 216
  metaphor use 134–35, 140
  see also affect; fear
empty chair 45
enactive experience 114
Escher, A. 118–19
ethical issues 5
experience-based approach 6
eye-movement desensitization
    reprogramming 26–27

family interventions 27
fear 35, 41–49, 54

agency 47–49
  boundary voices 43
  intentional control 48
  loss of reality 43
  modes of elicitation 41–42
  onset of voice-hearing 42, 48
  potentiality 43–44, 46–47
  realization 42
  working with 44–47
figurative language 134–41
  experiences 134–35
  metaphor 134–37, 138–40, 165
  simile 134, 136–37, 138–40
first appearance of voices
  anger 191
  emotional impact 214
  fear 42, 48
  memory of 214, 215
  sleep deprivation 33
first-episode psychosis (FEP) 22, 27–28
flashbulb memory 214–15
Fludernik, M. 114
food taboos 84–85, 89
frame narration 109–10
Frankfurt, H. 74
fused hallucinations 66

Gallagher, S. 77
ghost/houses 173–74
ghosts 153–60, 206–8, 234–35
glasshouses 173–74
Godric 94–96, 98
Graham, G. 76–77
grandiosity 61
grounding 137–38
Guattari, F. 122–23
Gurney, E. 157
Guthlac 94–95, 96, 97, 98
gyrification 224–25

hagiography 93–100
hallucinogens, ritual use 194–202
Handsome Lake 82–83, 89
head–heart lag 44–45
Hearing the Voice 4, 7–9
  phenomenological interview 8, 29, 54
  see also interviewees
Hearing Voices Movement 4
heart-beat detection 60
Heidegger, M. 162–63
Holt, L. 84
home/homelessness 169–75
  bughouses 173–74
  doll's houses 173–74
  dreamhouses 173–74

ghost/houses 173–74
glasshouses 173–74
safety 169–70, 171–72
sovereignty 178
unhoused 173–74
homosexuality 87–88
Horgan, T. 78–79

Illusions (Sully) 157
imagery re-scripting 45
inferior frontal gyrus 223
inner speech 170–71, 221–22
insula 223
intentionality 132
interdisciplinary approach 7–9
interoception 59, 60–61, 62, 63, 64
interviewees
  Alex 32, 33, 54–55, 94–95, 96, 104, 129, 148,
    171–72, 217, 232, 236
  Anthony 63, 103, 104–5, 169–70, 173–74, 199,
    215, 231–32, 233–35
  Bill 41–42, 43, 75–76, 78, 94, 95–97, 102, 103,
    129, 139–40, 162, 171–72, 214, 217, 220,
    226, 227, 236–37
  Brad 75–76, 78, 169–70, 221, 225, 233–34
  Carl 44, 105, 140, 147, 159, 233–34
  Chris 199, 215, 217, 234–35, 236–37
  Dan 75–76, 78, 83, 85–89, 94, 95–97, 102,
    110–11, 130–31, 142, 147, 170, 171–72, 213,
    217, 220, 222, 225, 232–35
  Dawn 59, 169–70, 199, 234–35
  Emma 4–5, 103, 159, 169–70, 171–72, 203–4,
    206–8, 233–34, 235–36
  Eric 94, 95–97, 171–72, 205, 215, 233–34
  Fran 43–44, 50, 215, 234–35
  Fred 33, 95–96, 139–40, 170–71
  Gail 34, 43, 94, 96, 103, 105, 106, 139–40,
    170–71, 204, 205–6, 220
  Grace 55b, 139–40, 161, 190–92, 204,
    221, 233–35
  Harry 32, 55b, 234–35
  Hugh 105, 145, 147, 169–71, 233–36
  Ian 94, 95, 146–47, 226
  Iris 55b, 161, 234–35
  Isaac 32–36
  Jade 54–55, 105, 217, 233–34
  Jane 33, 171–72, 204, 216, 231–32, 234–35
  Kate 64, 94, 103, 105–6, 140, 232, 233–34
  Kath 231–32, 233–34
  Leah 42, 71b, 94, 95, 96–97, 104–5, 111–12,
    113–14, 117–24, 170–72, 173–74, 176–83,
    215, 226, 231, 234–35, 236
  Liam 54–55, 204, 231–32, 234–35
  Matt 95, 96–97, 199, 234–35
  Mike 4–5, 234–35, 236–37

interviewees (*cont.*)
  Neil 103, 106, 162–63, 169–70, 236–37
  Nina 55*b*, 188–90, 216, 234–35
  Olivia 44, 80, 111–12, 114, 170–71, 214, 231–32, 233–36
  Orla 70*b*, 94, 106, 140, 165, 173–74, 233–34, 235–36
  Page 61–62, 70*b*, 75–76, 78, 169–70, 171–72, 225, 231–32
  Ryan 83, 85–89, 145, 146, 169–70, 174–75, 232, 234
  Sean 33, 42, 55*b*, 94–95, 96–97, 131, 171–72
  Toby 42, 220, 232
  Ulrich 199
  Ulrik 5, 140
  Violet 4–5, 64, 94, 171–72, 199, 200, 203–4, 226
  Will 74, 75–76, 103–4, 146–47, 153, 159, 199, 214, 215, 231–32, 233–34
  Xander 102, 106, 145, 146, 159, 161, 199, 200, 215, 225, 233–35
  Yan 94, 104–5, 106, 233–34, 236–37
  Zara 70*b*, 96–97, 148, 215, 232
intra-action 104

Jakes, S. 135
James, M. R. 153–54
Jaspers, K. 52–53
Jones, N. 121
Julian of Norwich 229–30, 233–36

Kalsched, D. 166–67
Kempe, Margery 229–30, 231–32, 233–36
Kerr, I. 187–88
Kestenberg Movement Profile 164
keyness analysis 143
keywords 143–44
Knoll, E. 56
Kraepelin, E. 50–51, 52–53

language processing 6–7
Levin, S. 134–35
Liebert, R. 206, 207–8
linguistics 142–50
  keyness analysis 143
  keywords 143–44
  negation 142, 143–44
listening 5
'lived' space 43, 163–65

McGorry, P. 18
McGurk effect 71–72
Maelstrom (Napthine) 239–47
magnetic resonance imaging 223–24
medial prefrontal cortex 223

medications 25–26
medieval perspective
  hagiography 93–100
  narratives 229–38
memory 213–19
  autobiographical 213, 214, 216–17
  childhood amnesia 216–17
  conformity 214
  disappearance of voices 217–18
  first appearance of voices 214, 215
  flashbulb 214–15
  recognition of importance of voices 215
  reconstruction 101, 213, 215–16
  trauma 215, 216–17, 218
  of voices 214–15
  voices as 216
  voices sparking memories 217
Merleau-Ponty, M. 163
metacognition 53
metaphor 134–37, 138–40, 165
movement 161, 162
  agency 163–64
  dance movement psychotherapy 161, 163–66
  lived space 163–65
  symbols and metaphor 165
  time as 164–65
multimodal hallucinations 6, 34, 66–73, 94, 233–34
  agency 71
  classification framework 69–71
  cognitive neuroscientific underpinnings 71–72
  distress caused by 72
  integration of identity 68–69, 71, 72
  phenomenology 68, 69–71
  temporal synchrony 68, 69–71
  variation 68–69
Multi-Modality Unusual Sensory Experiences Questionnaire (MUSEQ) 67–68
Myers, F. 157
mytho-poetic experience 161, 164, 165–67

Nagel, T. 114–15
narratives
  blending 115
  conspirations 103–5
  frame 109–10
  medieval voice-hearing 229–38
  psycho-analogies 113
  subtracting 115
  unnatural narratology 111–13
naturalization 111–13
negation 142, 143–44
neoshamanic practices 194–95, 200–1
neural mechanisms 6–7, 71, 223–25

neuroimaging 223–24
NICE guidelines 25–26, 27
Nichols, S. 78–79
non-distressing voice-hearing 6, 21
non-literal language 134, 135, 136
North East Visual Hallucination Interview 67–68

O'Donoghue, J. 136–37
olfactory perceptions 94
onset of voices *see* first appearance of voices
Oswald 98

Pacherie, E. 77
panopticon 205
paracingulate sulcus 223–25
Pargament, K. I. 181
Parnas, J. 135
peer support groups 200–1
Perry, A. 188
personality of voices 130–31
personification 6–7, 8–9, 153–60, 200
Personification Across Disciplines
    conference 8–9, 120–21
Peruvian Amazon, shamanic
    tourism 195, 196–98
phantasmata 229
Phantasms of the Living 157
phenomenological interviews
    enactive experience 114
    Hearing the Voice 8, 29, 54
    interviewing frame 109–11
    readerly dimension 108–16
    unnatural narratology 111–13
    see also interviewees
phenomenology 6–7, 127–33
    affect and voice-hearing 53–57
    agency 76–77, 78–79
    helpfulness in first-person reports 127
    intentionality 132
    multimodal hallucinations 68, 69–71
    open-ended questions 127–28
    paradox in voice-hearing 131–32
    similarity 137–38
    space 162–63
    two concepts of voice 128–31
physical health care 25–26
physical symptoms *see* bodily sensations
Podmore, F. 157
pollution model 83, 84–85, 86, 88
Positive and Negative Syndrome Scale
    (PANSS) 20–21
posterior superior temporal sulcus 71
posterior Sylvian fissure 225
potentiality 43–44, 46–47
presences 203–9

being watched 205–6
    as ghosts 206–8
    liminal space 204
    spatial distinctions 204
psychedelics, ritual use 194–202
psycho-analogies 113
psychosocial interventions 26–27
Psychotic Symptom Rating Scale
    (PSYRATS) 29, 67–68
psycurity 206
punishment 82–90, 106, 180, 181
    appraisal of voices 83–84
    functions 82–83
    pollution model 83, 84–85, 86, 88
    sexual orientation 87–88
    suicide 86–87, 88–89
    unholiness, 84–85
purification rituals 89–90

Quickening, The (Allnutt) 39–40

reality, loss of 34–35, 41–42, 43
reality monitoring 220–28
    brain folding 224–25
    hallucinations and 221–23
    measurement 222
    neural substrates 223–25
    source monitoring framework 221–22
realization 42
reappraisal 62–63
reciprocal roles 184, 186–87, 188–90, 192
Relating Therapy for Voices 200
relational therapy 45–47, 120, 200–1
relationships with voices 117–24, 192, 199–200
religion 105–6, 176–83, 194, 197, 230–34
Report on the Census of Hallucinations 157
Rhodes, J. 135
Rhys, J. 207, 208–7
rich perceptual experience 129–30
right superior temporal sulcus 225
Robertson, J. 157–58
roleplay 45
Romme, M. 118–19
rubber-hand illusion 63
Ryan, M.-L. 110–11
Ryle, A. 184

salience network 223
Satan (devil) 93–95, 97, 177, 180, 181, 231,
    232, 234
schizophrenia
    brain folding 224–25
    DSM 53
    interoception 61, 62
    McGurk effect 71–72

schizophrenia (*cont.*)
    multimodal hallucinations 66–67
    reality monitoring 222
    stigma 57
    visual hallucinations 66–67
    voice-hearing 6, 66–67
Schreber, D. P. 122–23
self-harm 41–42, 95, 232
self-help groups 194
Seneca people 82–83
sexual orientation 87–88
shamanic tourism 195, 196–98
sharing experiences of voices 36, 99–100,
    146, 200–1
silence 142–50
    meaningful 142–43
    power and control 142–43
    self-silencing 146
    silent voices 144–45
    social relationships 142–43, 146
    voice-hearer silenced by voices 146–47
    voice-hearer silent about voices 145–46
    voice-hearer silent with the voices 147–49
simile 134, 136–37, 138–40
sleep problems 33, 36, 44, 234
socialization of hallucinations 199–200
social movement 23
social power 142–43, 146
social relational role of voices 200, 217
sociocultural processes 6–7
socio-economic issues 25
somaesthetic perceptions 94
soundless voices 130
source monitoring framework 221–22
sovereignty 174–75
space 161–68, 204
    home 169–75
    'lived' space 43, 163–65
    phenomenology 162–63
    plasticity 169–70
speech-like voices 128–30, 131–32, 144, 200,
    220, *see also* whispering voices
spirituality 105–6, 176–83, 194, 197, 230–34
Stephens, G. L. 76–77
stigma 57, 218, 227
storytelling 239–47
stress-related voice-hearing 32, 33, 35–36
string hallucinations 66

subcultural contexts 6–7
subjectification 111–13
substance use 25
suicide/suicidal thoughts 41–42, 86–87, 88–89
Sully, J. 157–58
superior temporal gyrus 223
Sylvian fissure 225

tactile sensations 34, 64
Takiwasi community 196–98
talking with voices 45, 46–47, 236
Teale, P. 207
thought insertion 76
thought suppression 78–79
threatening voices *see* fear
threshold phenomena 203–9
    being watched 205–6
    as ghosts 206–8
    liminal space 204
    spatial distinctions 204
Tickle, A. 84
time
    movement and 164–65
    multimodal hallucinations 68, 69–71
trauma 6–7, 25, 33, 178–79
    medieval voice-hearers 230
    memory of 215, 216–17, 218
    mytho-poetic experience 165–67
    trauma-focused therapy 26–27
    of voice-hearing 236

unhoused 173–74
unnatural narratology 111–13

visual hallucinations 66–67, 68, 94
visual imagery (visualization) 194
Voice Club 7–8, 9
Voices in Psychosis (VIP) study 7–9, 17, 28–29
Vosgerau, G. 78–79
Voss, M. 78–79

Wegner, D. 76–77
whispering voices 75–76, 94–95, 129, 156–57,
    170–72, 177, 235–36
white matter tracts 6–7
Wilkinson, S. 84, 120–21
Woods, A. 84
word pair task 222